Office Politics

Office Politics
Computers, Labor, and the Fight for Safety and Health

Vernon L. Mogensen

Rutgers University Press
New Brunswick, New Jersey

Library of Congress Cataloging-in-Publication Data

Mogensen, Vernon, 1952–
    Office politics: computers, labor, and the fight for safety and health / Vernon Mogensen.
        p.   cm.
    Includes bibliographical references and index.
    ISBN 0-8135-2286-2 (cloth : alk. paper). — ISBN 0-8135-2287-0 (pbk. : alk. paper)
    1. Electronic data processing personnel—Health and hygiene—United States. 2. White collar workers—Health and hygiene—United States.   3. Video display terminals—Health aspects.   4. Electromagnetism—Physiological effect.   I. Title.
HD7269.D372U65   1996
363.11'9004'0973—dc20   95-46829
                                                                          CIP

British Cataloging-in-Publication information available

For permission to reproduce any portion of this work, except "fair use" as defined by U.S. copyright law, please contact the publisher, Rutgers University Press, Livingston Campus, Bldg. 4161, P.O. Box 5062, New Brunswick, New Jersey 08903.

Manufactured in the United States of America

To Carol

Contents

Acronyms

ABLI: Association for a Better Long Island
AFL-CIO: American Federation of Labor–Congress of Industrial Organizations
AFSCME: American Federation of State, County and Municipal Employees
ANPA: American Newspaper Publishers Association
ANSI: American National Standards Institute
AT&T: American Telephone and Telegraph Corporation
BIFMA: Business and Institutional Furniture Manufacturers Association
BLS: Bureau of Labor Statistics
BRH: Bureau of Radiological Health
CBEMA: Computer and Business Equipment Manufacturers Association
CDC: Centers for Disease Control
CIRRPC: Committee on Interagency Radiation Research and Policy Coordination
CLUW: Coalition of Labor Union Women
COSH: Committee for Occupational Safety and Health
COT: Center for Office Technology
CRT: Cathode Ray Tube
CTD: Cumulative Trauma Disorder
CWA: Communications Workers of America
CWT: Coalition for Workplace Technology
DEC: Digital Equipment Company
DED: (Connecticut) Department of Economic Development
DEMA: Data Entry Management Association
EC: European Community
ELF: Extremely Low Frequency
EMF: Electromagnetic Fields
EPA: Environmental Protection Agency
EU: European Union
FCC: Federal Communications Commission

FDA: Food and Drug Administration

FTC: Federal Trade Commission

GAO: General Accounting Office

HFS: Human Factors Society

IAM: International Association of Machinists

IBM: International Business Machines Corporation

IEEE: Institute of Electrical and Electronics Engineers

IPA: Illinois Press Association

ITC: Investment Tax Credit

LED: Light Emitting Diode

LIFT: Long Island Forum for Technology

MNPA: Massachusetts Newspaper Publishers Association

MPRII: Swedish National Board for Measurement and Testing Guidelines

NAS: National Academy of Sciences

NBOSH: Swedish National Board of Occupational Safety and Health

NCCI: National Council on Compensation Insurance

NIH: National Institutes of Health

NIOSH: National Institute of Occupational Safety and Health

NLRB: National Labor Relations Board

NOW: National Organization for Women

NRC: National Research Council

NSC: National Safety Council

NYCOSH: New York Committee for Occupational Safety and Health

NYNEX: New York, New England Telephone Corporation

OA: Office Automation

OIRA: Office of Information and Regulatory Affairs

OMB: Office of Management and Budget

OPEIU: Office and Professional Employees International Union

OSHA: Occupational Safety and Health Administration

OSH Act: Occupational Safety and Health Act of 1970

OTA: Office of Technology Assessment

PSI: Professional Secretaries International

RSI: Repetitive Strain Injuries

SAB: Science Advisory Board

SEIU: Service Employees International Union

TCO: Swedish Confederation of Professional Employees

TNG: The Newspaper Guild
UAW: United Auto Workers
UFCW: United Food and Commercial Workers
USWA: United Steel Workers of America
VDT: Video Display Terminal
VDU: Visual Display Unit
VLF: Very Low Frequency

Introduction

$\mathcal{T}$his book is about the political constraints on social regulatory policy making in the information age economy. Although there is considerable literature on the use of computers to automate and control the office labor process,[1] and the attendant occupational safety and health problems that affect those who work with video display terminals (VDTs),[2] little attention has been paid to the efforts of workers to address these problems in the political arena.[3] This book also examines the corporate counterattack to maintain nineteenth-century market conditions in the white-collar workplace as we approach the twenty-first century. The corporate community's opposition to VDT safety and health regulation is part of a larger attack on the welfare state itself and has had a constraining effect on the government's response to this public health crisis.

When they were first introduced in the 1970s, many business and technology forecasters claimed that VDT use would liberate clerical workers from repetitive, segmented tasks. In the computer-automated "Office of the Future," workers would be free to do more creative work, opening new opportunities for career advancement. However, these optimistic predictions have not panned out for most full-time VDT workers, the bulk of whom are unorganized women working in low-paid, dead-end jobs. For the most part, VDTs are being used to automate jobs and deskill workers, monitor employee productivity and behavior, and export work via satellite to low-wage, non-union offshore offices.

The widespread use of VDTs has precipitated the development of serious safety and health problems in the office workplace. Vision-related ailments, which are the most commonly cited group of problems, affect ten million workers and account for 14 percent of all eye exams in the United States.[4] Although office work is not usually thought of as being stressful, the National Institute of Occupational Safety and Health (NIOSH) found that

VDT workers experience high rates of stress, higher than air traffic controllers.[5] The routinization of tasks, work speedups, job insecurity, the lack of control and creativity, and computer monitoring contribute to stress-related health problems. Medical studies have documented that occupational stress contributes to psychiatric and heart-related illnesses in VDT workers.

Many VDT workers also suffer from musculoskeletal illnesses, such as cumulative trauma disorders (CTDs). CTDs, such as tendinitis and carpal tunnel syndrome, are caused by repetitive motions, and VDT workers are often expected to perform repetitive tasks for long hours, with few breaks. CTDs have become such a pervasive problem among VDT workers that the Occupational Safety and Health Administration (OSHA) called it the "occupational illness of the decade."[6] Tendinitis affects 4 million VDT workers, and carpal tunnel syndrome, a painful injury of the wrist's carpal tunnel that can lead to a significant loss of hand strength, afflicts 1.9 million computer users.[7]

The most controversial health problems reported by workers are associated with the electromagnetic fields (EMFs) emitted by the VDT's flyback transformer. The prevailing scientific view is that the nonionizing radiation emitted by VDTs is too weak to cause health problems, but female VDT workers around the world have reported cases of reproductive problems—such as infertility, birth defects, stillbirths, and higher than normal incidences of miscarriages—thought to be caused by the EMFs. Computer workers have also developed skin rashes, caused by electrostatic field buildup in front of the screen, and angina. A small, but growing number of studies links extremely low frequency EMFs, which VDTs emit, to health problems.[8]

Moreover, workers in the computer-automated office report an ongoing deterioration in safety and health conditions and in the quality of work. A 1991 Louis Harris poll of full-time office workers found that 36 percent thought nonionizing radiation emissions from the VDT were a problem, up from 27 percent in 1989; 47 percent considered eyestrain a serious concern, up from 44 percent in 1989; and one-third cited CTDs as a serious health risk. In 1989 the Harris organization considered the CTD problem so insignificant that questions regarding it were not asked.[9]

Another result of the introduction of computer-automated office systems has been a dramatic decline in job satisfaction among office workers: only 44 percent of office workers in the Harris poll said that the quality of work life improved in 1991, down from 70 percent in 1978.[10] The stressful, speeded-up, working conditions—and resultant occupational safety and health problems—faced by many VDT workers have become so pervasive that observers have likened the modern office to an "electronic sweatshop."[11]

Women workers are the mainstay of the electronic sweatshop. The postindustrial economy perpetuates the gender-based, two-tier employment pattern, with women, a steady source of inexpensive labor, filling most of the lower-paid positions.[12] It is on the lower rung that women's work is most closely linked with VDTs. The largest group of working women is concentrated in lower-paid clerical occupations—four out of five clerical workers are women.[13] Nationally, women office workers earn only 78 cents for each dollar made by their male counterparts.[14] Although other opportunities have emerged in recent decades, the U.S. Department of Labor forecasts that women, especially minorities, will continue to fill the bulk of these routinized, low-wage positions.[15] Moreover, there is a class and gender bias to the distribution of social costs in the postindustrial economy. Women working in these low-wage occupations, especially VDT workers, are more likely to suffer from occupational safety and health problems.[16]

The market system's tendency to produce workplace safety and health hazards along with material wealth led to the passage of the first state factory inspection and workers' compensation laws during the latter half of the nineteenth century and the Progressive era, respectively. Political recognition that the ravages of industrial enterprise required a federal regulatory presence came in 1970 with congressional enactment of the Occupational Safety and Health Act (OSH Act). The OSH Act established OSHA with the purpose of protecting the safety and health of virtually every working American.

Since the late 1970s, organized labor, women's groups, and others have petitioned OSHA, Congress, and numerous state and local legislatures to promulgate protective regulations governing VDT workers. Despite the serious nature of the problems faced by office workers, OSHA, Congress, and the states have failed to regulate the workplace use of VDTs.

The government's failure to regulate the safety and health problems of office workers raises a number of questions for investigation. Given its mission to protect the safety and health of workers, why has OSHA not acted to promulgate protective regulations for VDT workers? Why did Congress not act to pass VDT legislation or prod OSHA into action? What are the political consequences of trying to make occupational safety and health policy on a piecemeal basis at the state and local levels of government for a problem that is national in scope? Does government's collective failure to respond to VDT workers' problems indicate that the real power to make occupational safety and health policy lies elsewhere?

These questions will be investigated with the help of some analytical tools dealing with the concepts of power and participation. Most studies of occupational safety and health policy focus on OSHA's decision-making track record. They examine OSHA's effectiveness in areas that it has targeted for standard setting, enforcement, and education.[17] This approach often fails to consider the extent to which the areas OSHA targets for decision making are constrained by factors beyond its control, including underfunding, understaffing, political efforts to limit its jurisdiction, and administrative undermining of the agency's mission. The approach taken by this study differs in that it examines the political dynamics of the decision by OSHA and other public officials not to regulate an acknowledged occupational safety and health problem. In addition to the pluralistic focus on decision making, this study uses the analytical concepts of mobilization of bias and non-decision making.

As many analysts have observed, the game of politics is not carried out on a level playing field. E. E. Schattschneider points out that the ability of powerful interests to control the "mobilization of bias" around policy issues and to "define the alternatives" for decision making effectively limits the ability of less powerful groups to challenge the status quo.[18] Peter Bachrach and Morton Baratz describe the mobilization of bias as "a set of predominant values, beliefs, rituals, and institutional procedures ('rules of the game') that operate systematically and consistently to the benefit of certain persons and groups at the expense of others. Those who benefit are placed in a preferred position to defend and promote their vested interests."[19] The mobilization of bias influences and, in turn, is further sustained by a "second face of power" (i.e, nondecision making)—beyond the pluralists' "first face of power" (i.e., decision making)—which operates to block challenges to those in positions of authority.[20] Nondecisions, write Bachrach and Baratz, are "a means by which demands for change in the existing allocation of benefits and privileges in the community can be suffocated before they are even voiced; or kept covert; or killed before they gain access to the relevant decision-making arena; or, failing all these things, maimed or destroyed in the decision-implementing stage of the policy process."[21]

The unlevel nature of the policy-making playing field is further sustained by structural barriers. A key structural barrier of the U.S. political system is its fragmented design. Distrustful of democracy, the Constitution's framers laid out a political system whose purpose was to limit timely and effective majoritarian decision making. These features included the separation of governmental powers into three branches, with each branch having checks and balances on the others, shared powers between the national and state governments, a bicameral national legislature, staggered and indirect elections with differing term lengths and eligibility requirements, and an independent judiciary. This political labyrinth imposes a tremendous structural constraint—more elaborate and extensive than in other industrial democracies—on efforts to make democratic reforms in response to changing economic and social circumstances. Although the OSH Act established a national agency to monitor occupational safety and health conditions, it was grafted onto—rather than designed to replace—the preexisting and ineffective structure of state-made policy. The resulting patchwork quilt of federal and state policies mitigates against a clearly articulated and implemented national policy, and provides opponents with additional opportunities to block or weaken OSHA's regulatory powers.

Historically, the welfare state came later and has remained more limited in scope in the United States than in most of its industrial counterparts. Limited government and states' rights have been strategically invoked by conservatives and business interests to block policy initiatives to use the social welfare state to address societal needs created by an unregulated market system. These doctrines have been used to justify the evisceration of OSHA's powers since its inception in 1971 and have been used most recently by the Republican-controlled Congress to cut OSHA's budget and force an end to work on its proposed ergonomics standard. The governmental void has meant a larger role for market interests in shaping occupational safety and health policy making than in most other industrial countries. Private organizations with quasi-governmental authority play a major role in shaping occupational safety and health policy. In addition to the corporations and trade associations with direct interests in the outcome of the VDT safety and health issue, the American National Standards Institute, the Human Factors Society, the Institute of Electrical and Electronics Engineers, and the National Safety

Council played important roles in shaping and legitimating private alternatives to governmental regulation. As a result, the privatization of occupational safety and health policy leaves workers with little protection against the vicissitudes of market conditions. Complaints that occupational safety and health protections are too expensive to justify their expense are, in effect, calls to transfer more of the cost of production to workers and society in the form of increased incidences of illness, injury, and death.

The economic stakes involved for corporate interests in defeating the regulation of VDT sales and use are immense. The growth of the post-industrial economy is signified by the computer's supplanting of the smoke-stack as the symbol of economic progress. The computer industry occupies a commanding position in the postindustrial economy, facilitating the rapid growth of the VDT-dependent information economy. Today, an estimated 75 million computers are used in American workplaces.[22] Millions more are used at home. The United States is the world's largest computer market ($159 billion in 1994), accounting for more than 39 percent of worldwide sales.[23] It is also one of America's strongest performers in the highly competitive global economy. Worldwide sales, which have grown at an annual rate of 8 percent for the last decade, reached $646 billion in 1994.[24] The computer industry forecasts that more than 15.3 million units will be sold annually by 2003, nearly double the number sold in 1992.[25]

This book will argue that the mobilization of bias in favor of a large private-sector role in shaping occupational safety and health policy enabled corporate interests to dominate the VDT public policy debate and defeat organized labor's campaign for regulation. This was accomplished in several ways. By redefining the VDT ergonomics crisis as only an employee "comfort" problem, corporate interests succeeded in downgrading the seriousness of the problem in the eyes of many public officials. Computer industry control over and/or funding of domestic research into EMFs, and the corporate media's dismissal of troubling EMF studies, effectively limited debate on the need for further research into this important public health question. The ability of corporate interests to shape the policy agenda was strengthened by the federal government's failure to collect data on the true scope of VDT-related illnesses despite their tremendous growth. The Office of Management and Budget (OMB) interfered on behalf of affected corporate interests in scientific research into VDT use and reproductive problems, stripping a potentially embarrassing study of its usefulness. As the engine of the postindustrial economy, computer manufacturers and the information industry provide much-needed sources of tax revenues and jobs. Because economic prosperity helps public officials stay in office, most have been disinclined to regulate the workplace use of VDTs. As a result of this mobilization of bias, neither the federal nor state governments have regulated the workplace use of VDTs in the private sector. Finally, these decisions and nondecisions were made against the backdrop of the federal government's mobilization of bias against a strong occupational safety and health policy and equal treatment of women's health problems.

The plan of the book is as follows. Until fairly recently, the office was considered a hazard-free workplace. Chapter 1 discusses the development and scope of occupational illnesses associated with VDT work. Management has used VDTs to automate work, export work overseas, and exert greater control over both the work process and the worker. Chapter 2 analyzes the power relationship between labor and capital in the office that produced the hazards of VDT work. Organized labor's largely unsuccessful attempts to organize female office workers and negotiate occupational safety and health agreements with business is the subject of chapter 3. The corporate community was quick to mobilize a campaign to counter organized labor's attempts to broaden the scope of the conflict to the public arena. Chapter 4 shows how corporate interlocks and cooperation with the corporate media helped the computer industry get its message out. After largely unsuccessful attempts to bargain with business, organized labor took its campaign for VDT safety and health to the federal level of government, where it hoped to get a more sympathetic hearing. Chapters 5 and 6 discuss how both corporate and governmental use of nondecision-making tactics kept ergonomic and nonionizing radiation issues from being fully addressed and resolved at the federal level. Corporate interests were able to redefine the ergonomics crisis as an employee comfort issue that did not require action by OSHA, and the federal government contributed to this perception by not collecting data on the problem. Similarly, the ability of corporate interests to influence much of the domestic research on EMFs, combined with the corporate media's dismissal of foreign studies that questioned the safety of EMFs, enabled corporate interests to persuade government officials that further research was not needed. Under the Reagan administration, the treatment of science and technology issues became highly politicized. Chapter 7 explains how the Reagan administration used OMB to interfere with

NIOSH's epidemiological study of VDT workers and subordinate safety and health policy to its goal of deregulating business. The federal government's policy of inaction restricted the scope of conflict to the state and local levels. Chapter 8 examines why many state government officials considered VDT regulations a drag on their competitive efforts to attract high-technology investment, and its consequences for labor's legislative campaign. Finally, chapter 9 presents my conclusions and recommendations for reform.

Chapter I

The Hazards of Working with Video Display Terminals

The electronic office . . . makes much more efficient use of the current labor force. It gives more satisfaction to people who work in the electronic office, except for some poor person who has to sit in front of a CRT eight hours a day.
—Charles A. Jortberg, president, Jortberg Associates, an office automation consulting firm.

For many years white-collar work was considered to be safe and hazard-free, but the introduction of computers has given rise to safety and health problems in the office on an unprecedented scale.[1] Studies show that those who work with video display terminals (VDTs) experience more safety and health problems than non–VDT workers in control groups.[2] The National Institute of Occupational Safety and Health (NIOSH) reports that "the VDT imposes physical stressors that other office machines or hand work do not."[3] With millions of people using computers in both workplaces and homes, the VDT safety and health problem has become a public policy issue of major magnitude. As Dr. Steven Sauter, director of motivation and stress research at NIOSH, said, "We have millions of people using VDTs . . . and when you have even a small proportion of millions of people complaining, then you've got a public health problem."[4] Ailments reported by VDT workers fall into two categories: those attributed to the nonionizing radiation emitted by the computer terminal's flyback transformer and the vision, stress, and musculoskeletal problems that can be dealt with by the science of ergonomics.

The Problem of Nonionizing Radiation

The most controversial of the VDT-related safety and health hazards are associated with nonionizing radiation emitted by the video display terminal.

The conventional scientific wisdom is that electromagnetic fields (EMFs) are too weak to damage human cells; however, a small but steadily accumulating body of scientific literature indicates that nonionizing radiation does pose a risk.[5] Two types of nonionizing radiation on the electromagnetic spectrum are involved in the VDT controversy: very low frequency (VLF) waves emitted by the flyback transformer and horizontal deflection coil and extremely low frequency (ELF) waves produced by the vertical deflection coil. VLF and ELF radiation produce both electric and magnetic fields. Studies show that sixty-Hertz pulsed ELF waves, like those emitted by VDTs, can interfere with the immune system's defenses, altering cell structure and promoting leukemia, lymphoma, and brain cancer (tumors).[6] A Finnish study, for example, found that women who worked with VDTs that emit high levels of magnetic ELF fields experienced "a significantly increased odds ratio for spontaneous abortion" compared to women who used VDTs emitting low levels of magnetic fields.[7]

Health problems include reproductive hazards, such as infertility, birth defects, stillbirths, and higher than normal incidences of miscarriages. Allergic reactions to the electromagnetic fields emitted by VDTs—nausea, fatigue, hyperactivity, headaches, skin rashes on the face and upper extremities, and angina—have also been reported. EMFs of the same frequency as those emitted by VDTs have also been linked to leukemia, Alzheimer's disease, and brain tumors.[8] Some cases of premature eye cataracts have also been reported, but studies have not been conducted to see if there is a link to VDTs.

Numerous clusters of miscarriages among VDT workers have been reported in the United States, Canada, and Europe since 1979. Given the fact that many workers are unaware of the potential dangers of VDTs, it is likely that other clusters have gone unreported. A "cluster" is an epidemiological term designating the higher than normal coincidence of medical ailments in concentrated groups. A 1988 epidemiological study of 1,583 pregnant women conducted by the Kaiser Permanente Medical Care Program of California found that those who worked more than twenty hours a week at VDTs during the first three months of pregnancy had statistically significant increases (80 percent) in miscarriages.[9] More research is needed to clarify the extent to which extremely low frequency EMFs present a public health problem.

Ergonomic Problems

Since the rise of the industrial revolution, the work process has used workers as cogs in the larger wheel of production, requiring that they physically adapt themselves to the organization of the process without regard for the safety and health problems that might result. For example, assembly-line workers, who are expected to perform the same simple tasks over and over, suffer from high rates of repetitive strain injury. Ergonomics, sometimes called "human factors," involves the study and redesign of the workplace to address the safety and health needs of the worker. Most ergonomic-related problems result from the design and introduction of VDTs into the workplace without proper regard for the physiological needs of the individual. Professor Don B. Chaffin of the University of Michigan's Center for Ergonomics estimated that 98 percent of engineers have no background in ergonomics.[10]

Unlike the typewriters they replaced, VDTs are used by a greater variety of workers for longer hours. Managers often introduce VDTs into the office using a one-size-fits-all approach without taking the physiological differences between workers into account. VDT users are then forced to contort their bodies to the dictates of unadjustable VDTs—which do not have adjustable screens or detachable keyboards—and standard-issue chairs and desks. The human body is not designed to remain in a sedentary position for long periods of time, yet many VDT workers are expected to sit for hours on end. Denying workers the discretion to take rest breaks when needed puts them at greater risk of musculoskeletal illness. Failure to address ergonomic-related problems virtually assures that workers will experience vision problems, stress, and cumulative trauma disorders.

Stress, one of the most dangerous health hazards associated with VDT work, is the scourge of the information age—so much so that it has given rise to the term *technostress*.[11] Most workers experience some stress on the job from time to time, but the computerization of office work means that many VDT users are continuously exposed to highly stressful working conditions. A study of female data-entry workers in Quebec found that those who performed highly repetitive tasks and suffered from work speedup-induced stress experienced more psychiatric problems and were more dependent on prescription and over-the-counter drugs than other working women. Finding that they were more alienated from their jobs than auto assembly-line workers, the report's authors concluded that VDT data-entry work is a "high-risk occupation."[12]

Because workers using VDTs can process more information much faster than ever before, managers expect employees to produce more. In a nation-wide survey of office workers for Steelcase, Inc., one of the nation's largest manufacturers of office furniture, Louis Harris and Associates concluded that "the speed and efficiency of computers have no doubt raised produc-tivity pressures for everyone."[13] NIOSH observed that the number and severity of safety and health problems, such as visual and musculoskeletal ailments, increase, as do stress levels resulting from increased production pressures. Another NIOSH study concluded that "VDT operators reported higher levels of job stress and health complaints" than those who did not use them, and that "the job stressors showing the greatest impact on the clerical [VDT] operators dealt with workload, workplace, lack of control over job activities, boredom and concerns about career development."[14]

All these factors contribute to increased levels of occupational stress, which have been linked to angina (an early sign of heart disease), heart attacks, fatigue, gastrointestinal illness, headaches, and psychosomatic disorders, such as nervous tension and depression.[15] Working at a VDT for more than four hours a day, or twenty hours a week, greatly increases the number of health complaints.[16] For example, secretaries have reported higher rates of stress working with VDTs than typewriters.[17] NIOSH investigators were sur-prised to find that some VDT workers experienced the highest levels of stress they had ever measured, including among air traffic controllers.[18] In 1980, NIOSH examined the job stressors that affected three groups of employees: clerical workers who used VDTs, those who did not, and professionals who used VDTs. They found that the jobs performed by clerical workers using VDTs were designed in such a way that they were the most highly routinized and required the least amount of creative input. The result, NIOSH reported, was a higher rate of stress:

> When the job features of the various groups are examined we see
> that the clerical VDT operators held jobs involving rigid work pro-
> cedures with high production standards, constant pressure for per-
> formance, very little operator control over job tasks, and little
> identification with and satisfaction from the end-product of their
> work activity. In contrast to the clerical VDT operators, the profes-
> sionals using VDTs held jobs that allowed for flexibility, control over

job tasks, utilization of their education and a great deal of satisfaction and pride in their end-product.[19]

The problem of speedup-induced occupational stress is compounded by the computer monitoring of VDT workers, especially stressful when done on an ongoing basis. Jobs are often routinized in ways that make computer monitoring easier.[20] Medical researchers have observed that stress increases as an employee's control over the job decreases. Workers doing repetitive tasks report higher incidences of high blood pressure, nervous tension, depression, job dissatisfaction, sleep disturbances, and cardiovascular disorders.[21]

Vision problems, such as eyestrain, visual fatigue, and headaches, are the most commonly reported complaints of VDT workers. Approximately ten million Americans experience VDT-related vision problems, accounting for 14 percent of the people who get eye exams annually.[22] The American Optometric Association, which urges VDT users to get eye examinations, estimates that anywhere from 50 to 75 percent of these workers suffer from vision problems.[23] A survey of two thousand secretaries by Minolta Corporation's Business Equipment Division found that 52 percent suffered from eye strain.[24] Bright office lighting and sunlight create screen glare and reflections that cause vision problems. The prevention of glare on VDT screens requires light levels that are two to three times lower than those in offices without VDTs. Screen glare also contributes to musculoskeletal problems by forcing workers to contort themselves in the attempt to see screen images more clearly. The monotonous and repetitious nature of VDT data-entry work is another cause of vision problems.[25]

Inflexible and poorly designed VDTs and furniture and improper lighting contribute to musculoskeletal ailments of the lower back, shoulders, neck, arms, wrists, fingers, hands, and nervous system. Cumulative trauma disorders (CTDs), also known as repetitive strain injuries (RSIs), include musculoskeletal disorders such as carpal tunnel syndrome, epicondylitis, ganglion, tendinitis, and tenosynovitis. CTDs are progressive illness that manifest themselves over time. They are caused by the continuous unnatural bending motions of the arms, wrists, elbows, fingers, neck, and back in the worker's effort to compensate for the inflexible design of the VDT, chair, desk, and lighting.

Prior to the VDT, office workers typically performed a variety of tasks in the course of a day's work, such as writing, typing, filing, taking dictation, making mathematical calculations, and writing correspondence. The mix of tasks, interspersed with pauses, helped to give the musculoskeletal system a break from repetitive strain. The incorporation of these functions in the computer eliminated the need to stop typing to change paper, make corrections, or perform a different task. The lack of spontaneous work breaks and the speeded-up pace of VDT work contribute to the repetitive motion strain that causes CTDs. Those who are afflicted with CTDs can experience severe pain in the arms and wrists that may leave them unable to lift light objects or open drawers.

Carpal tunnel syndrome is the most common type of cumulative trauma disorder suffered by VDT workers. A 1989 study conducted for NIOSH by Ambulatory Sentinel Practices Network of Denver revealed that VDT workers had the highest percentage (21 percent) of cases of carpal tunnel syndrome of all occupational groups.[26] The syndrome results from the repeated bending of the tendons and the median nerve, which travel through the wrist to the hand. Symptoms include numbness, weakness, and a tingling sensation in hands, wrists, forearms, and fingers. If left untreated, surgery of the wrist ligament may be needed. At this stage, "it is important that the worker is not returned to the same job or tasks that precipitated" the problem.[27] On average, it takes longer for injured workers to recover from carpal tunnel syndrome than from any other type of occupational injury. The fact that VDT workers share this debilitating affliction with meat and poultry packers, automobile workers, postal service letter sorters, and supermarket checkout clerks illustrates the extent to which office work has been routinized and automated.

CTDs have been the fastest growing category of occupational illness for more than a decade.[28] CTDs accounted for only 18 percent of all reported occupational illnesses in 1981, but the disorders have skyrocketed to more than 60 percent of all reported cases by 1993.[29]

Although the problem's existence and scope has been documented for more than a decade, the Bureau of Labor Statistics (BLS) still does not keep detailed data on the number of CTDs resulting from VDT work. But the scope of the CTD problem among VDT workers can be pieced together from other sources. In 1989, Gerard F. Scannel, administrator of the Occupational Safety and Health Administration (OSHA), attributed much of the sharp rise in CTDs during the past decade to the increase in computer work. NIOSH concurred:

"The rise [in CTDs] is due in part to new, high-tech workstations," said Daniel Habes, an industrial engineer with the institute.[30] NIOSH's and OSHA's assessment of the severity of the CTD problem is supported by a number of studies. Analyses conducted by the Newspaper Guild and Communications Workers of America indicate that as many as 50 percent of the workers in the newspaper and telecommunications industries suffer from CTDs, and the Minolta study found that 46 percent of the 2,000 secretaries interviewed complained of back or neck problems.[31] The Massachusetts Coalition of New Office Technology, an organization of more than forty unions and community groups, surveyed 314 full-time VDT operators at NYNEX and found that 29 percent experienced the symptoms of CTDs.[32]

Reporters developed CTD problems after they switched from typewriters to VDT work stations. NIOSH and a team from the University of Michigan conducted a health hazard evaluation at Newsday and found that "working as a reporter was significantly associated with hand/wrist, elbow/forearm, and neck symptoms." Of the 834 employees studied, 40 percent suffered from CTDs; of these, 23 percent were afflicted with hand and wrist problems, 17 percent experienced neck pains, 13 percent suffered from elbow and forearm pains, and 11 percent had shoulder problems. Their report concluded that the "percent of time typing or typing speed was significantly associated with symptoms in each of the four upper extremity joint areas."[33]

Many of these ailments can be prevented, or alleviated, by implementing ergonomic knowledge; for example, lower levels of ambient lighting (to eliminate screen glare), ergonomically designed furniture, periodic rest breaks, alternative work after long stretches at the VDT, and redesign of the work process. Purchasers should take variations in body size into account when buying VDT work stations, rather than following the one-size-fits-all approach. Most VDT users are women, but many office work stations are designed for the longer leg and arm reach of men. "The value of adjustable work stations is not to make everybody fit," says Roger Stephens, OSHA's ergonomist, but to allow workers to change their positions during the day. He adds that workers are more likely to follow ergonomic recommendations if they are included in their preparation.[34]

Prevention of ergonomic problems is often hampered by the fact that the workers who need the ergonomically designed furniture the most (e.g., secretaries and clerical workers using VDTs) are not included in the planning process and are usually the last to get the proper equipment. As one ergonomist put it, "Executives get the best chairs, and secretaries get the worst, which is too bad, because secretaries spend more time in them."[35] Including workers in the ergonomic planning process, and redesigning the work process to give workers greater creative leeway, is important for many reasons: it results in better implementation of ergonomic proposals, helps to prevent health problems, improves productivity, and gives workers greater on-the-job responsibility.

Despite their tremendous growth since the early 1980s, VDT-related occupational safety and health problems remain a low priority for both federal and state governments.

Chapter 2

The Office of the Future Meets the Factory of the Past

The industrial revolution now comes to the office much faster than it did to the factory, for it has been able to draw upon the factory as a model. —C. Wright Mills,
White Collar: The American Middle Classes

Since its introduction in the early 1970s, the video display terminal has been heralded by office automation advocates as the technology that would transform office work.[1] The computer-automated office, these enthusiasts said, would not only be user-friendly but also improve the quality of work by liberating clerical workers, secretaries, and typists from routine tasks. As a result, office workers would be free to learn new skills that would upgrade and enrich their jobs. In a "special executive briefing" on the "office of the future," *Business Week* reported that computerized "office automation has emerged as a full-blown systems approach that will revolutionize how offices work."[2] Adia Personnel Services, the world's second largest supplier of both temporary and full-time workers, issued a report forecasting that "as the office becomes increasingly automated, routine tasks will become the province of these machines [i.e., VDTs] which extend human intellect, freeing staff and managers alike to expand their personal and professional roles."[3] Writing in the *Sloan Management Review,* Michael D. Zisman predicted that the VDT "will relieve workers of the mundane and routine functions and turn these over to computer control."[4] "New gadgetry, better jobs, less monotony—all are part of the office of the future," proclaimed *U.S. News & World Report.*[5] IBM advised its corporate clients that "centralizing and automating [VDT] network operations help eliminate routine operator tasks and errors, freeing skilled operators and programmers for more productive tasks."[6] Adia's report went so far as to suggest that VDT-empowered office workers might threaten corporate control of the workplace: "Today's machines require much more human input and are capable of much more than merely performing a repetitive task. The person at the keyboard can input data, control, interpret and creat [sic] patterns. If knowledge is power, then today's office workers have the ability to shape a very powerful system. And, the acquired ability to use these machines can lead to changes in the balance of power within an organization."[7]

Others, however, have maintained that the VDT is being used to increase management control over the work process and create routinized jobs that require less skill than the ones they have replaced. Labor and technology analyst Harley Shaiken observed that "it is ironic that a technology such as word processing, which theoretically requires more skills than the typewriter it replaces, can be used in a way that *deskills* the secretary or typist; used in a way that increases the monitoring or control and decreases the independence of the worker involved."[8] Jon E. Seidel, president of EDP Consulting, Inc., argued that office automation was leading to more monotonous work. "It is a very, very significant issue," he said. "It is the issue of control, the ability of the machine to dictate the pace of work that the human does."[9] The same *Business Week* story that heralded the office of the future also intimated that the transition would not be smooth and painless for office workers. IBM vice president, William F. Laughlin, was candid: "People will adapt nicely to office systems—if their arms are broken . . . and we're in the twisting stage now."[10]

Scientific Management and Automation Come to the Office

In many respects, the computerized clerical workplace more closely resembles a postindustrial version of the factory of the past than the utopian vision of the office of the future. Although VDT technology is relatively new, the corporate quest to adapt office work to the industrial ideal of the work process dates back to the Progressive-era concept of scientific management. The expanding volume of paperwork during that time forced firms to take a closer look at controlling costs and work flow. But the search for increased office productivity was hampered by the difficulty of gauging clerical work output. Unlike the factory, where the assembly line and automation rationalized the work process, the problem of how to measure the intangible nature of office work—the decisions, delivery of services, and information that constitute the finished product—remained a constant challenge.

William H. Leffingwell, a Progressive-era management consultant and president of the National Office Management Association, adapted Frederick W. Taylor's principles of scientific management, or Taylorism, to the study of the office work process. Scientific management requires that each task be studied in order to establish the most efficient way of doing it in the shortest possible time. Just as Taylor painstakingly held a stopwatch over laborers to find the one best way of shoveling coal, Leffingwell tried to find the most efficient way for an office worker to open an envelope and remove its contents. This process involved the standardization of tools as well as the worker's motions. That all workers used the right shovel or paper cutter was just as important as the amount of coal lifted per shovel, or the way the contents of an envelope were removed. Once the one best way was established, it became the standard by which managers measured the efficiency of other workers performing the same task. Dr. Harlow S. Person, the managing director of the Taylor Society, neatly summed up Leffingwell's approach: "The mental attitude of scientific management . . . must govern the management of clerical as well as of processing operations; in fact, desk activities *are* processing operations as surely as are activities at machine and bench."[11]

From management's standpoint, one of Taylorism's most important benefits was that standardized production procedures increased its control over the work process. As Leffingwell made clear: "Effective management implies control. The terms are in a sense interchangeable, as management without control is not conceivable." Like Taylor, Leffingwell believed that too much discretion was left to the worker in the non-scientifically managed workplace. Leffingwell asserted that the purpose of scientific management is to assure that "the balance shall be very much in favor of the manager, and not against him."[12] Unions, which might insist on having input into how efficiency standards were established or question other aspects of Taylorism, were viewed as impediments to greater efficiency.

The mechanization of office work was the development that permitted managers to start emulating the Taylor/Leffingwell model. Machines for taking dictation and simulating stenography; for punching, sorting, and tabulating data on cards; for bookkeeping, accounting, addressing, and billing; and for photocopying and data processing facilitated the creation of office factories.[13] Writing at midcentury, C. Wright Mills observed the effects of Leffingwell's legacy in what he referred to as the "managerial demiurge":

> The introduction of office machinery and sales devices has been mechanizing the office. . . . Since the 'twenties it has increased the division of white-collar labor, recomposed personnel, and lowered skill levels. Routine operations in minutely subdivided organizations have replaced the bustling interest of work in well-known groups. Even on managerial and professional levels, the growth of rational bureaucracies has made work more like factory production. The managerial demiurge is constantly furthering all these trends: mechanization, more minute division of labor, the use of less skilled and less expensive workers.[14]

From his vantage point in the early 1970s, Harry Braverman reported that the mechanization of clerical work made it possible for managers to train clerical workers more quickly, thereby making them more interchangeable and expendable: "The recording of everything in mechanical form, and the movement of everything in a mechanical way, is thus the ideal of the office manager. But this conversion of the office flow into a high-speed industrial process requires the conversion of the great mass of office workers into more or less helpless attendants of that process."[15]

Neither Taylor nor Leffingwell took human factors, that is, the design of work to give meaning and responsibility to the worker, into account. They expected workers to adapt to the requirements of the work process; job satisfaction and human fulfillment were considered irrelevant. The omission of the humanistic element was noted at the time by critics, including John Dewey, who wrote: "Much is said about scientific management of work. It is a narrow view which restricts the science which secures efficiency of operation to movements of muscles. The chief opportunity for science is the discovery of the relations of man to his work—including his relations to others who take part—which will enlist his intelligent interest in what he is doing."[16]

Despite increases in productivity achieved by efforts to mechanize office work, the limited capabilities of business machines could not keep pace with the expanding information economy's increasing volume of paperwork. Office costs increased from 20 to 30 percent of expenses in the 1960s to 40 to 50 percent of expenses by the early 1980s. With the total cost of U.S. business operations hitting the $1 trillion mark in 1981, that amounted to $400–500 billion spent annually on office expenses.[17] But 1980 automation investment figures showed that U.S. businesses still spent an average of $12.50 per factory worker for each dollar invested per office worker.[18]

Although factory productivity increased 85 percent during the 1970s, the small gains in office productivity (only 4 percent) were overshadowed by the doubling of operating costs.[19] Vincent E. Giuliano, an office automation consultant at Arthur D. Little, Inc., wrote that "the highest cost activities in manual correspondence are making multiple copies, filing them and retrieving them."[20] A *Fortune* magazine advertorial stated the problem succinctly: "The office [is] the jugular of the low productivity problem that faces business today."[21]

As the crisis of office productivity deepened, the business community came to see computerization of the work process as the answer to its dilemma of how to manage the burgeoning flow of paper and cut labor costs. With VDTs, management could exert much greater control over the office work process and routinize it along industrial lines. IBM told employers that VDT-based automation would bring "manufacturing and production lines into the office" by having clerical "work divided [and] specialization introduced."[22] John Naisbitt also saw the postindustrial workplace in terms of its industrial predecessor: "We now mass-produce information the way we used to mass-produce cars. In the information society, we have systematized the production of knowledge and amplified our brain power. To use an industrial metaphor, we now mass-produce knowledge and this knowledge is the driving force of our economy."[23]

Corporate America's reliance on the "industrial metaphor" as a model to achieve its automation goals was best exemplified by an influential *Harvard Business Review* article by Richard J. Matteis, a Citibank senior vice president. He wrote that America's largest bank, like many of its labor-intensive competitors in the banking, finance, real estate, and insurance industries, was faced with an overwhelming paperwork crisis in the 1960s and early 1970s. Labor accounted for 70 percent of Citibank's costs, whereas expenditures on computers and their programs amounted to only 10 percent. For Matteis, Citibank's solution to the paperwork crisis was "to flip the ratio entirely . . . until labor and other operations costs constituted only 30 percent, while [computer] hardware and software made up the rest."[24]

Matteis acknowledged that the "management program of controls, forecasting, and accountability" used in banking were "borrowed from production management," and its implementation was made possible by the introduction of VDT-based computer technology:

The recognition that a new technology was needed was also borrowed from the manufacturing industries. The production management disciplines that ensure the smooth running of mass production plants had been born alongside the introduction of machine tools that could produce more at less cost. In the Industrial Revolution, machinery and the development of modern management techniques were two strands of the same thread. In banking, however, the equivalent of the machine tool is the computer.[25]

In short, VDT-based automation brought office managers closer to their goal of exerting the kind of control over the office work process that their industrial counterparts did. But automation of the office, without regard for the human factor, created new job hazards. As NIOSH reported:

This is a serious concern since the persons who design systems such as these, and thereby the work activities of VDT operators, are typically computer scientists and systems analysts who have no concept of the human element in such a work process. *This leads to a dehumanization of the work activity that is similar to that produced by the introduction of assembly lines in manufacturing industries. In fact, such offices become "paper factories" with clerical assembly lines in which the work content is simplified to increase "thru-put" and capitalize on computer capabilities. This leads to jobs that produce boredom and job dissatisfaction. As such, the machinery becomes a source of misery rather than a helpful tool as it is for the professionals using the VDTs.*[26]

The computerization of work is contributing to the social stratification of American society. It is creating a two-tier work force, with an upper level of highly skilled and educated workers and a much larger, lower level of those who are less skilled and educated. A U.S. Senate study of new job creation from 1979 to 1987 found that 90 percent of all new jobs were created in the white-collar sector, but more than 50 percent of the new jobs paid less than the U.S. government's 1987 poverty threshold of $11,611.[27] The VDT's versatility has even led to a streamlining of the management hierarchy, mostly among midlevel managers and professionals. The automation of midlevel management duties means that, as with clerical workers, fewer employees are expected to do more work. In terms of job loss, however, the biggest impact of office automation is on the lower-tier, clerical workers. The economic boom in the information industries made clerical work the fastest growing occupation during the 1970s, but computer automation slowed the growth rate during the 1980s, and this trend is expected to continue into the next century.[28]

Controlling Employees by Computer Monitoring

Computer technology can automatically monitor VDT workers' production, which gives managers greater control over the work process. As William R. McAlister, vice president of Xytec Corporation, a manufacturer of computer monitoring devices, explained, these devices obtain results "much more thorough 'than [those] that used to be gotten by some guy with a clipboard jotting things down.' "[29] The increasing availability of cheaper and more sophisticated computer technology has made employee monitoring a pervasive phenomenon. 9 to 5, The National Association of Working Women estimates that ten million VDT workers were being monitored.[30] Among the many companies monitoring their employees are Blue Cross–Blue Shield, Equitable Life Assurance, MCI Telecommunications, NYNEX, the *New York Times,* and the *Washington Post.* At the White House Conference on Productivity in 1982, President Reagan urged business leaders to be more innovative in their efforts to boost productivity. One of the innovations managers turned to was computer monitoring. Further encouragement for computer monitoring came from Reagan's attorney general, Edwin Meese III, who exhorted corporate executives to "take responsibility for surveillance" of their employees. As a result, the Reagan administration's exhortations to increase productivity legitimated management's increasing use of computer monitoring.[31]

The process of computer monitoring involves recording the keystrokes of VDT workers, who are expected to keep pace with the fastest workers (e.g., the top 10 percent) in the group. Employee productivity figures are posted on a bulletin board at the end of the week as a means of peer pressure to induce the slower operators to work faster. Those who cannot are warned, exhorted to work faster, and, perhaps, docked a percentage of their pay. Many VDT operators are pieceworkers, whose pay is directly linked to their output. The system of computerized work pacing has the effect of disciplining workers and speeding up work, just as the assembly line does in the factory. "In the worst sites," notes management consultant Ronald Rice, "centralized [word processing] . . . is designed as an industrial assembly line, emphasizing line counts and time spent on line."[32]

Employers not only count how many keystrokes a VDT operator makes but also calculate how many mistakes are made, how long it takes to do the assigned job, and the amount of idle time between tasks. Telephone operators are monitored to ensure that they don't spend more time than management prefers answering each caller's inquiry, and airline reservations operators are monitored to see how well they make the sell. Computer programs can also be used to monitor employees' telephone conversations for key words and phrases that may indicate signs of union or political activities, drugs, and personal problems. Managers can even attempt to stimulate workers with subliminal messages that appear instantaneously on the screen, such as "work faster" or "I love my job."[33]

Professionals are also being monitored, a sign that the extension of management's control of the work process is not limited to lowly word and data processors. According to *The Electronic Supervisor*, a report by the Office of Technology Assessment (OTA), management's surveillance of VDT work "is increasingly being directed to higher level, more skilled technical, professional, and managerial positions. Even the most complex work has its routine elements, and given sufficient analysis, those elements can be identified, grouped together, and counted. The jobs of commodities broker, computer programmer, and bank loan officer . . . could lend themselves to monitoring."[34] Another example is that of newspaper reporters and journalists. The newsroom was one of the first work locales to switch from the typewriter to the VDT. A profession requiring superior skills, journalism doesn't seem to be the typical candidate for computer monitoring, job pacing, and piecework. But journalists' productivity is now being monitored, and some newspapers have started using the results to force reporters to produce more and have even experimented with pay on a piecework basis.[35] The overall effect of the automation and monitoring of many professional tasks is to level out the work hierarchy, making the job characteristics of many professionals less distinct from those of lesser-skilled workers.

Corporate management argues that computer monitoring is essential to the efficient operation of a productive office, helps them determine who is the best person for the job, and guards against employee theft of corporate services.[36] Corporate managers realize that computer monitoring is an unpopular and controversial practice, so they have attempted to redefine what the political debate is about by arguing that the issue is productivity, not invasion of privacy. Understanding that the way issues are defined often determines who wins the debate, they prefer euphemisms, such as "work measurement" for the more onerous sounding computer monitoring, "incentives" for piecework, and "service observation" for surveillance of employee telephone conversations. Employers claim that these monitoring systems are "objective," that is, they judge all employees by the same standard. If Equitable Life Assurance Company officials are to be believed, "workers like the objectivity" of computer monitoring, and "any stress" they feel "is self-imposed," not the result of an omnipresent electronic surveillance.[37] But the power to decide what information will be collected, and how it will be used, gives management a potent tool to control labor. "Jobs are often simplified just so they can be monitored, just so productivity can be kept track of," reports Sharon Danann, 9 to 5's research director. The American Civil Liberties Union reports that employers have subjectively used and distorted data to harass employees, especially those engaged in union activity, and those with alternative life-styles.[38]

The irony of computer monitoring and its attendant piecework/incentive pay system is that it usually doesn't achieve its stated goal—increased productivity. Many supervisors believe that "posting keystrokes . . . salary increases based on keystrokes, and incentives [are] key motivators" of employees, but a poll of data-entry managers conducted by the Data Entry Management Association (DEMA) revealed that "statistical results showed that *incentive programs do not necessarily improve employee performance.*" These results led DEMA president Norman Bodek to comment: "I guess if an incentive program is putting too much pressure on the operators it should be eliminated. Probably, good management is the answer."[39]

Rather than improving productivity, computer monitoring tends to increase employee stress—which contributes to occupational illness. It lowers employee morale and productivity and increases turnover. Monitoring increases stress levels, especially when it is used on a continuous basis or for disciplinary purposes. In fact, stress due to VDT work has become so prevalent that a new term, *technostress,* has been dubbed to describe it.[40] The Connecticut Union of Telephone Workers surveyed telephone operators using VDTs at Southern New England Bell and found that 75 percent of those who were monitored suffered from muscle aches, headaches, and dizziness. At Bell Canada, keystroke monitoring of individuals' productivity resulted in high levels of job-related stress. Two-thirds of the operators studied reported "high" or "very high" stress levels. As a result of union pressure, management switched to group keystroke monitoring.[41]

From Typewriter to VDT: Women and Office Automation

A good example of the structural segregation of women workers along technological lines is provided by the introduction of the typewriter to office work. At the outset, the positions of typist and secretary were male-dominated. But as demand increased, the position of typist became a mass occupation considered by managers to be more suitable to the "dexterity" of women's fingers. As typewriting became more of a low-pay, dead-end position, it became increasingly sex typed as women's work. Women were working at one-third of the two million typewriters in use in 1910. By 1930, 96 percent of all stenographers and typists were women.[42] Today, women constitute nearly 80 percent of the nation's administrative support and clerical workers. The Women's Bureau expects women to make-up the overwhelming majority of office workers for the foreseeable future.[43]

As with the typist of the past, the majority of female VDT workers in the office of the future are stuck in jobs with little chance for job enrichment or career advancement. Women are the production workers of the postindustrial economy. A poll conducted for Honeywell, Inc., revealed that women were twice as likely as men to be assigned to jobs requiring them to spend more than half their work time at the VDT.[44] An examination of the occupations in which this new technology is widely used reveals the extent to which women's work and VDT work are intertwined (see table 1).

Besides being heavily dependent on women workers, the VDT-based occupations shown in table 1 have three things in common. First, all the occupations in which women predominate have median annual earnings well below the 1994 national median of $24,284. Conversely, women are in the minority in the highest paid, higher skilled occupation in which VDT use is prevalent—editors and reporters. Second, with the exception of secretary, which is virtually an all-female occupation, women earn less than men in all the lower-paid VDT-using jobs, even where they constitute the majority of workers. Although female office workers have narrowed the pay gap over the last decade, they still earn only seventy-eight cents for each dol-

Table 1
Occupations in Which VDT Use is Prevalent

Occupation	Number Employed (in thousands)	Percentage of Women Employed	Median Annual Earnings	Percentage of Men's Pay Made by Women
Data-entry keyers	499	83.4	18,876	85.3
Editors and reporters	202	44.6	31,928	86.9
Financial records clerks	1,455	88.9	19,552	92.1
General office clerks	476	80.5	19,344	91.1
Records processing clerks*	633	79.5	20,592	90.0
Secretaries	2,604	98.8	19,916	100.0
Telephone operators	120	86.7	20,384	NA
Transportation ticket and reservation agents	185	77.8	21,164	84.5

SOURCE: U.S. Department of Labor, Bureau of Labor Statistics, *Employment and Earnings*, table 39.
NOTE: Percentages were calculated by the author.
*Except financial records clerks.

lar their male co-workers make.[45] The persistence of this structural pattern of pay inequity also helps employers keep labor costs down.

Finally, all these jobs, with the exception of editors and reporters, have become more automated, routinized with increased workloads since the introduction of the VDT. They provide little room for employee creativity or variation in the work process. For example, a computer program dictates that telephone operators take no more than twenty-four seconds per call. At this rate, they may handle as many as twelve hundred calls a day. This involves a continuous process of repetitive motions at the VDT that creates physiological stress and can lead to the development of painful CTDs such as carpal tunnel syndrome.[46] OSHA has cited computerization as contributing to the deskilling and routinization of office work. Gerard F. Scannel, administrator of OSHA, said: "We seem to be asking people to do their jobs faster and in smaller, more finely defined tasks."[47]

Ironically, the deskilling of white-collar work is occurring at a time when more Americans are going to college to increase their occupational skills. The decline of occupations requiring college-level skills means that those with less of an education are being pushed out of jobs they otherwise would be capable of doing. As the *New York Times* reports, the Department of Labor has found that "hundreds of thousands of jobs," including secretarial, bookkeeping, clerical, data- and word-processing positions, "once creditably performed without a college degree, are going to college graduates as employers take advantage of an oversupply of them."[48]

Performing jobs that require little skill is a common source of stress. A survey of 2,000 secretaries by Minolta Corporation found that 50 percent were frustrated by a lack of responsibility on the job and 40 percent felt overqualified for the work they were doing.[49] Kelly Services, Inc., the nation's largest supplier of temporary secretarial and office workers, polled 504 corporate secretaries and found that the "level of education also influences stress. Those secretaries with the highest education reported the least amount of job satisfaction and were the least capable of preventing work-related stress from affecting their personal lives."[50]

The high levels of occupational stress suffered by secretaries and clerical workers is due in large part to the fact that VDT use has not lessened their workloads as office automation advocates expected. VDT workers have heavier workloads than their counterparts in non-automated offices.[51] In a nationwide survey of office workers for Steelcase, Inc., one of the nation's largest manufacturers of office furniture, Louis Harris and Associates found that the percentage of office workers who felt they were overworked increased with VDT use—from 42 to 49 percent between 1978 and 1989.[52] Likewise, the Kelly Services survey found increasing numbers of secretaries spending more time tied to their VDTs. Fifty-eight percent spent more than half their time using VDTs during any given work week. Forty percent of the secretaries under the age of twenty-five were using VDTs for 70 percent of the day, and 30 percent said that "all" the secretaries did word processing. Most of the secretaries interviewed said that "word processing equipment is in use for a large portion of each day."[53]

Office automation has not resulted in increased career opportunities for office workers. IBM predicted that secretaries and clerical employees would have "their job status raised" as a result of the computerization of office work.[54] But after two decades working in the office of the future, secretarial and clerical earnings—the market's measure of job status—remain low (see table 1). Using educational level as a measure of job status, the Louis Harris survey found that those who use VDTs for more than five hours a day "tend to be less educated than office workers overall (37 percent are college graduates, compared with 46 percent overall). They are more likely than average to be women (61 to 53 percent), and show distinctly lower levels of personal income (73 percent report their own income as falling in the $35,000—or less—category, compared with 62 percent of office workers overall in this income group)."[55]

The Minolta survey revealed that two-thirds of the two thousand secretaries interviewed doubted they stood a fair chance of career advancement and commensurate salary increases.[56] The Kelly Services survey of corporate secretaries found that there was very little room for career advancement to management positions. "When asked what new positions or careers open up as a result of word processing, very few name positions which could be considered middle level management or higher," the Kelly survey reported. It added: "When asked to identify new decision-making responsibilities that they see as a result of word processing, most name duties which are essentially the same as the traditional tasks done before the introduction of automated equipment." T. E. Adderley, the president of Kelly Services, said that "secretaries' career expectations in the automated office have not all been fulfilled," but added that "they are beginning to see real benefits in terms of increased productivity and reduced stress."[57] However, the Kelly survey painted a different picture, concluding, "Stress is a very real problem for many secretaries, as indicated by the large number (eighty percent) who claim that their job is stressful." The Kelly survey also found that secretaries under twenty-five suffered "more stress and a low level of job satisfaction" and were "inclined to find meeting deadlines and being overworked to be very stressful."[58]

Computer automation is also altering the secretarial-managerial relationship. As a result, many secretaries now work for more than one boss. According to Sylvia Kurop, the director of placement for the Katherine Gibbs School of New York, "It is very seldom now that you have a one-on-one situation." Many secretaries using VDTs have seen their workloads increase without commensurate pay raises.[59] The Kelly Services report found that although 88 percent believed that their increased workloads merited pay increases, only 30 percent had actually received one as a result. The median annual earnings for secretaries in 1994 was only $19,916, more than $4,000 below the median for all full-time workers.[60] Perhaps the most telling commentary on the declining status of the occupation in the postindustrial economy came from secretaries themselves: 55 percent would not recommend the job to their daughters.[61]

Nor has IBM's prediction of raised job status proven to be true for data-entry workers using VDTs. John Maxwell Hamilton, a World Bank official, explains: "In the data-entry business, one of the essential ingredients is a dependable supply of low-wage workers." Put another way, says Faye Duchin, director of New York University's Institute for Economic Analysis, data entry "remains a dead-end job where the worker is even more specialized" than before the VDT's introduction.[62]

Reinventing the Office: Contingent, Home, and Offshore Workers

The routinization and deskilling of office work wrought by computer automation, coupled with the growth of internationally linked labor markets, have enabled employers to hire more contingent workers and parcel out tasks to those working at home and abroad. This development has made it possible for employers to conceive of office personnel as interchangeable parts for which they have minimum responsibility. As the OTA put it: "When back-office work (the routine processing of standardized data or text) is rationalized and deskilled, investment in training is minimal, and the value of experience and continuity is also minimal."[63] Consequently, the practice of lean staffing lessens information industries' dependence on permanent employees.

The permanent labor bill (i.e., salary and benefits) is the single largest component in the cost of doing business for information industries. The automating ability of VDTs, coupled with slower rates of economic growth, has prompted the corporate trend toward lean staffing in an effort to maximize profits. The OTA notes that contingent workers "are usually a bargain for the employer . . . because [he] pays only for actual productive work hours." In this laissez-faire environment, the computerized office enables employers to save on such overhead items as social security, workers compensation, medical and dental benefits, and pension plans. These economic advantages resulted in tremendous growth rates for the temporary service business since the 1980s, with 60 percent of its business coming in the clerical occupations.[64] The shift to lean staffing has helped make Manpower, Inc., a temporary work agency, the nation's largest employer. The trend toward contingent work is likely to have a negative effect on efforts to close the wage and career advancement opportunity gap between men and women. This is because women, who constitute 87 percent of the nearly 3.3 million part-time administrative support and clerical workers and 75 percent of temporary workers, will be hired to fill the vast majority of these low wage, dead-end jobs.[65]

Although contingent workers using VDTs are being employed throughout the white-collar world, they are most likely to be found in the banking, insurance, real estate, and financial sectors. The financial industry's reliance on temporary workers is now one of the fastest growing in the nation. William Olsten, chairman and chief executive officer of the Olsten Corporation, one of the nation's largest suppliers of temporary secretarial and office help, saw an opportunity for growth in the business slump: "It's regrettable that the market collapsed the way it did, but from our perspective, I feel that it could be beneficial to the temporary service business."[66]

The flexibility of VDTs has enabled managers to reinvent and expand the office's locale by farming out office tasks to full- and part-timers working at home. Employers tout the advantages: the time, money, and aggravation saved by not having to commute and pay for child care, working in the friendly confines of one's home, and being able to adjust one's work schedule to take care of personal matters. However, many clerical homeworkers, or *telecommuters* as they are sometimes called, must lease their terminals from their employer, take personal responsibility for any health hazards that might arise, feel under constant pressure to work, and are divorced from the employee work culture in the office. In 1992 it was estimated that 6.6 million workers were telecommuting.[67] As rapid advances in computer technology continue, and business costs increase, telecommuting may become a major work option in the next century. If so, organizing VDT workers by traditional means would become all the more difficult, if not impossible.

VDTs are giving corporations a truly global reach. With the aide of satellite signals, employers are now beaming work to "offshore" offices in the Caribbean, the Pacific Rim, India, and Ireland. Banking, insurance, publishing, and transportation, in the United States, Japan, and Europe, are among the industries engaged in exporting office work.[68] Companies such as Saztec International, based in Kansas City, Missouri, act as service bureaus for corporate clients by electronically shipping their data-entry and word-processing work to both home and offshore workers. Wages, as low as 10 percent of the U.S. rate, make it very attractive for American employers to export data-entry work overseas.[69] Moreover, there are no unions to bargain for wage increases or safer working conditions.

The offshore office, just like its onshore counterpart, is modeled on the industrial work pattern. As the *New York Times* declared, the "new technology lets services follow the route taken by manufacturing."[70] In business parlance the offshore office is referred to as "office sharing." Office sharing, adapted from the industrial practice of "production sharing," combines, in the words of Kevin P. Power, a Washington-based international business consultant, "the higher labor skills and technology available in the developed countries for the manufacture of materials and components with lower-cost labor available in developing countries for processing and assembly operations to produce finished goods for the market." Writing in the *Wall Street Journal,* Power advised information-sector executives that they could emulate their industrial counterparts by moving office work overseas: "Application of the office sharing concept in developing countries can revitalize companies in banking, insurance, publishing and other industries facing rising operating costs and increasing competition." He also argued that office sharing is beneficial for developing countries: "The application of office sharing to these economies can provide employment within a relatively short period of time, diversifying the skills of the labor force and familiarizing it with computer technology."[71] But the rapid employment of unskilled workers is made possible because the available word- and data-processing jobs are deskilled, simplified occupations, not the more sophisticated programming jobs that would familiarize this new labor force with computer technology.

While Power was proclaiming the benefits of office sharing, the reality of the offshore office unfolding in the Caribbean was more disturbing. The Satellite Data Corporation set up offshore office operations in Barbados to take advantage of its cheap and plentiful labor supply. Based on an interview with its chairman, George R. Simpson, *Business Week* reported that "the average pay for Caribbean data-entry personnel is about $1.50 an hour ... compared with up to $9 an hour in New York. This low-cost labor will more than offset the $10,000 monthly charge for the satellite channel, he says, and allow him to realize a 50 % aftertax profit-three times the domestic industry average." As Simpson exclaimed, "We can do the work in Barbados . . . for less than it costs in New York to pay for floor space."[72]

American Airlines move of two hundred ticket-processing jobs from Tulsa, Oklahoma, to Barbados in 1983 provides another example of how the transnational reach of computer technology is creating global labor markets at the worker's expense. "With technology where it is now," said a corporate official, "we had no reason to keep this operation in America." That is, the same work could be performed in Barbados for one-third the amount earned by U.S. workers, and the government sealed the deal with generous tax incentives.[73] The new subsidiary, named AMR Caribbean Data Services, soon branched out to do work for insurance and medical companies. One of the reasons AMR Caribbean was successful at attracting outside business was its policy of keeping client's names confidential. As an executive explained: "If you were an insurance company and were firing data-entry people in the States, would you want anyone to know you were hiring them in the Caribbean?"[74] Power concluded that "office sharing holds the potential to be a powerful development tool in bridging the technological gap that exists between industrialized and developing nations."[75] But the more likely prospect is the expansion of corporate power in an increasingly global labor market. The ability to disperse computer-based work beyond local and national borders via satellite on short notice is an enormous aid to transnational corporations in their efforts to find the cheaper labor markets, seek better tax breaks and other incentives, and avoid union organizing attempts.

Despite the utopian promise of liberation from drudgery, the reality of the computerized office has been deskilling, employee monitoring, lean staffing and job loss, lagging pay and the lack of career opportunities, and occupational safety and health hazards. Ultimately, the question of how office computers will be used involves the issue of power. Monitoring abuses and VDT-related health hazards are not an aberration of the system; they are the logical outcome of a system that lacks effective checks and balances and an independent voice for workers. NIOSH monitored the stress levels of three groups—clerical workers using VDTs, those who don't, and professionals using VDTs—and found that "the comparison of the working conditions for the various groups demonstrates that those working conditions that led to the stress problems reported by the clerical VDT operators are not entirely related to the VDT use, *but are also related to the entire work system that goes along with using VDTs.*"[76]

The VDT's introduction to the office was accompanied by predictions that it would liberate workers from drudgery. Instead, many workers found that this new technology was being used to extend management's control over the workplace. Faced with an authoritarian management structure that was unresponsive to the growing VDT safety and health problem, office workers sought to organize in order to socialize the conflict and seek policy solutions in the political arena.

Chapter 3

Organizing Office Workers for Occupational Safety and Health

The development of safety and health problems among workers using VDTs provided unions with a compelling issue to enlist unorganized office workers and prompted them to launch a political campaign for protective regulations. However, workers in other industrialized countries have had greater success at gaining protective measures than their counterparts in the United States. This is due, in part, to the presence in other industrialized nations of labor/left parties, higher rates of unionization (especially among white-collar workers), and a stronger tradition of state intervention in the economy.[1]

Commenting on the relative weakness of organized labor in the United States, labor and technology analyst Harley Shaiken observed: "In the U.S., it is only management which decides on technological changes." He added that safety and health problems created by office automation were "being buried to speed up technological change," and that for management, the "bottom line is return on investment."[2]

Regulating the Workplace Use of VDTs around the World

Labor's global struggle to secure VDT safety and health protection began in Europe during the 1970s. Swedish workers were the first to report health problems (musculoskeletal and vision problems) related to VDT use, and in 1985, Sweden became the first country to regulate the workplace use of this new technology. Health Directive 136 amends Sweden's Work Environment Act of 1978 to regulate office lighting, glare levels, and visibility of screen characters; ergonomic factors such as adjustability of chairs, desks, keyboards, and terminals; and employer-paid eye exams and glasses. It also provides for rest breaks, limits of four hours a day on VDT work, and says that VDT work "involving severe control or constraint or monotonous routine work shall be avoided or restricted." Moreover, Sweden limits computer monitoring of workers' productivity to a monthly (not daily) basis, and on a departmentwide (not individual) basis. In 1990, the Swedish National Board for Measurement and Testing (MPRII) established guidelines for low electromagnetic field monitors, which have become the de facto standard for the European Union (EU) and the world. They were developed as a result of the combined pressure of the Swedish labor movement and the Social Democratic Party. The Swedish Confederation of Professional Employees (TCO) pushed the standard further in 1992 by developing its own guidelines, which are tighter than MPRII's and include an energy-saving feature that turns down power when the VDT is not in use. This feature saves money and eliminates EMF exposure while the VDT is dormant.[3]

Sweden's ergonomic standard became the basis for the 1990 directive by the EU (then called the European Community) on VDT use in the workplace. The directive went into effect in 1993 and covers 80 percent of office workers in the fifteen member countries: Austria, Belgium, Denmark, Finland, France, Germany, Greece, Ireland, Italy, Luxembourg, the Netherlands, Portugal, Spain, Sweden, and the United Kingdom. EU directives establish minimum policy requirements, which give member states considerable flexibility in the way they meet the standards. For example, the United Kingdom has opted for some of the weakest standards permissible under the EU directive. Nevertheless, the EU regulations are the most comprehensive in scope ever promulgated and are bound to have an impact on both market and public policy that reaches beyond the European Union. The EU regulations include: free vision exams before starting VDT work, and periodically thereafter; free corrective lens if needed; training to enable workers to use VDTs in an ergonomically wise manner; and the mandate that workers have the right to know the content of EU regulations. The regulations also direct that newly purchased computer terminals and chairs be adjustable for height. VDTs must be equipped with detachable keyboards and have glare-free screens that can be tilted up and down and turned from side to side to suit the user's needs. The EU standards require that nonionizing radiation levels be "reduced to negligible levels" and also cover such work environment factors as work surfaces, noise, lighting, and glare.[4]

The EU directive was the result of nearly two decades of labor activism on the VDT safety and health issue around the world. Although Norway is not an EU member, it has some of the strongest VDT regulations in the world. Norway's Working Environment Act of 1977 was amended in 1995 to require employers to provide detachable keyboards and adjustable VDTs. It also requires that terminals be grounded to prevent skin rashes caused by electrostatic charge buildup in front of the screen and provides for both workers' input during the planning stages of VDT installation and ergonomics training. Norwegian unions have also won maximum two-hour shifts and half-day limits on VDT use, which helps to alleviate and prevent stress, vision problems, and RSIs.[5]

In Canada, workers called for alternative work and other safety and health provisions after a group of VDT operators at the *Toronto Star* experienced adverse pregnancy outcomes in 1979–80. As a result, the Canadian government issued VDT guidelines for its employees. In 1979, seventy-five translation workers walked off their jobs at the United Nations in New York in protest over VDT-related work speedups and uncertainties regarding the nature of the radiation emitted by the machines.[6] French VDT workers charged the Post and Telephone Office with sacrificing their safety and health in the name of increased efficiency. As they saw it, management's attitude was "give us your health—in return you will get a modern word processing machine, a bonus and a pair of spectacles."[7] Subsequent labor pressure forced the French government to add VDT work to its list of jobs that are monitored for safety and health problems.

Fears that computer automation would eliminate printers jobs and turn journalists into word processors brought the International Federation of Journalists and Graphic Trade Unions together in November 1978 to plot strategy. They resolved that VDT work should be limited to four hours a day with periodic breaks, and that computers should not be used to put printers out of work. In 1980, Germany amended its technical standards, known as the Deutsche Industrie Norm, to include the ergonomic aspects of VDTs employers and manufacturers must meet. Broad in scope, the standards covered screen character size and luminance, keyboard and VDT design, and work rules. With VDTs in widespread use, the German standards spurred the development of ergonomic research and design in Europe. In Austria, VDT operators who work overnight are given breaks and other benefits required under the government's "strenuous" work laws. The government also adopted Germany's VDT design recommendations. Some Austrian unions negotiated collective bargaining agreements that put a four-hour limit to continuous work on the VDT.[8]

In the United Kingdom, the Printing Industries Committee of the Trade Union Council reported in 1978 that its members were suffering from VDT-related stress, vision, and musculoskeletal problems and called for a half-hour of alternative work after two hours of continuous work, rest breaks, and daily time limits. In 1985, British trade unions organized the "VDU Workers' Rights Campaign" in an attempt to amend the vaguely worded Health and Safety at Work Act (1974) to protect VDT workers. They criticized the Health and Safety Executive's laissez-faire policy for assuming that "employers would seek to minimize the harmful effects of prolonged VDU usage without Government or Trade Union intervention."[9] Blocked by the ruling Conservative Party, the unions were forced to fall back to the position of lobbying within the Labour Party in the "hope that a future Labour government in this country will take up our cause."[10]

Some of the earliest reports of cumulative trauma disorders, especially carpal tunnel syndrome, came from Australia. In 1983, the Trade Union Council issued model contract language for VDT work and journalists won the right to ten-minute rest breaks after two hours of continuous VDT work. Subsequently, an arbitrator ruled that the Australian government's introduction and use of VDTs increased its employees workload, which warranted an 8 percent pay increase. Japan has had ergonomic workplace guidelines in place since the 1960s. In 1984, the Japanese Ministry of Labor released guidelines calling for adjustable VDTs and furniture, ambient lighting, glare reduction, hourly rest breaks, and medical exams for workers. In New Zealand, an arbitrator ruled that insurance workers had the right to advance notification of the introduction of VDTs, to play a part in their implementation, and compensation for those who jobs were eliminated by automation.[11] In December 1987, the New Zealand journalists' union negotiated hourly ten-minute work breaks, limitations on computer monitoring, and employer-provided glasses when prescribed during periodic eye exams. Putting the agreement in international perspective, a union spokesman said: "The health and safety code, work breaks and guarantees of continued employment were better than anything negotiated in Australia, the U.S. or Britain."[12]

The enactment of VDT standards and guidelines around the world testifies to both the extent of safety and health hazards faced by VDT workers and the market's failure to keep pace with developments in ergonomic research and design. The challenge for U.S. unions was to secure VDT regulations in the country where organized labor was weakest and market forces were strongest.

Organized Labor and Unorganized Women Office Workers

The VDT safety and health issue gave the U.S. labor movement a tremendous opportunity to organize new members in two interrelated areas in which it was poorly represented: among office workers and women workers. At the start of organized labor's VDT campaign in 1979, only 6.5 percent of the nation's office workers were organized.[13] Because 80 percent of office workers are women, championing safety and health regulations for VDT workers provided organized labor with an excellent opportunity to expand its membership among this underrepresented group.[14] Women constituted 46 percent of the work force in 1994, and the percentage is expected to continue to increase. The Bureau of Labor Statistics projected that women, many of them minorities, will be 65 percent of the new entrants into the labor pool between 1985 and 2000.[15] Many women are, and will continue to be, employed in low-wage clerical and service occupations in which VDTs are used. Ninety percent of all full-time VDT workers are women.[16]

Since the 1880s employers have steered women into marginal white-collar occupations, characterized by lower-pay, non-career-path, and routinized work. As Margery W. Davies has documented, the job of secretary was originally a male-dominated field with management opportunities, but it diminished in importance when the typewriter was introduced and employers hired women to operate them. Designated as women's work, neither the position of secretary nor typist offered a career path to management.[17] The educational system trained men to be managers and administrators and young women to be clerical workers and secretaries. Linda Valli notes that sex-typing in education continues to steer many women into clerical positions.[18] Like typing, VDT work is now sex-typed as women's work.

For years, labor unions focused their organizing efforts on the male-dominated industrial workplaces, leaving the vast majority of the predominantly female office work force unorganized. Like employers, many labor leaders viewed working women as being marginal to the labor force.[19] In addition, organizing drives were made more difficult because many companies encouraged office workers to believe that they were part of management's team.[20] In the few instances in which white-collar workers were organized, as Sharon Hartman Strom notes, it was not uncommon to find locals established along gender lines. In the insurance industry, there were separate locals for the male-dominated sales force and the predominately female clerical work force. In sum, writes Alice Kessler-Harris, "Limited labor-force opportunities, protective labor legislation and virtual exclusion from labor unions institutionalized women's isolation from the mainstream of labor. Not accidentally, these tendencies confirmed traditional women's roles, already nurtured by many ethnic groups and sustained by prevailing American norms."[21]

Many labor unions continued to view women office workers in the post–World War II economy as unworthy of organizing, assuming that most women were temporary participants in the work force. Women, so the rationale went, were a more fluid pool of workers who would be more difficult to organize due to high turnover and greater employee reluctance to take risks for a job they did not intend to hold for long. Added to this was the view of many union officials that women's lower wages could not generate enough union dues to make an organizing drive worthwhile.[22] Women have made advances in low and midlevel leadership positions since the 1960s, but few have reached the level of union president.[23] As a result, the labor movement had little or no structure of support for working women's issues when the VDT issue arose in the late 1970s. Unions have had a poor organizing record among office workers. When unions did organize clerical workers, it was often as an afterthought. Clerical workers whose jobs were near industrial work sites were among the easiest to organize.[24] But these efforts were the exception. As a rule, sustained efforts to organize clerical workers were few.

During the 1970s and 1980s the information and service sectors experienced tremendous growth in employment while the industrial sector shrank. The transformation from industrial to postindustrial economy eroded labor's traditional organizing base, resulted in the loss of tens of thousands of members from its industrial unions, and put the labor movement on the defensive. Membership declined from a high point of 35 percent of the work force in 1954 to only 15.5 percent in 1994.[25] A more telling indicator of organized labor's weakness is that only 10.9 percent of private-sector employees are union members.[26] The decline in labor's membership has been paralleled by its weakening influence in the political arena.

The structural shifts in the economy that have resulted in declining union membership have also resulted in a decline of labor's influence within the Democratic Party. The decline of the industrial work force and the globalization of capital have combined to create a new post–New Deal political economic order in which the Democrats have recast themselves as a more conservative, probusiness party. Since the 1970s, unions have been unable to persuade Congress to pass key pieces of labor/consumer legislation, such as OSHA reform and national health care, or to stop probusiness measures, such as the North American Free Trade Agreement and the recent amendments to the General Agreement on Tariffs and Trade.[27]

Although many women's groups, such as 9 to 5, The National Organization of Working Women; the Coalition of Labor Union Women (CLUW); and others had been calling for an organizing drive of the predominantly female clerical work force since the 1970s, organized labor's leadership was slow to focus on the need for a white-collar organizing initiative. By the early to mid-1980s, however, the AFL-CIO began to emphasize the need to organize white-collar workers, especially women and minorities. At an AFL-CIO conference in 1984, Secretary-Treasurer Thomas Donahue stressed the need to organize white-collar workers, especially women, and this was reflected in the report he directed, *The Changing Situation of Workers and Their Unions.*[28]

Labor's greatest success at organizing white-collar workers has been achieved in the public sector. In 1994, 38.7 percent of government employees were organized.[29] But its success was due in large part to factors that are peculiar to the public sector. These factors included a tradition of employee associations that served as a ready-made base for the transition to unionization, President Kennedy's 1962 executive order permitting federal employees to organize, and similar reforms at the state and local levels of government, which were experiencing a boom in job growth.[30] Added up, these factors created a more favorable negotiating climate than could be found in the private sector. In the process of organizing public sector workers, many women, especially blacks and Latinos, were organized. As Deborah Bell notes, this opened the door for the treatment of women's concerns such as pay equity, child care, and the VDT issue. However, the public sector experience is not a good model for organizing the private sector, where employer resistance to unions is much stronger.[31]

If organized labor was to reassert itself, a campaign among clerical workers on the scale of the Committee for Industrial Organization's efforts to organize unskilled and semiskilled industrial workers during the 1930s was needed. Unions, such as the International Association of Machinists, International Brotherhood of Electrical Workers, International Brotherhood of Teamsters, the United Steel Workers of America (USWA), and the United Auto Workers (UAW) all launched campaigns during the late 1970s and 1980s to organize office workers and push for collective bargaining agreements that included VDT safety and health provisions.

In doing so, they joined unions such as the American Federation of State, County, and Municipal Employees (AFSCME), the Communications Workers of America (CWA), the Office and Professional Employees International Union (OPEIU), and the Service Employees International Union (SEIU), which had traditionally represented office and service sector workers. In 1981, 9 to 5 joined forces with the SEIU, the nation's fifth largest union, to form District 925, a union affiliate established to organize office workers.[32] For the first time, traditional unionists and women's rights activists came together to organize women clerical workers, a group whom conventional labor wisdom had regarded as unorganizable. In a merger that symbolized the coming together of industrial and service sector unions, the Amalgamated Meat Cutters Union and the Retail Clerks merged in 1979 to form the United Food and Commercial Workers (UFCW) and began organizing bank workers.

Labor's Efforts to Organize around the VDT Issue

During the mid- to late 1970s, unions began to press employers for collective bargaining language that included periodic eye exams, regularly scheduled rest breaks, time limits on daily VDT use, shields to block the nonionizing radiation emitted by the display unit's cathode ray tube (CRT), alternative work assignments for pregnant women concerned about the possible harmful effects on the fetus, ergonomically designed furniture and equipment, and glare-reducing screens and lighting.

The Newspaper Guild (TNG) was the first union to actively address VDT-related safety and health problems experienced by its members. This was a reaction to the newspaper industry's pioneering switch to VDTs in 1970 and the resultant workplace problems. The most commonly cited problems VDT workers faced were vision impairment and musculoskeletal strain. Screen glare from lighting and windows, and fuzzy characters, created eye strain and headaches. Straining to read the characters on the screen, in turn, produced neck and arm pains. In 1976, a TNG survey found that 50 percent of its VDT-using members at the Associated Press and 33 percent at United Press International suffered from musculoskeletal and vision problems. In 1977, the National Institute of Occupational Safety and Health reported that "complaints of eyestrain . . . often are voiced. And, with the many VDTs in use, the number of complaints could be quite large."[33] Subsequently, TNG's annual convention took up the issue, adopting a resolution calling for regular employer-provided eye exams for VDT operators.

By 1980, TNG had negotiated deals for paid eye exams with seventeen newspapers, paid eyeglass prescriptions with seven others, and rest breaks with four Minneapolis/St. Paul dailies.[34] Vision-related ailments had become a pervasive problem in the newspaper industry. *Association Trends,* a publication of the American Newspaper Publishers Association (ANPA), remarked in 1984 that the "latest employee benefit in many newspapers is yearly eye exams and free prescription glasses for those working at video display terminals." It attributed this development to a combination of employee fear and employer compassion, saying: "Lingering but probably irrational fears about radiation from VDTs make computer jobs a morale problem, and several newspapers have countered with the added benefits."[35] But collective bargaining struggles, as much as employer empathy, was the reason for many of these safety and health gains.

By 1979, the growing volume of worker complaints reached the point where TNG and OPEIU asked NIOSH to investigate VDT working conditions at the *San Francisco Chronicle,* the *San Francisco Examiner,* the *Oakland Tribune* and Blue Cross–Blue Shield of California. NIOSH issued its report in June 1980, finding that VDT clerical workers suffered from the highest levels of workplace stress they'd ever recorded, blurred vision, loss of color perception, musculoskeletal ailments, numbness in hands, and loss of strength in their arms. But David Cole, the *Examiner's* systems editor, was not impressed by NIOSH's report. "I recall that there were complaints when you had pencils and paste pots too," he said. By the beginning of 1981, working conditions at Blue Cross–Blue Shield worsened to the point that OPEIU workers went out on strike.[36]

In November 1979, TNG and OPEIU formed organized labor's first VDT coalition and were soon joined by seven other unions: the CWA, the Graphic Arts International Union, the International Association of Machinists (IAM), the International Typographical Union, the National Association of Broadcast Employees and Technicians, the Transport Workers Union, and twenty-five AFSCME locals. The coalition's plan was to publicize the problems surrounding the workplace use of VDTs, promote the inclusion of VDT safety and health provisions in collective bargaining agreements, and launch a national campaign for federal enactment of VDT regulations.[37]

COSH and Women's Groups Organize VDT Workers

During the 1960s increasing environmental awareness produced a growing concern among workers over safety and health issues in the workplace. This concern manifested itself in the safety and health movement that helped produce the landmark Occupational Safety and Health Act of 1970. The occupational safety and health movement was institutionalized in labor unions that broadened, or created, their own units, and in the formation of COSH (Committee on Occupational Safety and Health) groups. COSH groups—coalitions of labor unions, industrial hygienists, activists, and academics—were started in New York, Boston, Chicago, Philadelphia, and many other locales across the nation in order to advise labor and lawmakers about on-the-job dangers and to advocate corrective and preventative measures. The New York group, NYCOSH, established a VDT action committee during the late 1970s, held the first conference on VDT-related workplace ailments in January 1980, and has lobbied for passage of laws at all levels of government.

The women's movement of the 1960s and 1970s profoundly altered the way many working women viewed their jobs. Emphasizing equality with men, it gave female clerical workers the conceptual basis around which to organize and protest their subservience in the office hierarchy. Discriminatory practices, such as paying women less than men for the same work performed, sexual harassment, and racism, were institutionalized management practices in many offices. Moreover, women had to fight the stereotype of the secretary as office wife/mother, who was expected to fetch coffee and run domestic errands, as well as type and take dictation. These injustices gave rise to support groups that strove to educate, organize, and empower women office workers in order to overcome their disadvantaged situation.[38]

Some of the more successful support groups formed during the 1970s were the Municipal Women's Project in Boston, Women Employed in Chicago, Women Organized for Employment in San Francisco, Women Office Workers and the Women's Action Alliance in New York City, and Working Women in Cleveland. The National Organization for Women (NOW) established a Committee on Women in Office Work to help coordinate these efforts on a nationwide basis. CLUW, organized in 1974, and Union WAGE were also instrumental in raising women's issues in labor circles. In 1984, CLUW broadened its role by establishing a task force to address VDT-related safety and health and worker retraining issues.[39]

The most important labor group to emerge from the women's movement was 9 to 5, The National Association of Working Women. Founded in Boston in 1973, 9 to 5 later merged with Working Women of Cleveland to form the present-day organization with thirteen thousand members in twenty-five chapters. The organization has taken a leading role in educating women office workers about the safety and health hazards associated with VDT use. It has prepared a book and numerous reports on VDTs, ranging from its health effects to the employment prospects in face of computer automation, and established a "VDT hotline" for working women concerned about their safety and health.[40] On National Secretaries' Day, when managers are encouraged to give flowers to their secretaries, 9 to 5 held demonstrations and letter writing campaigns to emphasize the point that working women want "Raises and Roses!" They also drew up a Bill of Rights for the Safe Use of VDTs, which calls for giving workers a greater say in decisions on how new technologies are introduced and used in the workplace, fifteen-minute rest breaks every two hours (every one hour for intense work), a limit of four consecutive hours per day of VDT work, the elimination of stress creating keystroke pacing and computer monitoring, alternative work for pregnant employees, shielding of terminals to protect operators from nonionizing radiation, and ergonomically designed VDT work environments.[41] Karen Nussbaum, cofounder and former executive director of 9 to 5, has become the leading spokesperson on the VDT issue, writing articles, giving interviews and press conferences to the media, and speaking at demonstrations and academic conferences. In 1985, the *Wall Street Journal* cited her as "part of a small but growing nucleus of women wielding real power," in the labor movement.[42] When Jane Fonda became interested in its work on the VDT issue, 9 to 5 received nationwide publicity. Fonda included a four-page section on VDT and other office safety and health problems in her best-selling *Jane Fonda's Workout Book* (1981) and starred in the 1980 motion picture entitled *9 to 5* (which served as the basis for a television series). As a result, her husband, Assemblyman Tom Hayden, introduced VDT bills in the California state assembly.[43] Despite 9 to 5's relatively small membership, it has succeeded in generating considerable publicity on the VDT issue.

Getting Equity at Equitable

District 925 faced an early challenge in 1982 when it received a call from some workers at the Equitable Life Assurance Company's claims office in Syracuse, New York, who said they wanted to form a union. Working conditions at Equitable's Syracuse office made it a prime candidate for an organizing drive. One VDT worker said it "looks and operates like a factory."[44] Excepting a fifteen-minute morning break and the lunch hour, workers were confined to their computer screens for eight to ten hours a day processing medical and dental insurance claims. Management ignored their complaints of glare-induced headaches, musculoskeletal aches, and skin rashes. In addition, Equitable used computer monitoring to keep track of every keystroke, set the pace of work, and determine wages (which averaged only $12,000 in 1984) accordingly. Wages were set according to management's assessment of each employee's productivity and "attitude" toward the job.[45]

Like many employers, Equitable introduced VDTs to the office without consideration of the social costs that accompany the computerization of office work. As one of the VDT workers, Rebecca Alford, told a House Subcommittee: "We were left to master it ourselves. Made to work on a system that determined the pace and content of our work, we were stripped of any autonomy or job satisfaction. We asked for information on safety and health risks and were assured there were none."[46]

When its employees petitioned the National Labor Relations Board (NLRB) for a union representation election in February 1982, Equitable responded by bringing in Ray Mickus Associates, a consulting firm specializing in defeating union organizing efforts. Management then threatened to close the Syracuse office, lay off employees, and electronically reroute work to other locations. Regina Canuso, a District 925 organizer, said: "We can't strike Equitable. . . . With this technology, they could flick a switch, and the work could be in Kansas City. This changes the whole nature of organizing."[47] Although the union won the election, Equitable dragged its feet by challenging the validity of the results before the NLRB. Despite the NLRB's conclusion that the election had been fairly won and that Equitable had filed a frivolous challenge, the insurance giant refused to bargain with District 925. The NLRB failed to compel Equitable to negotiate with the union in a timely manner. Vice President John H. Goddard defended Equitable's stalling tactics, saying that the company was "merely following a course set by hundreds of employers."[48]

The SEIU responded to Equitable's intransigence by calling a national boycott. NOW endorsed the boycott, as did the AFL-CIO, whose member unions were asked not to invest their $1 billion worth of pension funds with Equitable. Boycotts thrive on publicity, and District 925's effort to get Equitable's attention was no exception. It succeeded in focusing public attention —including a congressional hearing—on the conflict. Embarrassed by the negative publicity (its advertising campaign portrayed Equitable as an insurer that cared about women's issues), Equitable agreed to enter into collective bargaining negotiations with the union in September 1983. Still, another fourteen months went by before a settlement was reached. The agreement called for rest breaks every two hours, eye exams, and anti-glare screens. It gave pregnant employees a limited right to alternative work, established a grievance procedure for soliciting employee input on the extent of computer monitoring, included a wage increase, and guaranteed that the office would remain open for the duration of the three-year contract.[49]

Although only fifty-four workers were covered by the contract, union observers saw the Equitable victory as a major breakthrough. Charles McDonald, the AFL-CIO's assistant director of organizing, hailed it as "a tremendous step for unions." District 925's success marked the first time that office workers at any insurance company in the United States had been organized around the issues of monotonous work, speedups, computer monitoring, and safety and health hazards. Historically, the insurance industry has been an anti-union stronghold with only 3 percent of its workers (mostly salesmen) organized.[50] The U.S. situation stands in stark contrast to that in the rest of the world. In the Scandinavian countries, 95 percent of finance and insurance workers are organized, and a majority are organized in many African, Asian, European, and Latin American countries. Many of these white-collar workers belong to unions affiliated with the nine-million-member International Federation of Commercial, Clerical, Professional, and Technical Employees, which includes two and a half million bank and insurance workers.[51]

The Blue Cross Blues

The Syracuse victory produced a spate of collective bargaining activity, but nationwide, unions failed to generate and maintain a consistent organizing effort. Nor did the Syracuse victory attract the major commitment from the AFL-CIO that the organizers expected.[52] Although the occupational shift from industrial to service sector was well established by 1984, the year the drive for VDT protection was in full swing, and the advantages of organizing white-collar workers were well known—labor's success rate was 52 percent compared to only 40 percent among industrial workers—only 25 percent of all organizing efforts were directed toward white-collar workers. As *Business Week* commented in 1984, "Only about ten percent of service-industry and office workers have been organized, in part because major unions have not concentrated on signing them up."[53] Despite a sizable war chest, and the favorable publicity generated by its victory at Equitable, District 925 organized only six thousand workers from 1981 to 1986.[54]

Inspired by the success at Equitable the year before, AFL-CIO president Lane Kirkland announced an ambitious plan to organize the nearly forty thousand eligible Blue Cross–Blue Shield workers in 1985. After years of neglect, it seemed as though the AFL-CIO was ready to commit the necessary time and resources to organize private sector clerical workers. The organization established a special office to help the lead unions—CWA, OPEIU, SEIU, UAW, and UFCW—pool their resources and coordinate organizing activities. Following their lead were AFSCME, the International Union of Electrical Workers, and USWA.[55]

However, the AFL-CIO's one broadly coordinated attempt to organize clerical workers resulted in failure. Union activity was uncoordinated: even with the help of the AFL-CIO's advisory office, it took nearly a year to resolve jurisdictional disputes over which union would organize which workers. The campaign relied on traditional organizing tactics when a new approach was needed: male organizers used traditional tactics more suitable to the male-dominated industrial work force than to the female-dominated clerical workplace. The campaign lacked a maximum effort by the participating unions: although the campaign was chaired by the SEIU's John J. Sweeney, his union continued to place much of its organizing emphasis elsewhere. The campaign also relied on a public relations and top-down organizing approach rather than grass-roots effort focused around specific employee grievances. When the campaign was met by corporate intransigence, the unions failed to counter with additional rank-and-file organizing attempts. Moreover, organized labor, which had its medical plans with Blue Cross for many years, underestimated the degree of resistance its organizers would meet.[56] To be sure, this was labor's most ambitious effort to organize office workers. There was no guarantee of success. However, the lessons learned from the initial failure have not been incorporated into a follow-up campaign.

Moreover, there were serious limits to labor's collective bargaining efforts. Although some unions won pioneering VDT provisions through the collective bargaining process, there was no guarantee of victories in most union shops. As the Newspaper Guild reported in 1986: "Guild bargaining for VDT contract provisions continued to encounter strong publisher resistance."[57] The situation at TNG was typical for most unions. Moreover, collective bargaining agreements—which, at best, could only cover the minority of VDT workers who were organized—were no substitute for universal OSHA standards.

The weakness of U.S. labor stands in stark contrast to the power of their better-organized corporate opponents. Moreover, organized labor has been fighting against business on an unlevel playing field; the VDT issue arose at a time when the anti-union Reagan administration deregulated OSHA and tilted the NLRB in favor of business. The U.S. labor movement is more isolated from white-collar workers and political parties than their European counterparts. In Europe, Australia, and New Zealand—where white-collar workers are more organized than in the United States and where labor/left parties are the norm—workers have been able to win more VDT protections and research.

Although the AFL-CIO was slow in responding to issues affecting women office workers, it must be noted that it was taking up the challenge for millions of unrepresented workers. Often portrayed as a narrow special interest, the labor movement is the one organized group in the United States that fights for benefits—such as job safety and health—for all working people, whether or not they are organized. Labor's next step would be to take the campaign for VDT safety and health to the federal government. But first it would have to deal with the counterattack being organized by the corporate coalition opposed to VDT safety and health regulations.

Chapter 4

A Question of Business

$\mathcal{D}$istrict 925's victory at Equitable's Syracuse office sent a ripple effect through the business community, which feared that more clerical workers might follow suit and organize. Martin F. Payson, a prominent attorney and management consultant, told the *Wall Street Journal* that District 925's victory "sent a shock wave not only through the insurance community but every major white collar business." Writing in the *Personnel Journal,* he warned employers to preempt organizing drives by "audit[ing] your policies and procedures before the union does." *Computer Decisions* magazine cautioned its readers: "Let the manager beware. These working conditions promote the unrest that in turn causes low morale, high turnover, unionization fights, and worse. Your data-entry department could be a time bomb waiting to explode with serious consequences. And your management style could be at the root of the problem."[1]

A cottage industry of consultants specializing in white-collar workers sprang up to advise managers on how to maintain a "union-free" office. One of the leaders in the field, John G. Kilgour, advised information-processing managers that office work could now be deskilled and segmented so as to inhibit organizing drives. Office workers were to be treated as an impersonal commodity in the new postindustrial world order. If managers had any moral qualms about the new framework of employer-employee relations, he reminded them: "You are in the middle of something that is of the same magnitude as the industrial revolution. It's really not a question of good guys and bad guys, it's a question of business."[2]

Manufacturers and Users Unite

Corporate opposition to VDT regulation was spearheaded by the Computer and Business Equipment Manufacturers Association (CBEMA) and the

American Newspaper Publishers Association (ANPA). CBEMA represented forty-two computer and business equipment companies (accounting for 85 percent of all industry revenues) operating in an oligopolistic economic setting. Its members included the most important VDT producers, such as International Business Machines (IBM), American Telephone and Telegraph (AT&T), Apple Computer, Inc., Compaq Computer Corporation, Control Data Corporation, Digital Equipment Corporation, Hewlett-Packard, NCR Corporation, Unisys, and the Xerox Corporation. Based in Washington, D.C., CBEMA is the chief lobbying arm of the computer industry. A CBEMA pamphlet declares that "Congress, federal agencies and the Administration know that when CBEMA speaks, it speaks for its members."[3] In his study on corporate power, Edward S. Herman cites the computer industry as the primary example of a dynamic oligopoly. The newspaper industry is closely linked to the computer industry by its considerable investment in VDTs. ANPA represents approximately fourteen hundred newspapers, accounting for more than 90 percent of the nation's daily and Sunday circulation.[4]

Computer manufacturers and business users of office automation systems are united by a common interest in defeating VDT regulation. Manufacturers oppose regulations that would force them to revise the way they build VDTs, and corporate users oppose regulations that dictate purchasing standards and regulate VDT use in the workplace. Together, they form a powerful front line of defense. With VDTs being used in virtually every major industry in the nation, a formidable coalition has been mobilized against organized labor's drive for protective regulations.

Secret discussions in 1983 led CBEMA and ANPA to form the Coalition for Workplace Technology (CWT) in early 1984. Its purpose was to coordinate and plan their lobbying campaign against VDT regulation. Claudia James, ANPA's legal counsel, explained that the CWT's job "would be to provide greater credibility for business positions in dealing with the media and state legislators." CBEMA's Charlotte LeGates added that it would also serve "to correct the misinformation [about VDTs] being circulated by the press and word of mouth."[5]

Besides CBEMA and ANPA, the CWT included an impressive array of trade associations (twenty-two in all)—whose members were major VDT users—representing virtually every major sector of the nation's economy. Among them were: the Air Transport Association of America, the American Bankers Association, the American Council on Life Insurance, the American Electronics Association, the Business and Institutional Furniture Manufacturers Association, the Information Industry Association, the Motor Vehicle Manufacturers Association of the United States, the National Association of Manufacturers, the North American Telephone Association, the Printing Industries of America, and the U.S. Chamber of Commerce.

CBEMA members are also linked to corporate VDT users by their role as suppliers of VDTs and office equipment, and by corporate interlocks. As the U.S. Senate's 1980 study on corporate concentration said, "The most important interconnections in the . . . information processing and office equipment group lay in the seating of multiple competitors on the boards of the largest customers, suppliers, and financial institutions."[6]

The Coalition for Workplace Technology opposed the workplace regulation of VDTs on three grounds. First, it said that there was no scientific proof connecting nonionizing radiation emitted by VDTs and miscarriages, birth defects and eye cataracts suffered by users. Thus, the CWT charged that union calls for alternative work during pregnancy and shielding of CRTs were unwarranted.

Second, the CWT maintained that there were no ergonomic problems requiring government action, there was only a question of employee comfort. That, the CWT maintained, could best be dealt with by the voluntary efforts of employers. They argued that an OSHA ergonomics standard would be a hindrance to the flexibility employers needed to meet the particular comfort needs of each employee. After all, CWT argued, who knew employees' needs better, the manager in the workplace, or OSHA bureaucrats in Washington?

Finally, the CWT maintained that VDT regulations would increase employer operating costs, impede new technological developments, and slow economic development in the rapidly growing computer and information industries. The result, they argued, would place the United States at a competitive disadvantage with other countries at a time when both economic revitalization and national security depended on maintaining a comparative advantage in the fields of computers and information services.

The corporate coalition's use of the phrase "employee comfort problems" instead of "safety and health hazard" may seem like an exercise in semantics, but, as E. E. Schattschneider and Murray Edelman have pointed out, those who succeed in defining the terms of debate have a political advantage over their opponents.[7] If the problem is defined as one of "comfort" rather than "hazards," then it becomes much more difficult, if not impossible, to justify regulation of VDTs as an occupational safety and health problem. For example, the National Council on Compensation Insurance (NCCI), the workers compensation research and rate-making arm of the insurance industry, reported that there was "no statistically significant increase in workers compensation claims or payouts in the clerical sector" from 1981 to 1984. On this basis they concluded that "the workers compensation experience seems to add further support to the conclusion that most VDT problems are matters of *comfort,* rather than adverse health effects or disability."[8]

But NCCI's assessment was based on incomplete information. Despite the use of the word *national* in its title, the NCCI does not operate in eighteen states, including California, which has the nation's largest VDT-using work force. Data for the study was collected from only thirteen states.[9] Furthermore, the VDT was still relatively new to the office during the years studied (1981–84). Initially, there were few reported VDT-related worker compensation claims. But this is explained by factors such as: the lag time between the introduction of VDTs and the manifestation of widespread safety and health problems; delays caused by management's opposition to, and contesting of, employee claims; and the slow pace at which state workers' compensation systems add new occupational ailments to their lists of compensable illnesses and injuries.[10]

However, the number of VDT stress–related occupational disease claims increased from less than 5 percent in 1980 to 14 percent of *all* claims in 1988. CNA Insurance Company reported to the National Safety Congress in 1988 that the rise in these stress-related occupational disease claims was largely attributable to VDT work, in which operators experience a lack of control over the work process or fear that automation might put them out of work.[11] NCCI's conclusion was also contradicted by the *Wall Street Journal,* which reported in 1985 that "increasingly, computer workers are winning disability claims, causing concern among companies about soaring insurance costs."[12] The Bureau of National Affairs came to the same conclusion:

> In light of the successful claims filed to date, worker's compensation
> claims related to VDTs are likely to increase in the coming years.
> Although research on the terminals to injuries [sic] is incomplete,
> there now appears to be sufficient scientific and medical evidence to

support some claims. Moreover, the legal and medical precedents being established in these early cases are likely to encourage other workers to file similar claims.[13]

In 1991, the *New York Times* reported that the "soaring" cost of worker compensation insurance was due, in part, to the fact that "courts in some states have stretched the coverage to include treatments for stress, back pain and injuries from repetitive tasks at computers."[14]

Business interests launched a public relations campaign to discredit employee concerns about job loss and computer health hazards. They portrayed employee concerns about VDT safety and health hazards as just another case of an irrational fear of new technology. CBEMA's president, Vico E. Henriques, told a House subcommittee that "while the safety of the equipment has not changed, there is an element in the workplace that has changed. Today we have fear, and it is fear that comes from a rapid change in the way of conducting our work and our lives. It also comes from some zealous and self-interested parties who create fear for their own advantage."[15] Writing in *PC Week,* Renee S. Ross, the executive director of the corporate-funded Center for Office Technology (COT) said that "myths and new technology seem to go hand in hand. People once thought railroad trains passing through fields would make cows go dry. They also feared the freon in frozen food cases would harm food. . . . Most of the anecdotes we hear today concerning possible hazards from video display terminals . . . have the same roots."[16] Dr. Myron L. Wolbarsht, a professor of ophthalmology and biological engineering at Duke University, and a computer industry consultant, explained that people were the problem, not VDTs: "When a person is put in a position where he feels uncomfortable, he gets tired and achy. If people thought rationally, they'd realize it's the way they're sitting and it's the glare coming off the screen. But most people aren't rational; it's easier to blame mysterious radiation."[17] A report by Adia Personnel Services even blamed dead writers for encouraging workers' resistance to office automation (OA): "The newness of this technology, coupled with negative cultural impressions that have been perpetuated by such writers as H. G. Wells, Jules Verne, Aldous Huxley, and George Orwell, have contributed to an underlying suspicion and mistrust of OA. The only real answer to this residual fear is education."[18] The cumulative effect of these statements was to discredit VDT workers and their arguments without a debate over policy.

The Stakes Involved

The economic stakes in defeating labor's drive for regulation are high for both computer manufacturers and corporate users. Manufacturers maintain that VDT regulations will increase production costs and decrease sales. Business users argue that increased prices would discourage new purchases, which, in turn, would hinder their ability to take advantage of the latest models' productivity improvements. The U.S. is the world's largest computer market ($159 billion in 1994), accounting for more than 39 percent of worldwide computer sales. An estimated 75 million computers are in use in American workplaces.[19] Moreover, the computer industry forecasts that more than 15.3 million units will be sold annually by 2003, nearly double the number in 1992.[20]

Desktop computers are the fastest growing segment of the new integrated information technology industry, with 27 percent growth in sales—compared to 15 percent for all industry sales—from 1993 to 1995. From negligible sales in the early 1980s, they now account for 66 percent of all expenditures on computers.[21] The globalization of information markets and rapid advances in computers means that corporations are engaged in a never-ending quest for quicker and more efficient modes of communication. Worldwide sales of the U.S. computer industry increased from $278 billion in 1983 to $602 billion in 1993. The computer industry expects sales to reach $1.19 trillion annually by 2004.[22]

At first, computer manufacturers dismissed ergonomic modifications as unnecessary and too expensive. The *New Scientist* described this attitude: "One representative of a major manufacturer conceded that salesmen are reluctant to encourage buyers to design a better environment before plugging in their machines, because that would cost too much."[23] Ironically, it was organized labor's insistence that poorly designed VDTs be improved that led manufacturers to introduce ergonomically designed terminals into the market. Organized labor's efforts were crucial to generating public awareness of the need for ergonomically designed computer work stations, which, in turn, generated greater sales—and profits—in this new and lucrative market.

For computer manufacturers, it was the best of both worlds: greater demand for more expensive machines without regulations that might limit corporate autonomy. However, some corporate VDT users in the Coalition for Workplace Technology were uneasy about the computer manufacturers dominance of the group. With organized labor's drive for VDT legislation gaining momentum during the early 1980s, they feared that VDT manufacturers "might find it beneficial to sell out" to proponents of VDT regulations and "stick the [business] users with a whole bunch of rotten ergonomics proposals in exchange for having machine proposals."[24] Such a deal, business users feared, might include office ergonomic guidelines that would add to their operating costs but leave the design of VDTs untouched. To guard against this possibility, corporate users demanded a greater say in the affairs of the manufacturer-dominated CWT. This crisis was resolved in 1985 by the creation of the Center for Office Technology, which was governed by a board of directors weighted in favor of trade associations representing corporate users, such as the Air Transport Association of America, the American Council of Life Insurance, the American Insurance Association, the American Newspaper Publishers Association, and corporations such as Aetna Life and Casualty Insurance, American Express, AT&T, CIGNA, Prudential Insurance, and St. Paul Fire and Marine Insurance. Computer manufacturers were represented by the American Electronics Association, CBEMA, Digital Equipment Corporation, Hewlett-Packard, IBM, NCR, and Xerox.[25] The corporate coalition's reincarnation as the Center for Office Technology illustrates its member's skill and determination to subordinate internal conflicts in the name of achieving their common goal of defeating VDT legislation.

The Media Connection

ANPA's opposition to VDT regulation stemmed from both its staunch conservatism and its dependence on the computer terminal.[26] During the 1970s, ANPA members across the country began to invest millions of dollars in the conversion to VDTs. The newspaper industry's use of VDTs grew from twenty-three in 1970 to sixty thousand by 1987.[27] ANPA's leadership position among corporate users grew out of its lengthy experience fighting the Newspaper Guild on the VDT issue. ANPA acted quickly to use its power to shape reportage of the VDT debate to its advantage—both on and off the editorial page.

    1983 was the turning point in ANPA's mobilization against the labor movement for VDT legislation. In June, George Cashau, ANPA's director of technical research, briefed members of the Newspaper Personnel Relations Association, a professional association closely linked to ANPA. He warned them to be on the lookout for those who would exploit the VDT issue in their quest "for shorter work weeks, longer rest breaks, more people hired, or [those] who have something else to gain."[28] In December, ANPA convened a meeting of its state associations at its Reston, Virginia, headquarters to discuss how to defeat organized labor's campaign for VDT legislation. ANPA instructed its state counterparts to closely monitor the content of stories on the VDT issue. In its successful effort to defeat the 1984 state VDT bill, the Massachusetts Newspaper Publishers Association (MNPA) advised the editors of its member papers to "carefully screen" all VDT stories for anti-employer or anticomputer industry bias before publication. MNPA warned editors and publishers to watch out for reporters who hadn't yet learned to put its slant on VDT stories:

> Unions, particularly the 9 to 5 organization, have been distributing
> propaganda conjuring up all kinds of perils to safety of operators,
> and some of the information is being fed to young reporters who do
> not understand all the elements involved in the dispute. . . . The
> ambition of young reporters to achieve a page-one by-line by
> stretching or embellishing the facts is ever present and the conse-
> quences can cause serious damage.[29]

Why did professional reporters, who were considered competent to cover other stories, need to be put on a tight editorial leash when it came to reporting on VDTs? MNPA's sudden interest in maintaining the strictest standards of journalistic objectivity was motivated by two concerns. First, reporters had been suffering from ailments related to VDT use since the early 1970s, and the union to which many belonged—the Newspaper Guild—was pressing publishers to include VDT regulations in its collective bargaining agreements. As a result, publishers tended to view reporters with the suspicion that they might have more than a casual interest in the VDT story. Second, the profession of concern for objectivity served as a smoke screen, deflecting the public's attention from the publishers economic interest in opposing an open inquiry into the VDT issue. Given the newspaper industry's massive investment in the conversion to VDTs, MNPA did not have to belabor the point that the VDT safety and health coalition's alleged "misinterpretation of facts and statements is . . . dangerous, especially to business interests."[30] But MNPA's policy of censorship was doubly damaging to the public interest. The major media's control of VDT news flow gave MNPA and its allies a strategic advantage in their effort to defeat Massachusetts's VDT bill and, simultaneously, hindered the public's and government officials' ability to assess the pros and cons of the issue.

The attempt by publishers to limit news coverage of the VDT story was repeated in other states considering VDT legislation. Publishers, however, did not always need to remind editors and reporters that they, like any business enterprise, had economic interests that must be considered. As media critic Ben H. Bagdikian observed: "Some intervention by owners is direct and blunt. But most of the screening is subtle, some not even occurring at a conscious level, as when subordinates learn by habit to conform to owners' ideas."[31] As a result, the computer industry's perspective on the VDT issue has been promoted by much of the mainstream and business press. When mainstream news media did cover the story, accounts generally reflected a skepticism of the health hazards associated with the use of VDTs. Not even a letter written to *Newsweek,* the *Wall Street Journal,* and *American Health* by a Research Triangle Park–based IBM employee, which implicated the company's 3279 terminal as the cause of serious safety and health problems, stirred concern among the major media. Except for a local television station in Raleigh, the story was ignored by the major media.[32]

More commonly, the major news media did not report the VDT story at all. When the *Columbia Journalism Review* ran an article on the mystery of the missing VDT news coverage in 1981, it was aptly titled "VDTs: The Overlooked Story Right in the Newsroom."[33] Revisiting the story three years later, it found that the VDT safety and health issue was still not being covered by the major media: "We have been troubled for years about indications that VDTs *may* cause health problems—and equally troubled by the fact that the press as a whole seems unwilling to report in any depth on the nagging questions about safety."[34]

The *Columbia Journalism Review* charged the "major news media" with practicing a policy of "benign neglect," but the neglect was not always so benign. Although two of its young copy editors developed cataracts while working at VDTs in 1976, the *New York Times* refused to report the story. Although the *Times* published two stories (in 1977 and 1980) on the growing concern of some scientists that nonionizing radiation might be harmful to humans at levels lower than previously thought, it failed to mention the VDT controversy on its own premises.[35] Its policy of silence was made public by a 1978 *Wall Street Journal* story, which revealed that NIOSH had inspected the *Times*'s VDTs for radiation leakage.[36] The *Times* did not mention the VDT safety and health controversy for five years, and, then, it was only to say that its terminals had passed a test for radiation leakage.[37] Given that this article never mentioned the reason the VDTs were tested in the first place, the reader was left to wonder why the *Times*'s terminals being cleared of any danger was a newsworthy event. The paper did not run a story addressing office automation for another year and a half.[38] In all, more than six years elapsed from when the *Times* first learned of the VDT controversy and when it first reported on it.

The *Times* record of reporting on the VDT safety and health issue showed little improvement during the 1980s. In 1990, Louis Slesin, founder and editor of the authoritative *VDT News,* wrote: "The *New York Times* has a reputation for ignoring news items on VDT health risks, especially radiation effects."[39] Nor did the *Times* address the growing cumulative trauma disorder problem that affected one in six newsroom employees until senior executive editors were afflicted in 1991.[40]

Similar situations occurred at other major dailies. At the *Baltimore Sun,* where two journalists developed cataracts while working with VDTs, only one brief wire service story had been run on the safety and health issue as of early 1981. When Mary Knudson, the *Sun*'s medical writer, suggested writing a story on VDTs in February 1980, her editor refused. He cited Knudson's position as head of the local Newspaper Guild's health and new technology committee as a conflict of interest. " 'He said he would assign it to another reporter,' Knudson said, 'and that's the last I heard about it. The story hasn't been written.' "[41]

In March 1980, the *Chicago Sun-Times* pulled a story on Dr. Milton M. Zaret, the ophthalmologist who diagnosed the cataracts in the *New York Times* copy editors who used VDTs, after it appeared in the limited circulation early edition.[42] The only other coverage of the story was provided by the *Chicago Reader,* a small circulation, alternative press weekly. Stuart Loory, the *Sun-Times*'s editor, killed the story because, in his opinion, Zaret's theory that cataracts might be caused by continuous exposure to nonionizing radiation emitted by VDTs was not shared by his peers.[43] More significantly, however, was the fact that the publishers' aversion to reporting the VDT story came at the same time they were investing millions of dollars to computerize their newsroom and business operations.[44]

The media's reluctance to report the VDT story hadn't changed much by the late 1980s. "The media has been . . . neglectful in not focusing on this issue," said Mark Pinsky, who has investigated the VDT issue since the early 1980s. He added: "As the evidence [of safety and health dangers] has built they sort of lost interest in this story. I'm hard pressed to understand that short of the fact that the [computer] industry has been effective at getting out its message" to the media.[45] The effort by ANPA and its state affiliates to control VDT news coverage did not prevent stories from appearing in the nation's media, but it did limit the scope of coverage, skew story content, and delay the emergence of public debate on VDT safety and health issues. The public's limited awareness of the issue greatly aided computer manufacturers' and corporate users' efforts to define the contours of the VDT debate to their political advantage.

IBM's Economic and Political Influence

IBM is synonymous with computers. The company released its first desktop computer in 1981, just as labor's campaign for VDT regulations was getting under way. As a leader of the computer industry, and one of the nation's leading manufacturers of VDTs, IBM has had a direct interest in defeating organized labor's drive for VDT regulations. With considerable economic power and high-placed political connections, it amounted to a formidable foe. IBM has maintained a network of close contacts with many businesses through numerous corporate interlocks. The Senate's 1980 study on corporate concentration found that the computer giant had 20 direct and 733 indirect interlocks with 99 corporations, second only to AT&T.[46] With 73 subsidiaries based in 54 countries, IBM ranks as one of the most influential transnational corporations in the world.[47] It is also a perennial top ten member of the *Fortune* 500.[48] Considered by many analysts and traders to be the bluest of all the blue chip stocks, IBM's impact is so massive that fluctuations in its economic fortunes influence market direction. The *New York Times* called it the one stock that "dozens of traders check even before checking the Dow to see where the market is going."[49]

Despite three antitrust suits, both Thomas J. Watson Sr. and Thomas J. Watson Jr. (each in his capacity as chief executive officer) maintained open and cordial relations with Washington for more than fifty years. Watson Sr. had personal contacts with every president from Coolidge to Eisenhower.[50]

He was appointed by President Franklin D. Roosevelt to serve on the newly created Business Council in 1933. Composed of the nation's top corporate executives, the Business Council served "as a clearing house for industrial views on governmental matters which affect business."[51] His son and successor, Thomas J. Watson Jr., was instrumental in establishing closer links between the Business Council and the Kennedy and Johnson administrations. In return for his long and generous financial support of the Democratic Party, President Carter made Watson ambassador to the USSR in 1979, the most important post in the diplomatic corps.[52]

IBM has recruited many important, former high-ranking, federal government officials in its efforts to influence public policy. The list is impressive and represents most recent administrations. It includes former secretary of defense Harold Brown (Carter administration), former secretary of transportation William T. Coleman Jr. (Ford administration), and former attorney general (and retired IBM vice president) Nicholas Katzenbach (Johnson administration), who represented IBM in its successful effort to stave off the Justice Department's eight-year antitrust prosecution. Its advisory board has included such political luminaries as former secretary of state Cyrus R. Vance (Carter administration), former Federal Reserve Board chairman William McChesney Martin Jr. (Truman to Nixon administrations), and William W. Scranton, former governor of Pennsylvania and ambassador to the United Nations (Ford administration). Former undersecretary of state Kenneth W. Dam (Reagan administration) has served as IBM's vice president for law and external relations.[53]

Through interlocking directorates, IBM has also maintained close links with major media firms that shape the news and share its opposition to VDT regulations. Scranton was a longtime New York Times Company board member, and Vance, a former member of the *Washington Post*'s board, is now one of the *New York Times*'s directors. Besides its authoritative position as the nation's paper of record, the *Times* influences news coverage via its twenty-six daily and nine nondaily newspapers, five television stations, two radio stations, and numerous magazines.[54] Katzenbach sits on the *Washington Post*'s board and served as one of Time Inc.'s directors before that. Martin served on the board of the Times Mirror Company, which publishes the *Los Angeles Times, Newsday,* the *Baltimore Sun,* the *Hartford Courant,* and numerous magazines and owns four televisions stations and a cable network.[55] Former chairman Watson Jr. served on the board of Time Inc. for many years and then on the board of Dow Jones and Company, Inc., which includes the *Wall Street Journal* and *Barron's* among its many business publications and twenty-three smaller daily newspapers.[56]

IBM's relationship with the *Washington Post* has been particularly close, giving it another avenue of influence in the seat of government. Four of the *Post's* nine outside directors have ties to IBM. Joining Katzenbach are IBM board member James E. Burke, former IBM executive Ralph E. Gomory, and IBM World Trade Americas/Far East board member Donald Keough. A national institution in its own right, the Washington Post Company also publishes a national weekly edition, owns *Newsweek*, co-owns a national wire service with the *Los Angeles Times,* and holds large shares in the *Minneapolis Star Tribune* and the *International Herald Tribune.* It also owns four television stations and is involved in cable television. As a member of ANPA with an antilabor attitude regarding its own employees, the *Post* shares CBEMA's concern that the VDT safety and health issue remain privatized.[57]

John F. Akers, former IBM chairman of the board and chief executive officer, is one of the Times Company's directors, and both Hewlett-Packard board member Donald E. Petersen and Xerox board member Vernon E. Jordan Jr. sit on Dow Jones's (i.e., *Wall Street Journal's*) board.[58] IBM maintains an elite relationship with two other media giants—Time Warner Inc. and Capital Cities/ABC Inc.—through one-for-one exchanges of inside directors. Both products of media mergers, Time Warner Inc. bills itself as "the world's leading direct marketer of information and entertainment," and Capital Cities's American Broadcasting Company is the leading source of network news for American television viewers.[59] Former IBM chairman of the board Frank T. Cary and Capital Cities/ABC Inc.'s chairman of the board (and retired chief executive officer) Thomas S. Murphy served on each other's board, as did IBM's chairman of the Executive Committee, John R. Opel, and Time Warner Inc.'s chairman of the board/chief executive officer, J. Richard Munro.[60]

Media corporations and the computer industry have also been linked in opposition to safety and health regulations by virtue of their business relationship concerning the buying and selling of VDTs. As Edward S. Herman states in *Corporate Control, Corporate Power:* "The concern about interlocks has focused on their centralizing and anticompetitive potential—their possible use as instruments of command and as means of communications between competitors and as devices making for community of interest among competitors and establishing privileged positions for suppliers, banks, and customers."[61] As mentioned earlier, ANPA members more than doubled their investment in the newsroom use of VDTs—from 1981 to 1987 —at the same time labor's campaign for VDT regulations was heating up. Besides the many computers and VDTs needed for their numerous newsrooms and bureaus, media giants also purchase them for use in their many information service subsidiaries, including television and radio, computer data base news retrieval, financial newswires, and customer interactive services.[62]

Computer manufacturers and business users of computer-automated systems formed an impressive coalition to oppose organized labor's drive for VDT safety and health regulations. Despite the intrabusiness conflict between manufacturers and users, the corporate coalition against VDT regulation held. Moreover, the major media's limited and skewed coverage of the VDT story helped it succeed. Without adequate media coverage of the issue, the public's knowledge was limited. In this political vacuum, the corporate call for "education" instead of regulation seemed to be a reasonable policy position. As a result, public pressure on government to act was limited. Moreover, the globalization of the computer and information services markets encouraged the federal government to deregulate the industry, oppose safety and health regulations, and construct a new policy framework supporting the integration of computer hardware, software, and telecommunications. As long as their coalition held, computer manufacturers and business users of VDTs had good reason to believe that neither the federal nor state governments would intervene on behalf of workers.

Chapter 5

The Federal Politics
of Ergonomic Inaction

[OSHA is] one of the most pernicious of the watchdog agencies.
—Ronald Reagan, 1979

Ronald Reagan's statement was not just campaign rhetoric. Once in office, the Reagan administration severely weakened the Occupational Safety and Health Administration's congressionally mandated enforcement powers by emphasizing "voluntary compliance," "consultation," and a "nonadversarial relationship" with business. President Reagan's evisceration of OSHA's powers was the culmination of a decade-long attack started by business and conservative critics with the agency's inception in 1971.

Since the computer manufacturing and computer-using service sectors are growth industries in an otherwise sluggish economy, many public officials view regulating the workplace use of VDTs as a measure that will hinder economic growth. In his 1983 State of the Union address, President Reagan told the nation that "keeping America the technological leader of the world" through support for "the miracles of high technology" was one of his administration's highest priorities.[1] Economic growth means greater tax revenues and job creation, which helps incumbents stay in office. As elected official's fortunes are tied to business prosperity, there is an inherent motivation to manage the economy in ways that facilitate business enterprise, especially during economic downturns. Political support for economic growth initiatives places a severe constraint on occupational safety and health funding because a strong OSHA is perceived as adding to the cost of doing business and stifling growth.

In this political economic environment, the possibility that funding will be forthcoming to address new occupational safety and health problems, such as the ailments suffered by VDT workers, is slim. The federal government's policy of inaction on VDTs is demonstrated by its failure to: adequately fund NIOSH and independent research on VDT safety and health problems, promulgate OSHA regulations governing the ergonomic aspects of VDT work, adequately fund research on women's health problems, and establish a comprehensive system of recordkeeping on office and VDT-related occupational illness. Federal inaction, in effect, blocks the recognition of the full scope of the growing office safety and health problem and prevents the timely development of a public policy to address it.

The Computer and Business Equipment Manufacturers Association, which represents VDT manufacturers, and the Center for Office Technology, a coalition between CBEMA and corporate computer users, adamantly opposes the idea that VDTs present an occupational safety and health problem.[2] Although former CBEMA president Vico E. Henriques allowed that working with VDTs could cause ergonomic "problems in what we call the comfort area," he has denied that they were serious enough to warrant regulation by OSHA.[3] Moreover, the computer industry's and corporate users' campaign to limit news coverage of the VDT safety and health issue succeeded in reinforcing the perception of many public officials that it was not a serious problem. The regulatory vacuum that has been created by the federal government's policy of inaction has been filled by the computer industry and corporate computer users. Left in a strong position to dominate the VDT issue, and, in effect, make policy, they drafted voluntary ergonomics guidelines that serve to stave off governmental regulation.

Labor's Uphill Battle on Capitol Hill

Collectively, organized labor has not been a very effective voice for VDT workers. Its efforts to secure federal regulations protecting VDT workers have been sporadic and relatively uncoordinated and have occurred within the larger framework of a declining labor movement and growing hostility to unions. The AFL-CIO has concentrated most of its political lobbying and organizing resources on the male-dominated, industrial unions. With the exception of the Service Employees International Union, the Newspaper Guild, the Communications Workers of America, and the American Federation of State, County, and Municipal Workers, most unions were neither adequately prepared nor inclined to take advantage of the opportunity to organize the predominantly female clerical work force around the VDT safety and health issue. In addition, it was labor's misfortune to have the VDT issue gain momentum—during the late 1970s, early 1980s—just as political support for protecting the safety and health of workers was waning and anti-OSHA sentiment in the business community was growing.

Organized labor's efforts to bring the VDT issue to Congress's attention peaked during the early 1980s, when four House subcommittees held six hearings addressing the issue of VDT safety and health in the span of four years.[4] Collectively, these hearings represent the high water mark of federal governmental attention to the VDT issue. Of the six hearings, Congressmen Joseph Gaydos's 1984 hearing was the most important in determining the course of the VDT debate. With manufacturing jobs declining and budget deficits increasing, organized labor had to show dramatic proof of a health crisis in order to convince Congress to regulate the booming computer industry, which was creating new information sector jobs and prosperity. It needed the medical equivalent of a "smoking gun."

However, the computer industry carefully cultivated an image of information-age prosperity dependent on the continued nonregulation of VDTs. Playing to fears of the growing global competition, Henriques warned Congress in 1984 that VDT legislation "simply raises the costs of the products, making U.S. companies less competitive with others around the world."[5] CBEMA's effort to stave off VDT regulations was made easier by the popular perception of the office as a hazard-free workplace and the computer as a "user-friendly" machine. As Congressman Tom Lantos (D, Calif.) said regarding cumulative trauma disorders, a painful wrist and arm ailment caused by VDT workers' repetitive motions: "When we think of occupational illnesses, we usually think of problems that are easily visible. Most of these problems are not easily visible. When you walk into a comfortable-looking office with people sitting in front of video display terminals, you don't see the problem."[6] These hidden health problems have given many public officials the impression that federal action is unnecessary. Congressman Cass Ballenger (R, N.C.), a leading opponent of OSHA, exemplified this shortsighted approach when he said, "No one ever died of ergonomics."[7] As a result, the hidden health nature of the problem has hindered efforts to publicize the problems of working with VDTs and has sustained the federal policy of inaction.

Vision and Voluntarism

Support for the computer industry's position came from the prestigious National Academy of Sciences' National Research Council (NRC) in 1983. The Panel on the Impact of Video Viewing on the Vision of Workers issued a report, based on its review of the scientific literature, stating that there was no proof that VDT use caused vision damage. The panel also advised against legislating European-style regulatory standards that it claimed would freeze computer technology in place while it was still evolving.[8] Overlooked by the NRC panel was a 1982 report by one of its own members, Harry L. Snyder, a VDT engineering specialist at the Virginia Polytechnic Institute. He stated that most cathode ray tubes on the domestic market were poorly made, causing them to lose their brightness after approximately one year's use. Increasing the brightness level to compensate for the decline resulted in blurred character resolution and contributed to vision fatigue. Snyder recommended that VDT manufacturers, few of whom informed their customers of the problem, be pressed to bring their CRTs up to European standards.[9] Ironically, he failed to dissent from the NRC panel's conclusion that the United States did not need European-level standards.

There was one dissenter on the NRC panel: Dr. Lawrence W. Stark of the University of California–Berkeley. He pointed out that much eye fatigue was due to the computer manufacturers' practice of adapting their visual displays from the CRTs used in televisions despite the differing display functions performed by the two electronic devices. Stark wrote: "Implicit in the appearance of video display terminals on the marketplace for office and clerical work is the manufacturers' claim that adequate legibility can be obtained from these terminals. I believe this not to be true. I have never seen a video display terminal that was nearly as legible as the ordinary pieces of typewritten paper or copied reports that circulate in our paper world." Although "adequate time and effort was spent" discussing each panelist's specialized perspective on the problem of VDTs and vision, Stark stated that "adequate time was not spent on consideration of policy questions by the group as a whole." He cautioned that the NRC report could be misconstrued "as supporting the status quo of no standards or guidelines for VDT work places and no clear concern with unacceptable levels of ocular discomfort and visual fatigue."[10]

As Stark indicates, scientific reports, including the NRC's literature review, are not conducted in a political vacuum. Their conclusions often are used to influence and justify policy makers' decisions as to whether to research and regulate technological devices and toxic substances that might be harmful to humankind and the environment. The NRC's enormous prestige—it was the most prominent body of the scientific establishment to examine the VDT issue to date—gave the report's conclusion an aura of authority that overshadowed its limitations. Union officials echoed Stark's concern. "The danger is that the study will be interpreted as saying that video display terminals pose no hazards to workers," said Charles Perlik of the Newspaper Guild. Margaret Seminario, then associate director of occupational safety and health for the AFL-CIO, feared that the NRC report would send a "signal to industry that there are no significant problems," which, in turn, could create "a false sense of security."[11]

Labor's fears about the political uses to which the NRC report would be put proved to be well founded. The panel's report was a literature review, not a new scientific study of the effects of VDTs on vision. Nevertheless, the NRC report was largely portrayed in the media and by opponents of VDT regulations as the definitive study on the subject. Moreover, its conclusion that VDT regulations weren't warranted had the effect of downplaying the significance of the problems faced by VDT workers and bolstered the computer industry and corporate users' position that voluntary efforts to improve employee comfort was the best way to proceed. With the battle on Capitol Hill heating up, the release of the NRC's report could not have come at a better time for opponents of VDT regulations.

The Gaydos Hearings

Held during the winter and spring of 1984, the Gaydos hearings represented the most important congressional standoff between labor and management on the VDT issue. Joseph Gaydos, who chaired the House Education and Labor Committee and its Subcommittee on Safety and Health, represented a blue-collar, steelworking district in western Pennsylvania. Representatives from AFSCME, CWA, SEIU, 9 to 5, the Newspaper Guild, the Office and Professional Employees International Union, and the Metal Trades Department of the AFL-CIO testified to the subcommittee that many of their members suffered from vision and musculoskeletal ailments. Noting that the United States lagged behind Europe, organized labor urged Congress to enact VDT regulations based on NIOSH's recently released recommendations: VDTs with detachable keyboards, chairs and desks designed for maximum flexibility, proper illumination of screen and work surface to control glare problems (i.e., less bright than conventional office lighting), rest breaks every two hours of continuous work (unions also asked for rest breaks after one hour of intense work), and vision exams for workers before commencing VDT work and periodically thereafter. David LeGrande, the CWA's director of occupational safety and health, noted that it would not be difficult for the computer industry to adjust, because IBM was already manufacturing computers to meet Sweden's stricter ergonomic standards.[12]

Opposing VDT regulations were representatives from a cross section of corporate America, including CBEMA, the American Newspaper Publishers Association, the Business and Institutional Furniture Manufacturers Association (BIFMA), the American Electronics Association, the Air Transport Association of America, the American Society of Travel Agents, the Printing Industries of America, AT&T, the Digital Equipment Corporation, and the *New York Times*.[13] Echoing the NRC's report, CBEMA's Henriques warned Gaydos's subcommittee that federally mandated VDT standards would freeze the technology's development in place, causing the U.S. computer industry to loose its edge against foreign competitors. In order to further discredit the case for VDT regulations, he depicted its supporters as unreasonable people who would "force" others to follow unnecessary rules. According to Henriques, they

> would force people to sit in special chairs, even if they were satisfied
> and comfortable in the present model; mandate covering windows
> with blinds even if there were no glare problem, or even if the glare
> problem came from another source. They would force low light levels
> in all working places using visual displays, even though such light
> levels might pose serious problems, such as on the factory assembly
> line, or might even be dangerous as in a hospital. They would reduce
> the number of hours people could work on displays to a maximum
> of four or five, ignoring the fact that millions of users would be
> forced out of full-time jobs and into half-time jobs, reducing their
> pay and, in many cases, removing many fringe [benefits]. They
> would force employers to pay for meaningless devices and activities,
> such as metal shielding for terminals and radiation inspections.[14]

He added that "legislative mandates force citizens to conform to a legislator's best guesses about what will make them feel better."[15] However, ergonomic regulations governing VDT design had been adopted by Australia, Austria, New Zealand, Norway, Sweden, and West Germany without "freezing" the technology's development, and they were leading the way in terms of technological innovation.

Henriques promised Gaydos's subcommittee that, in lieu of federal regulations, the computer industry would launch a publicity campaign to "educate people about the best use of visual displays in the workplace." He asserted that "with education people have the freedom to choose solutions to problems that are best for them as individuals."[16] Henriques's argument that voluntary, management-led education of office workers is superior to government regulation rests on the assumption that an open and trusting relationship exists between management and labor. However, the vast majority of VDT workers do not have a meaningful voice in management's decision about how the technology will be used. Given that almost 90 percent of full-time VDT workers are unorganized, occupational safety and health regulations are necessary to assure that all workers are protected.

Corporate-sponsored surveys of secretaries and office workers also challenge Henriques's assertion that workers are free to choose on the job. A survey of four thousand American secretaries, cosponsored by the Electronic Typewriter Division of the Panasonic Industrial Company and Professional Secretaries International (PSI), found that "many respondents feel isolated from their executives." It reported that 70 percent of secretaries experienced "a lack of communication from their supervisor and almost as many (68 percent) believe that they have little input into the decisions affecting them."[17] "In the face of fierce business competition," explained the PSI's Candace M. Louis, "managers are demanding even greater productivity from their secretaries. This expanded role is increasing the level of secretarial stress." The study linked much of the stress increase to poor communication on management's part; 41 percent of the secretaries attributed the increased work stress to "a lack of communication from their supervisors."[18]

Another survey conducted by Louis Harris and Associates for Steelcase, Inc., found that American office workers had a widespread distrust of management. It revealed that although 89 percent of office workers highly valued "management that is honest, upright, and ethical in its dealings with employees and the community," only 41 percent believed that this actually described their experience with management. Moreover, the fact that 72 percent of management felt that they had good relations with their employees indicated the extent to which they were ignorant of their workers' feelings. Furthermore, the Harris survey found that, on average, management over-estimated the contentment and satisfaction of their employees with work-ing conditions by anywhere from ten to seventeen percentage points. Although 76 percent of office workers felt that "a free exchange of information among employees and departments" was essential, only 35 percent said it existed in their workplace. Sixty-one percent of office workers said "a par-ticipatory management style at all levels of decision-making" was "very impor-tant" to them, but only 28 percent said it described the labor-management relationship in their company.[19] In sum, the freedom to choose that office workers lacked was due to their lower status and lesser power within the corporate culture, not proposed VDT regulations.

CBEMA launched a public relations campaign to disseminate their view on VDT safety. Stating that "our group is not an entirely appropriate group to sponsor public service announcements on this issue," Henriques hired the American Council on Science and Health (ACSH) "to work with us on the campaign."[20] ACSH's public service announcement, entitled "VDT Health," gave the mistaken impression that all VDT problems were relatively benign and within the power of the worker to control. It told viewers to "adjust the controls, move the screen to cut glare" and "have your vision checked," but said nothing about improper room lighting as the source of screen glare and the cause of eye strain, or the fact that many VDTs were not adjustable. It advised the viewer to "adjust your chair and move around during the day," but said nothing about the employer's responsibility to provide an ergonom-ically designed work station and chair. It omitted the fact that many VDT workers were not permitted to take breaks when they needed them—nor did it mention NIOSH's recommendations that VDT workers be given periodic rest breaks and ergonomically designed work stations.[21] Despite these omissions, the ACSH's imprimatur gave CBEMA's message the stamp of scientific legitimacy.

Henriques told Congress that the ACSH was an "independent scien-tific organization."[22] However, it is a private organization (not public as its name implies) that receives 70 percent of its funding from the corporate com-munity (including the computer and VDT-user corporations) and industry-supported foundations to provide them with scientific arguments against government regulation of business.[23] It was founded in 1978 by members of the scientific and corporate communities who objected to what they saw as the excessive influence that liberally oriented public interest groups exerted on public opinion and government officials. As an ACSH brochure states: "Many of the existing 'consumer advocate' groups weren't giving either policy makers or consumers the balanced, accurate, scientific information they needed."[24]

Short of government regulation, what would compel manufacturers and employers to incorporate the latest ergonomic advances into their computers, furniture, and offices? Defenders of the market perspective maintain that corporate consumers' demands for the latest ergonomically designed equipment will spur competition among manufacturers to provide the latest designs at the best prices. This argument is based on two assumptions: that corporate consumers and manufacturers are ergonomically informed and that manufacturers will produce ergonomically designed computers and furniture in quantities sufficient to make them competitive with cheaper, less ergonomically designed models. Both assumptions are questionable. There is no guarantee, short of mandatory federal regulations, that corporate purchasers will prefer the safer, more expensive, VDT equipment when their competitors can still buy the cheaper, less safe equipment. Likewise, without federal regulation, many, if not all, VDT manufacturers will continue to make the less expensive, less ergonomically safe equipment to meet the market demand.

Despite their assurances to the federal government that the voluntarist approach is the best method to ensure safe and healthful VDT workplaces, many employers have not seriously addressed the ergonomics crisis in their workplace. A survey of workplaces, released shortly after the Gaydos subcommittee concluded that employers were best suited to resolve occupational safety and health difficulties arising from computer use, found that 75 percent of VDT-related ergonomic problems were due to poor management.[25] Another survey, conducted by the *Wall Street Journal*, found that "only a few employers are concerned" about the VDT safety and health issue. It cited a handful of firms, including CBEMA members IBM and Kodak, as having vision and glare guidelines, but added that "none think they're a health hazard." TRW Incorporated declared that working with VDT's presents "no hazard." Several banking and financial sector firms, such as AmeriTrust Corporation, Chase Manhattan Bank, and the Security Pacific Corporation, were studying and designing ergonomic programs for their VDT employees to follow, but these companies were the exception to the rule.[26] "Most companies resist official VDT policies," the *Wall Street Journal* reported.[27] As a case in point, a spokesman for NCR, a major computer manufacturer, dismissed the VDT problem outright, saying: "We don't have any guidelines whatsoever."[28]

According to Laura Punnett, a research fellow at the University of Michigan's Center for Ergonomics, the voluntarist approach favored by business offers no guarantee that workers will benefit from the latest scientific advances in the field. She reports that many employers require that workers sit at the VDT for most of the working day in order to recoup their investment in the machines, but the human body is not meant to sit in one position for long periods of time. The resultant "static posture" problem causes musculoskeletal ailments. Many manufacturers, however, have not kept up with design changes in chairs to compensate for this problem. As a result, Punnett said, "Ergonomics has become a buzzword that can be used to sell furniture" rather than to address the safety and health needs of office workers.[29]

The development of VDT-related ergonomic problems spawned a new market for computer software aimed at informing workers when to take breaks and how to do aerobic exercises, but slow sales to corporate VDT users undermined CBEMA's and COT's claims that employers were making VDT safety and health a high priority. "We haven't found a lot of big time excitement from customers," Christian Banes, a marketer of these products said. Ironically, Banes found that many employers saw these automated take-a-break programs as a threat to their control over the pace of work. "Top level executives say, 'I'm not going to pay you money in order to have my work force not work,'" he explained.[30]

Too often, corporations shift the occupational safety and health burden to their employees. The *American Journal of Public Health* criticized companies that promoted employee "wellness" programs, which focus on what employee can do for themselves (e.g., proper diet and exercise, getting regular checkups, stopping smoking, etc.) instead of the more comprehensive, employer-supported occupational safety and health programs. The editorial's author, Dr. Charles Levenstein, wondered if "workers are being lulled into a false sense of security when occupational hazards are not mentioned or dealt with by work-site health educators." Jonathan Fielding, a Johnson & Johnson Company doctor, retorted that "wellness" programs are intended as a "supplement," not a "substitute," for occupational safety and health programs.[31] However, millions of VDT-using office employees work for information-producing companies that are not regulated by OSHA and do not maintain their own occupational safety and health programs.

The policy of IBM, which *Business Week* described as "the leader in ergonomics," is indicative of the problems involved in coordinating education and implementation efforts between manufacturers and corporate users. "We offer a certain amount of guidance from a human factors [i.e., ergonomics] point of view," said Vice President Lewis M. Branscomb, IBM's chief scientist. "But we regard that as a decision for the customer to make. There is little that IBM can do about a facility's layout."[32] Stephen D. Channer, executive director of BIFMA, a trade association representing companies controlling 90 percent of the U.S. office furniture market, allowed how the same problems existed between his industry and its corporate customers: "Ergonomic assistance on how to best fit the worker to the furniture of the work station is available from most of the major manufacturers of office furniture, but it is *rarely* asked for by companies buying such furniture."[33] The lack of communication between retailers of computers and office furniture is also a major problem. As the *New York Times* reported: "Part of the difficulty for shoppers is that computer dealers often know little about furniture, and furniture dealers often know nothing about computers."[34]

In the voluntarist system that now prevails, many employers do not buy ergonomic equipment for their workers. Many of the musculoskeletal ailments suffered by workers are caused by the daily use of VDTs without detachable keyboards and tiltable screens, and chairs and desks that are not adjustable to the particular height and reach requirements of each user. The CWA's David LeGrande told Gaydos's subcommittee that "all too often, VDT equipment is installed in traditional offices with little or no redesign of the work place. In many cases, workers have witnessed the VDT's introduction into their work environments without proper consideration of ergonomic factors." He added that federal regulations were needed, especially as the vast majority of VDT workers weren't organized and, therefore, were unable to avail themselves of the collective bargaining process. "It is the experience of the CWA and other concern organizations that employers of these workers have not and will not introduce ergonomic and protective VDT working conditions unless they are forced to do so," LeGrande remarked.[35]

Despite the documented growth of health hazards related to VDT work, and the existence of regulations in other industrialized countries,

Representative Gaydos stated that he would not introduce legislation regulating the safety and health conditions of VDT workers. "I'd like to see the industry regulate itself," he said.[36] Finally, the Gaydos subcommittee's staff report reflected the computer industry's and the NRC panel's contention that regulation was unwarranted: "It is unlikely that the legislative action at any level will do more than provide contradictory and, perhaps, more restrictive limits rather than encouraging the flexibility that is both desirable and necessary for worker health and safety in offices and other locales where VDTs are in prevalent use." The report also reflected congressional anxiety about the alternative work provision's implicit challenge to corporate autonomy in the workplace: "Is the Congress or any other legislative body prepared to tell an employer that an employee must be given other tasks to do as a form of respite from VDT work?"[37] The answer given by Congress was a resounding no.

The Invisible Woman

Overlooked by the Gaydos subcommittee were the cautionary remarks of Congresswoman Mary Rose Oakar (D, Ohio). Although not a member of Gaydos's subcommittee, she took a special interest in the problems of working women. Oakar charged that Gaydos's subcommittee had not fully appreciated the safety and health problems affecting VDT workers. She said that "33 million Americans work in office settings. More than 50 percent of all office workers are women. Every day, these employees are exposed to low-level radiation from viedo [sic] display terminals. . . . We don't know if it's safe for pregnant women to sit near video display terminal[s] all day."[38] Oakar added that "federally funded research into these hazards has been sparse. In addition, information about how to control their health effects is not readily available."[39] To reinforce her point, she cited a report by the Office of Technology Assessment showing that NIOSH's budget for office health hazards research in 1984 was only $300,000, or "less than 1 penny per office worker."[40] Karen Nussbaum, the executive director of 9 to 5, commented that "the figure is outrageously small."[41] "Not only is this not a priority for this Administration, it is not a concern," Oakar said, referring to President Reagan's veto of the appropriations bill containing funding for research on office hazards.[42] She added that "it is the responsibility of government—and employers—to undertake more serious research into office health and safety. Our health depends on it."[43]

The federal government's extensive record of inaction is illustrated by the paultry sums spent for VDT research by the Reagan administration. From 1981 to 1986 it spent only seven cents per office worker researching the hazards they faced. The figures were even worse for VDT research, only two cents per worker.[44] This concerted policy of neglect led a frustrated David LeGrande to accurately predict that the Reagan administration would never promulgate VDT regulations.[45]

Without adequate funding to collect accurate data and conduct thorough studies, it is impossible to determine the true extent to which workers suffer job-related health problems.[46] In 1979, the U.S. surgeon general, Julius B. Richmond, reported that, due to underreporting and lack of awareness of occupational illness among medical practitioners, the true extent of occupational disease probably exceeded NIOSH's estimates of 100,000 deaths from work-related diseases and 400,000 new cases of occupational disease per year. In 1985, the OTA reported that U.S. recordkeeping was so inadequate that estimating the magnitude of occupational illness was virtually impossible.[47] The same year, the House Committee on Government Operations concluded that "federal occupational health hazards surveillance is 72 years behind communicable disease surveillance" and "is decades behind . . . England, France, Germany, and Sweden."[48] Dr. Irving Selikoff, the nation's foremost authority on occupational illness put it bluntly: " 'We cannot expect to rapidly increase our knowledge' of workplace disease if only epidemiological evidence— 'in the vernacular, counting dead bodies on the street'—is used to the exclusion of laboratory findings." Lamenting the lack of worker surveillance studies, he added, "You talk about workers being guinea pigs, but at least guinea pigs are observed."[49]

Inadequate recordkeeping of occupational injuries and illnesses also makes it more difficult for critics to counter computer industry claims that VDT work involves only issues of employee "comfort."[50] The Bureau of Labor Statistics, for example, does not keep track of the number of CTDs that afflict VDT workers. Using worker compensation records instead of a sampling of employers, a study by Arthur Oleinick and Jeremy V. Gluck revealed that the BLS reporting system underestimates the true rate of occupational injuries by a factor between four and nine. It also suggests that occupational illnesses are also underreported, because the BLS uses the same system to collect data on them.[51] Given the poor quality of the BLS's data gathering for CTDs, it is safe to assume that its statistics are underestimates of the real magnitude of the CTD problem.[52]

The failure of the federal government to collect accurate statistics and epidemiological data on occupational illness is an example of a nondecision. That is, it serves to understate the true magnitude of the problem, denying the public the information they need to evaluate the extent of the problem and challenge the policy status quo. As a result, the debate is skewed in favor of corporate interests who view occupational safety and health as a relatively unimportant problem that does not require government intervention.

Another case of nondecision making is the federal government's pattern of bias against studying and regulating the health problems of women. OSHA's policy of targeting the highest risk workplaces, such as construction and manufacturing, which are male-dominated, means that female-dominated workplaces, such as the office, are neglected. Noting that inspections of female-dominated workplaces are "rare," the National Association of Public Health Policy's Women's Occupational Health Committee challenged OSHA's assumption that "women's work is safe" and urged it to promulgate a standard addressing the ergonomic and radiation aspects of VDT use.[53]

Just as the federal government has failed to adequately research the problems of VDT workers (the vast majority of whom are women), it has also failed to include women in its health studies.[54] As a case in point, the National Institute on Aging studied the aging process from 1958 to 1978 without including women in its study population. *Normal Human Aging* (1984) excluded the majority sex from its "representative" sample. It routinely recommended that the results of its male studies be applied to women, despite their hormonal and physiological differences.[55] In an ongoing study started in 1981, the National Institutes of Health (NIH) employed twenty-two thousand male doctors in a study of aspirin's ability to prevent heart attacks. When asked by the General Accounting Office (GAO) why women weren't included in the study population, NIH officials replied that doctors were chosen because they could be relied on to follow the requirement that they take an aspirin (or placebo) every other day for a long period of time. Dr. Claude Lenfant, director of the National Heart, Lung and Blood Institute, maintained that it would be too costly to locate a sufficient number of women doctors for a study population that size. At the very least, both objections could have been overcome by using female registered nurses.[56]

In June 1990, the GAO reported that the NIH routinely approved medical studies excluding women, despite its own 1986 directive to cor-rect this glaring omission. Admitting the NIH's failure to follow its own guide-lines, acting director William F. Raub told the House Subcommittee on Health and the Environment: "Those who received the word about the policy don't all seem to understand it, and most distressing of all from this morn-ing's testimony, some of those who have received this policy and understand it have demonstrated some arrogance or indifference with respect to it."[57] VDT work has been defined as women's work, and as with women's health policy in general, VDT health and safety issues have been neglected by the federal government.

ANSI's Ergonomic Action

In 1982, CBEMA members and the Human Factors Society (HFS), an industry supported association of professionals engaged in ergonomic research, began work on voluntary ergonomic guidelines for the American National Standards Institute (ANSI). ANSI is a private, industry-dominated organization that promotes the adoption of voluntary guidelines. However, ANSI's name, reputation, and the fact that its guidelines are widely used in lieu of (and provide the basis for) OSHA regulations gives it quasi-governmental authority. Six years in the making, the computer industry's voluntary guidelines were released in 1988; they suggested that manufac-turers follow uniform specifications for computer terminal and keyboard design, office lighting, temperature, and noise levels.[58] Because the guide-lines were voluntary, there were no penalties for noncompliance.

The development of a voluntary industry standard was politically important to CBEMA and COT for two reasons. First, it enabled them to tell policy makers and the public that they were addressing the ergonomic problem and, therefore, legislation was not needed. As Beth O'Neill, COT's executive director, explained, the guidelines provide the computer indus-try and corporate users with a "useful tool to show legislators that orga-nized professional bodies are concerned about VDT ergonomics."[59] Second, by preempting what CBEMA and COT considered to be the more onerous option of mandatory regulation, the voluntary guidelines helped to side-track organized labor's drive for VDT regulations. As a result, the volun-tary guidelines helped to solidify corporate control over the VDT occupational safety and health debate.

However, a hitch in the plan developed when organized labor announced that it intended to use the guidelines as the basis for state legislation. Although the guidelines were narrow in scope (e.g., they did not address concerns about shielding terminals for nonionizing radiation, workloads, rest breaks, and monitoring), some unions (such as the Newspaper Guild) and state legislators (e.g., in California) saw them as a model for legislation. They reasoned that if the voluntary standards were good enough to meet HFS's and ANSI's professional standards, why shouldn't their benefits be made available to all VDT workers in the form of mandatory regulations? Fearing this eventuality, the computer coalition withheld release of the VDT guidelines for eighteen months. COT's O'Neill said legislation would be a "nightmare," and added that "ANSI works because the standard is voluntary and allows flexibility. Why would we try to turn that into law?"[60]

CBEMA's and COT's solution, endorsed by HFS and ANSI, was to include a vaguely worded escape clause in the VDT guidelines that reserved to manufacturers the right to deviate from the stated specifications "if it is empirically demonstrated by substantive research conducted under accepted scientific practice that the system yields equivalent or higher levels of human performance without a decrease in comfort."[61] If organized labor attempted to enact ANSI guidelines into law, CBEMA and COT could insist that legislators also include the escape clause. Because most ergonomics research is carried out by the computer industry, in conjunction with the HFS and ANSI, they would effectively retain control over the interpretation of VDT standards even if legislation were enacted.

Through effective lobbying, however, CBEMA and COT were able to prevent the issue of enacting the ANSI guidelines into law from reaching a legislative showdown in California. With the failure of federal and state legislative initiatives, CBEMA became a quasi-government unto itself regarding VDT ergonomics standards. Public and union officials may be invited to comment, but the computer industry has veto power over the final result.

OSHA's Ergonomic Inaction

In May 1984, after more than four years of study, NIOSH issued its recommendations for VDT ergonomic regulations. But NIOSH's action had little impact on OSHA because the Reagan administration decided to ignore its recommendations. The low priority that the administration attached to the growing problem of ergonomic-related VDT ailments was further exemplified by the fact that it did not permit OSHA to hire its first ergonomist until the fall of 1985. After two years of administrative inaction on the NIOSH ergonomic recommendations, Dr. Roger L. Stephens, OSHA's only ergonomist, lamented that the agency "will never be able to force the needed job redesign or even lead the way."[62] When Reagan left office in 1989, OSHA's staff of approximately twenty-four hundred employees included five hundred lawyers but still had only one ergonomist.[63]

That policy makers in the Reagan and Bush administrations were insensitive to the rapidly increasing CTD crisis is further illustrated by their collective failure to seek the authority to hire additional ergonomists in either the fiscal year 1989 or 1990 budget requests.[64] The question of how OSHA under the Reagan and Bush administrations could keep on top of the exploding CTD crisis with only one ergonomist led Congressman Tom Lantos to hold a subcommittee hearing. Resultant public exposure forced the Bush administration to hire two new ergonomists in 1990, but this was a token response to the problem. OSHA's inability to handle the CTD problem with only three ergonomists was illustrated by Stephens's admission that the agency needed at least ten (one per region) ergonomists, plus a Washington-based team, just to start a rudimentary ergonomics program.[65] The Bush administration's indifference to the problem was illustrated by this exchange between Congressman Lantos and OSHA's only ergonomist, Dr. Roger Stephens, in 1989:

> Stephens: I've been coached in what to say if this question came and—
> Lantos: Tell us what they coached to tell you [sic] and then tell us the truth.
> Stephens: That they're aware of the fact that we need more people, and it's a resource allocation problem. But I, of course, would welcome the help.[66]

As a result of the Bush administration's "resource allocation problem," OSHA's influence was limited to Stephens's lone efforts to exhort corporate industrial hygienists to voluntarily follow NIOSH's ergonomics guidelines.[67]

The Reagan and Bush administrations' policies of inaction allowed the rise of cumulative trauma disorders in the workplace to go unabated. In 1981, CTDs accounted for only 18 percent of all reported occupational illnesses, but the growing use of VDTs helped it to swell to more than 60 percent of all cases by 1993.[68]

CTDs commonly afflict workers in industrial, assembly-line-type work processes that require the use of repetitive motions on the part of the worker but have spread to VDT workers, blurring the distinction between industrial and office work. Congressman Tom Lantos recognized this convergence when he called "cumulative trauma disorders the industrial disease of the information age." CTDs, he said, are "occurring in offices where more than 28 million people work at video display terminals as well as on assembly lines using the most up-to-date technologies."[69]

The Reagan and Bush administrations' policy of assessing headline-grabbing large fines against meatpackers deflected the public's attention from the rapidly increasing and unregulated problem among VDT and other service sector workers. NIOSH's statement that the rapid proliferation of VDTs is an "especially important factor" in the increase of the CTD problem, and OSHA's pronouncement that the use of this computer technology has "generated new and pervasive sources of biomechanical stress to the musculoskeletal system," were lost in the publicity generated by the large fines policy.[70] Untargeted corporations (the vast majority), such as those that use VDTs, were left to police themselves free of public scrutiny. Deprived of an accurate injury and illness reporting system by Reagan and Bush policies of underfunding, OSHA had no reliable means of monitoring the growing CTD problem. As a result, OSHA's institutional memory contained a significant blank space where VDT-related CTDs were concerned. Lacking the statistical data, OSHA director Gerard F. Scannel was forced to resort to generalities when asked by the New York Times in 1989 what percentage of CTDs were due to VDT work. "I don't think you can associate it all with the computer," he said. But the Times added, paraphrasing his words, "The proliferation of computer technology in many industries was a significant cause of the increase in repetitive motion disorders."[71]

OSHA's failure to respond positively to the development of safety and health hazards in the office was not due to either bureaucratic or cultural lag—it has been petitioned by organized labor and others to act for more than a decade. Rather, it was due to the Reagan administration's policy of inaction and the Bush administration's go-slow approach. Strong corporate support for Reagan's deregulatory policies and lack of sustained pressure from the Democratic-controlled Congress (many of whom were also recipients of corporate campaign largesse) also impeded the promulgation of an ergonomics standard during the 1980s and early 1990s. The Clinton administration was slow to finish work on the proposed ergonomics standard that had languished in the Bush administration since 1990. When the Republicans gained control of Congress in 1994 for the first time in forty years, the ergonomics proposal was at the top of their list of pending regulations to be killed. House Republicans slated OSHA for a budget cut of $16 million. OSHA responded with a much weaker version of the ergonomics standard, which did not require employers to identify the most dangerous jobs, and exempted many from compliance. This was not enough for House Republicans, who quickly cut another $3.5 million from OSHA's already paltry budget, in effect prohibiting it from completing work on the ergonomics standard. House Majority Whip Tom Delay (R, Tex.) said the additional budget cut was needed to discipline OSHA for "flouting the will of this Congress."[72]

Chapter 6

The Nonproblem of
Nonionizing Radiation

The most controversial aspect of the computer safety and health debate involves the question of whether continuous exposure to nonionizing radiation emitted by video display terminals is harmful to human health. The VDT's flyback transformer powers the electron ray gun that creates the visual display on the phosphor-coated backside of the cathode ray tube. In the process, it emits pulsed electromagnetic fields. Concern has focused on the lower nonionizing radiation portion of the electromagnetic spectrum, especial very low frequency (VLF) and extremely low frequency (ELF) fields. VLF and ELF fields are strongest at the sides and back, where the flyback transformer is located. Those who are working in close proximity to these positions might be at risk of exposure even though they are not working with a VDT. Pulsed EMFs are of particular concern to researchers because they can produce power increases five to ten times that of unmodulated fields.[1] Studies of children and workers exposed to sixty-Hertz fields, emitted by power lines and VDTs, have found that these fields can promote cancer—namely, brain cancer, leukemia, and lymphoma—disrupt cellular structure, and suppress the immune system.[2] There is also concern that EMFs might be responsible for reproductive problems, including miscarriages, suffered by female VDT workers. Some cases of premature eye cataracts have also been reported, but studies have not been conducted to see if there is a link to VDTs. However, extensive research on the EMF question has not been conducted in the United States. Because the theory of a link between nonionizing radiation and health hazards runs counter to the prevailing scientific theory that only ionizing radiation (not a serious problem with VDTs) is harmful, public officials have rejected health and safety advocate's appeals to authorize funds for EMF research.

In his seminal book *The Structure of Scientific Revolutions,* Thomas S. Kuhn maintains that the scientific establishment (practitioners of "normal science") stifles "fundamental novelties" that do not fit with its prevailing paradigms. Paradigms, in Kuhn's words, are the "universally recognized scientific achievements that for a time provide model problems and solutions to a community of practitioners." He adds: "Normal science, the activity in which most scientists inevitably spend almost all their time, is predicated on the assumption that the scientific community knows what the world is like. Much of the success of the enterprise derives from the community's willingness to defend that assumption, if necessary at considerable cost. Normal science, for example, often suppresses fundamental novelties because they are necessarily subversive of its basic commitments."[3]

Kuhn's analysis serves as a model for the nonionizing radiation controversy. Because the governing scientific paradigm holds that the nonionizing radiation waves emitted by VDTs are too weak to cause biological damage in humans, research to the contrary is treated as a fundamental novelty that is suppressed by practitioners of normal science. Thus, research in this field is viewed as unnecessary. U.S. scientists are more likely to support this view than their European counterparts, who have been encouraged by a history of state funding and nonionizing radiation research to explore the possibility that EMFs are harmful to humans. However, in the United States there is less of a tradition of state support for independent research. Since its fiscal and political fortunes are closely tied to the state of the economy—and the computer industry is one of the few bright spots in an otherwise sluggish economy—federal government officials are more likely to support research that leads to commercial applications (new product development) that can help restore the competitiveness of U.S. corporations in an increasingly global economy. Under the Reagan administration, "science was no longer to be treated as a public good but as a private commodity," David Dickson observed.[4] "At both ends of Pennsylvania Avenue," President Bush's science advisor, Dr. D. Alan Bromley, said, "there is a real sense that science and technology must play a more important role if we are to be competitive internationally." *Industry Week* reported that "the economic downturn has brought a recognition of the link between science/technology and long-term growth" to the attention of both the president and Congress.[5] This emphasis on gearing federal research to enhance the global competitiveness of U.S. business places severe budgetary constraints on the state's support of occupational safety and health research. Except for a relative handful of liberal Democratic members of Congress, there is little high-level political support for occupational safety and health research into the effects of nonionizing radiation on VDT workers. These factors explain why computer industry officials were able to convince federal government officials that state-sponsored research on nonionizing radiation emitted by VDTs was unnecessary and a waste of the taxpayer's money.

The "Catch 22" of Nonionizing Radiation Research

Concern about the radiation emitted by VDTs emerged as an issue in 1976 with the report that two *New York Times* copy editors had developed eye cataracts at the ages of 29 and 35. Eye cataracts in people that young are highly unusual. The Newspaper Guild, which represented the two copy editors, consulted Dr. Milton Zaret of Bellevue Medical Center, an authority on eye cataracts and radiation. Zaret diagnosed the two as having radiation-induced eye cataracts, which he attributed to their use of VDTs. The National Institute for Occupational Safety and Health (NIOSH) investigated and exonerated the VDTs, although it allowed that the eye cataracts might have been radiation-induced. NIOSH based its decision on the view that there was no conclusive proof that EMFs emitted by VDTs cause eye cataracts. However, NIOSH's investigation focused on the ionizing radiation (X-rays) and the higher end of the nonionizing radiation spectrum: infrared, radio frequency, and microwaves. NIOSH was not prepared to test VDTs for VLF and ELF emissions. Moreover, very little research had been done in the United States on VLFs and ELFs. As NIOSH's Wordie Parr said in 1980: "To be quite honest, nobody knows a damn thing about that low a frequency."[6]

Because VLF and ELF fields are too weak to create a thermal effect, they were assumed to be harmless. However, the Soviets and East Europeans, who had researched the subject since World War II, came to a different conclusion. Their research on the biological effects of microwave and radio frequency radiation on animals and humans found that prolonged exposure *at nonthermal* levels disrupted the operation of the nervous, cardiovascular, reproductive, immunological, and blood systems and had deleterious effects on vision. But, caught up in Cold War politics and methodological disputes, their work was largely ignored in the West.[7] "Apparently Western scientists have always thought the risks were only from thermal (high-level) radiation and simply concluded that the 15-to-125 kiloHertz [VLF] range was safe," said Ian Marceau, science advisor to the House Committee on Science and Technology in 1981. "So no one studied this radiation range until the military did it."[8] But the Defense Department's research on the nonionizing frequencies focused on their communications potential, not their effects on health and safety. It was not until Representative Al Gore Jr.'s (D, Tenn.) 1981 subcommittee hearings on VDTs that the military publicly admitted that a hazard to human health might exist at the lower end of the electromagnetic spectrum.[9]

Western science's failure to study the health and safety aspects of EMFs and the secrecy shrouding the military's research had the effect of circumscribing the VDT debate. When the Bureau of Radiological Health (BRH) tested VDTs in 1981, it found very low frequency fields, but lacking a prior body of health and safety research to refer to, "simply said it didn't violate any known health standards." But occupational safety standards for radio frequency and microwave nonionizing radiation in the Soviet Union and Czechoslovakia were one hundred times stricter than in the United States. The weaker—and for some frequencies nonexistent—U.S. standards were due in part to the lack of research in the field. Moreover, U.S. standards are based on the premise that microwaves are harmful only at high intensities, which can burn tissue. The East European standards are based on the conclusion that continued exposure at nonthermal levels over a period of time can do biological damage.[10]

The weaker, and nonexistent, U.S. standards gave computer manufacturers and corporate users a tremendous tactical advantage over health and safety advocates when they argued that there was no reason to worry, let alone spend large sums of money on nonionizing radiation research. Reacting to calls that the Radiation Control for Safety and Health Act of 1968 (which covers color television CRTs) be amended to include VDTs, Dr. Myron L. Wolbarsht, a Duke University professor of ophthalmology and biomedical engineering and computer industry consultant, said: "A label certifying that CRTs pass radiation measurements may be a good idea. Not because there's radiation coming out of them. But because there is a scare and a label might make CRTs more acceptable."[11] A label, however, would offer a false sense of security because there were no federal safety and health standards governing ELF and VLF waves—those suspected of causing health problems. The Computer and Business Equipment Manufacturers Association's president, Vico E. Henriques, assured Gore's subcommittee that there was nothing to be alarmed about: "In view of the work that has been going on in our industry for many years, it comes as no surprise to us that this recent FDA testing program and a similar NIOSH testing program conclude what we have known for some time, that radiation from VDTs is well within safe levels."[12]

However, NIOSH and the FDA take their cue from CBEMA and the American National Standards Institute, which work together to set voluntary occupational safety and health standards in the effort to forestall governmental action. ANSI is industry-supported but performs an important quasi-governmental role in lieu of federal action. Since ANSI had not established voluntary standards for VLF or ELF radiation (i.e., below three hundred kiloHertz), neither OSHA nor the BRH saw any need to act. Besides showing that VDTs can malfunction, the following exchange between Congressman Gore and the BRH's William Herman illustrates the extent to which the federal government follows ANSI's lead:

> Herman: We found measurements of 1,000 volts per meter, which were then compared to a standard of 200 volts per meter. That standard applies to a different frequency range, not the [VLF] range of the measurements that we made.
>
> Gore: Only because there is no standard in the other range, is that right?
>
> Herman: There is no standard in the frequency range where our measurements showed the emissions to be.
>
> Gore: OK. But if the standard in that frequency range did exist, and if it was the same level as the other one, then it would have been exceeded by a factor of five.
>
> Herman: Right, but that is a substantive question.
>
> Gore: I understand that.
>
> Herman: The absence of a standard in that [VLF] band may be a meaningful piece of information.
>
> Gore: Well, I think it certainly is no matter what side of the debate you are on.
>
> Herman: Right. The fact that the ANSI organization did not choose to extend it down to that level is significant.
>
> Gore: Well, there are no studies of radiation effects in that level—at that level, correct—in the United States?
>
> Herman: There are some animal studies, and there are physical models which we believe are reliable. There is not as much data as there are in the higher frequency ranges.[13]

Besides ANSI, the Institute of Electrical and Electronics Engineers (IEEE) also plays an important role in setting performance standards for electrical equipment. It has showed little tolerance for the view that nonionizing radiation emitted by VDTs may be unsafe. In 1984, the IEEE severed its connection with a contributing editor after his story on the biological effects of nonionizing radiation appeared in the *IEEE Spectrum*. Then, in 1986, IEEE killed an article on the VDT safety and health issue that was scheduled to appear in the *IEEE Spectrum,* telling the editor that work on the story was not to be continued.[14]

The argument that there is no need to study the effects of EMFs emitted by VDTs on human health has a circular "Catch 22" quality to it. The nonionizing radiation emitted by VDTs is harmless, the reasoning goes, because there is no scientific proof that it isn't. There is no scientific proof that nonionizing radiation is harmful because no scientific research has been done. No scientific research is needed because, theoretically, nonionizing radiation can not be harmful. BRH director John C. Villforth's testimony before Gore's subcommittee illustrates this Catch 22–like logic. Referring to his bureau's report, Villforth stated that VDTs "do not pose a significant radiation hazard." When Gore asked him if he was sure, Villforth declared that there is no proof of harm of VLF radiation. Pressed by Gore, Villforth admitted that studies had not been done to find out. Gore asked why. Villforth answered: "The voluntary scientific community has not felt a need for standards in this area based on non-observance of biological effects." To which Gore responded: "But you say, yourself, on page 7 of your statement 'Research on bioeffects for the 15-to-125 kilohertz [VLF] range is lacking.'" "Yes that is correct," Villforth replied. Then Gore told Villforth, "It may be that your reassurance is valid, but it does not appear to be based on any scientific evidence at all." Despite its congressional mandate to study products emitting EMFs, the BRH, and its parent, the FDA, have consistently refused to test VLF and ELF emissions from VDTs. Villforth dismissed those who called for VDT tests: "One of the beautiful things about radiation is that anyone who's paranoid can blame their problems on it." However, *VDT News* attributed the BRH's and FDA's policy of inaction more to "trying to avoid having to do anything that might rile the computer industry."[15]

In July 1983, the National Academy of Sciences' (NAS) panel on the Impact of Video Viewing on the Vision of Workers reported that there was no scientific proof that VDT use caused vision damage, including eye cataracts. However, the panel added: "Studies of long-term (years) exposure to radiation of the wavelengths and levels emitted by VDTs have not been done, and few studies of chronic exposure exist for radiation of any wave-length."[16] The significance of this proviso was lost in the print media's cov-erage, which generally gave VDTs a clean bill of health. The *New York Times's* lead was: Video Terminals Harmless to Eye, Study Asserts. The *Washington Post's* headline read: Eye Disease Not Caused By VDT Use, Panel Says.[17] As a result, CBEMA and the Center for Workplace Technol-ogy (CWT) added the NAS report to its arsenal of arguments against con-ducting research on VDTs, radiation, and vision.

Clusters of Concern: Reproductive Hazards

By early 1980, NIOSH officials were confident that they had laid to rest any fears that workers might have regarding VDTs and radiation. Wordie Parr, coauthor of NIOSH's *New York Times* study, said, "We don't particularly give a damn about them. It's not our responsibility to go out and test VDTs. We just don't think there's a radiation problem." Wolbarsht, the computer industry consultant, concurred: "There is no dangerous radiation coming out of these machines. In fact," he added, "if one wanted to shield oneself from all the radiation bombarding us from radio stations, space, luminous watch dials and other peoples' bodies, a good place to hide would be *behind* one of these machines." His comment was curious because that is where the electromagnetic fields are strongest. Moreover, it was made just as higher than normal incidences of reproductive health problems among women using VDTs began to be reported.[18]

Concern that EMFs might be linked to reproductive problems was first aroused when four clusters, or groupings, were reported among female VDT workers in the span of eighteen months. The first report came from the *Toronto Star,* where, during a one-year period starting in May 1979, four out of the seven babies born to VDT workers in the classified department had birth defects. This was quickly followed by other reports of clusters.[19] However, the federal government, which has a history of inaction on women's health problems, was slow to respond. Because most of these clusters were self-reported by women workers who made the association between reproductive health problems and VDT work, and had unions or support groups to back up their claims, it is likely that other clusters went unreported. The clus-ter at the United Air Lines reservation department in San Francisco came to light as a result of 9 to 5's VDT Hotline, established as part of its Campaign on VDT Risks. It received six thousand calls from VDT users over an eight-month period. As reports of new clusters mounted during the early 1980s, *Microwave News,* a respected publication covering the issue, observed that "it is impossible to know how many clusters exist."[20]

The Centers for Disease Control (CDC) and NIOSH attributed many of the clusters to statistical chance. But doubts continued to grow when NIOSH's health hazard evaluation of the General Telephone Company of Michigan's office in Alma found a statistical association between VDT work and miscarriage. The uncertainty was summed up by NIOSH's statement that "a small number of miscarriages was statistically associated with VDT work in the Alma, Michigan office," but "many of the necessary scientific links required to attribute this excess to VDT use are missing."[21] NIOSH did not test the terminals' VLF and ELF fields.

Understandably, many workers were distrustful of government and industry claims that VDTs were perfectly safe. They drew comparisons with asbestos workers, who were reassured by industry, government, and science officials for many years that the problem did not warrant effective regulation. A VDT worker at the *Toronto Star,* whose child was born "with a nearly fatal heart defect," said: "Any of those machines doesn't give off enough radiation at a time to harm, but I wonder about the cumulative effects of the radiation.... It just seems like we're going to be the asbestosis people of the future." *Computerworld* charged that CBEMA was playing politics with a very sensitive issue: "Who in the country would dare tell a pregnant woman that she shouldn't worry about the effects of low-level radiation on her fetus because conclusive evidence won't be available for another five years or so? ... The attitude that 'What hasn't been proven, simply does not exist' is the same attitude that coated the nation's schools in asbestos."[22]

Unions had some success in winning alternative work assignments for pregnant VDT workers through the collective bargaining process. Canadian unions won the first alternative work provisions in the wake of the reports of reproductive problems at the *Toronto Star.* District 65, UAW, won the first U.S. alternative work provision in its 1983 contract with Boston University. It called for the reassignment of pregnant operators to non-VDT work but, if no other work could be arranged, permitted her to take a personal leave. This breakthrough was followed by agreements at other workplaces, but most employers, especially where workers were unorganized, resisted calls for alternative work.[23] It was also viewed unfavorably by those, such as Dr. Jeanne

Stellman, executive director of the Women's Occupational Health Resource Center, who felt that it could be used as a means to isolate women in the workplace, much as the protective legislation of the Progressive era barred women from doing certain jobs for decades thereafter.[24] They argued that the solution to the radiation problem should focus on shielding VDTs, not barring women from work, but this approach was also unpopular with employers and VDT manufacturers. Still, CBEMA was concerned that employer grants of alternative work for pregnant women might be construed by observers as a tacit admission that VDTs presented reproductive hazards. CBEMA's LeGates ridiculed workers' requests for alternative work, saying it was "like protecting them from light bulbs. . . . It's like employees saying, 'the office is filled with cosmic rays and we need to fight them with balloons.' " She warned that employers were setting a bad precedent by "giving in to a baseless fear." The American Newspaper Publishers Association was also concerned that no cracks appear in the corporate coalition against VDT regulation. Claudia James, ANPA's legal counsel, said: "To permit this is almost to admit there's a problem." But workers' fears were not allayed by such statements, or industry efforts to block EMF studies of terminals.[25]

Delgado's Effect on the Nonionizing Radiation Debate

Although many continued to assert that VLF and ELF fields were harmless and did not warrant study, a team of Spanish researchers led by Dr. José M. R. Delgado found that chick embryos exposed to pulsed ELF magnetic fields (the same type emitted by VDTs) showed arrested or inhibited development in 80 percent of the cases. It contradicted the prevailing scientific view that the weaker the radiation's frequency, the less harmful it was, and indicated that further research of the teratogenic effects of ELF waves was needed. The teratogenic effect was produced by ELF fields, the weakest on the electromagnetic spectrum; stronger nonionizing fields did not produce this effect. This important study, which was published in the British *Journal of Anatomy,* went unnoticed in the United States for nearly a year. Follow-up experiments also implicated pulsed ELF magnetic fields in inhibiting the development of the chick embryos.[26]

U.S. interest in the "Delgado Effect," as it came to be known, increased in 1984, when Kjell Hansson Mild of the Swedish National Board of Occupational Safety and Health replicated it. IBM, one of the nation's largest manufacturers of computer terminals, hired Dr. Arthur W. Guy, an engineer at the University of Washington's School of Medicine, to study the Delgado Effect. He told IBM that "the levels of induced currents where Delgado, et al., (1983) observed teratogenic effects in chick embryos can be produced in human tissue exposed to magnetic fields."[27] But Guy counseled against shielding to block magnetic fields, "unless it can be shown that there is a real hazard due to the magnetic fields exposures."[28] Significantly, Guy's sixty-six-page report to IBM substantiated critics' charges that the electric fields emitted by unshielded terminals could reach harmful levels. It said in part that "it certainly is desirable to shield the cover of the VDT. Since such shielding is relatively inexpensive the benefit to cost ratio is large."[29] But IBM withheld this news from the public. Instead it released a six-page summary, which failed to mention Guy's recommendation that electric fields be shielded in older VDTs, and it downplayed the possibility that the Delgado Effect had any relevance to VDTs. IBM's summary also omitted Guy's statement that a *relationship could exist* with ELF fields produced by VDTs.[30]

When Guy's report became known, IBM assured the public that its terminals were shielded and tested. But this was done primarily to comply with a 1983 Federal Communications Commission (FCC) requirement that terminals be shielded to keep their electric fields from interfering with communication, not to protect safety and health. IBM's claim that its terminals were thoroughly tested for radiation emissions was contradicted by one of its own officials, who told visitors to one of the computer giant's manufacturing plants that only two terminals a month were tested.[31] Guy's findings raised some basic questions. Given the reported cases of eye cataracts and reproductive hazard clusters, might not the abnormally high readings recorded by Guy—and the *New York Times* and the BRH before him—be a factor worth investigating? Also, why couldn't NIOSH and the BRH conduct the same tests of electromagnetic fields emitted by VDTs that Guy had?

Guy's IBM study revealed the extent to which the computer industry and its paid consultants were ahead of the federal government on the issue of ELF fields and VDTs. Not only did IBM take greater interest—and action—in the issue than NIOSH, OSHA, and the BRH, but the greater extent of their knowledge gave them an edge in the public policy debates. It was five months before the public learned of the full extent of IBM's experiment through *VDT News,* a publication with a small circulation. Despite its importance to VDT users, the story was not picked up by the mainstream press. Guy's study prompted renewed calls for publicly sponsored research on the nonionizing fields emitted by VDTs. Karen Nussbaum, leader of 9 to 5, called upon NIOSH and the FDA "to begin at long last to investigate the pulsed magnetic fields and appropriate shielding mechanisms." A *Computerworld* editorial remarked: "Recent findings regarding radiation emissions from VDTs have opened the door once again for much-needed discussion on the potential health risks posed by these terminals."[32] However, budget cuts under the Reagan administration made it highly unlikely that NIOSH would have sufficient funds necessary to conduct research even if it had been willing to do so.

In 1982—two years before Guy told IBM that such shielding was unnecessary—Dr. Karel Marha and his staff at the Canadian Center for Occupational Health and Safety in Hamilton, Ontario, recommended that VDTs be shielded to block the pulsed VLF electromagnetic emissions. He was the first to suggest a link between the miscarriage clusters and VLF fields emitted by VDTs. As a simple remedy, Marha recommended that terminals be spaced at least forty inches apart and that operators keep at least twenty-eight inches from the screen. But Marha's recommendations were publicly dismissed by the computer industry and ignored by most of the major media.[33] At the same time, CBEMA threatened to file a complaint with the Federal Trade Commission (FTC) to halt shield advertisements that claimed to block the radiation emitted by VDTs. Objecting to the ads' inference that VDTs were hazardous to human health, CBEMA general counsel John Voorhees warned manufacturers that it would file complaints with the FTC "if we establish a pattern of false advertising."[34] CBEMA's tactic was effective in maintaining the view that there were no radiation hazards associated with VDTs. It forced shield manufacturers to think twice about the content of their ads and, in effect, limited the scope of the VDT safety and health debate.

Ignoring the News from Europe

Prompted by the findings of two recent studies, Sweden's National Board of Occupational Safety and Health (NBOSH) held a press conference on January 30, 1986, to announce that "low frequency pulsed magnetic fields of a kind similar to those appearing at VDUs and TV sets seem to have an influence on the pregnancy outcome of mice and rats."[35] One study was conducted in Sweden by Drs. Bernard Tribukait and Eva Cekan of the

Karolinska Institute, and Lars-Erik Paulsson of the National Institute of Radiation Protection; the other was done by the Institute for Industrial Medicine in Lodz, Poland. Calling for further research, NBOSH's medical director, Dr. Ricardo Edstrom, said: "There's a big step between animals and humans . . . but the findings mean we can no longer rule out the possibility that radiation [from VDTs] could affect fetuses."[36]

Although this was a very important story and was available on Reuters's wire service, the *NBC Nightly News* was the only major media outlet in the United States to mention it (ever so briefly). In contrast, the *Toronto Globe and Mail* and the *Toronto Sun* promptly reported it. CBEMA quickly dismissed the significance of NBOSH's announcement, issuing a press release the next day saying that the Swedish study "contradicts all other evidence."[37] CBEMA was already defensive about any indication, no matter how slight, of a link between VDT use and reproductive hazards. When the Office of Technology Assessment released a report a few weeks earlier saying that *"there is at this time no good basis for fear of VDT effects on reproductive processes,"* CBEMA promptly criticized OTA's use of the phrase *"at this time"* as being "needlessly alarming."[38] Lost in the dispute was the OTA's call for further research on the health hazards of VDT use. On February 6, the Center for Office Technology, established by CBEMA and VDT-user companies to combat labor's drive for protective regulations, sent a twenty-one-page press kit to editors and science writers, emphasizing that "it is premature to draw conclusions from this study."[39] COT's press kit was accompanied by a "Note to Editors" from Renee S. Ross, COT's executive director, that also downplayed the significance of the Reuters story. The press did not follow up on Reuters's story for nineteen days.

By then, NBOSH's governing board had done a surprising turnaround. In a hastily revised statement, it said that Tribukait, Cekan, and Paulsson's study was not as significant as it first thought. The controversy was heightened by NBOSH's implication that its decision was unanimously supported by the business, labor, and government representatives on its governing board.[40] But this statement ignored the objection by Monica Breidensjo, who represented the Swedish Confederation of Professional Employees, on NBOSH's governing board. She charged NBOSH officials with engaging in political "tricks and cheating" in order to downplay the study's importance. Breidensjo added that "NBOSH must go out and clearly admit that there actually are problems at workplaces, no matter at what stage the scientific investigations may be. . . . Now research is needed on a broader scale. It is not only a question of pregnancy risks. We have skin and eye problems, fatigue, stress and problems with work organization. The reports on workers' injuries are piling up at TCO." A Swedish scientist who was familiar with the study supported her charges, calling NBOSH's turnaround "political business."[41] NBOSH's sudden denial of the implications of EMF research for VDT users was the result of computer manufacturers' and European civil servants' "pressure on the Swedish authorities not to act . . . because of the economic implications."[42]

Despite the heated controversy generated by NBOSH's surprising turnaround, the story found virtually no coverage in the U.S. media. It was briefly mentioned in the *Wall Street Journal*'s "Labor Letter" column on February 18, but the *New York Times* and other major media outlets ignored the story. The lack of U.S. coverage moved the *Columbia Journalism Review* to comment that the NBOSH incident provided "further evidence of a blind spot in print journalism." It added that ignorance was no excuse, for the VDT safety and health "story had been there all along, right in front of every publisher's and editor's nose."[43]

The U.S. media also ignored an important study presented at the International Conference on VDTs, held at Stockholm in May. Jukka Juutilainen and Keijo Saali, researchers in the Department of Environmental Hygiene at the University of Kuopio, Finland, reported that sixty-Hertz extremely low frequency magnetic fields—the lowest frequency fields in the electromagnetic spectrum—emitted by the VDT's vertical deflection coil were actually stronger than the very low frequency fields, the next highest frequency in the spectrum. This finding confounded the scientific view that frequencies become weaker in sequential order as you go down the electromagnetic spectrum, and supported the view that ELF fields did not behave according to the accepted theories of normal science. They also found sixty-Hertz magnetic field strengths of eight milligauss one foot from the VDT (one milligauss is considered acceptable). This was significant because epidemiological studies had found that children who lived in close proximity to sixty-Hertz magnetic field strengths of only two to three milligauss had higher than normal incidences of cancer than those who did not.[44]

In 1987, the Swedish University of Agricultural Sciences announced that research conducted by professors Gunnar Walinder and Hakon Frölen found a statistically significant increase in fetal abnormalities among mice exposed to pulsed ELF electromagnetic fields. Tribukait observed that their study was in accord with his findings. In 1988, the U.S. Office of Naval Research announced that its "Henhouse Project" (so named because it involved exposing chicken eggs to pulsed ELF magnetic fields) had replicated the Delgado Effect.[45] A subsequent study by two researchers involved in the project found that embryonic development is most susceptible to pulsed ELF magnetic fields during the first twenty-four hours.[46] Taken together, these research results amounted to a growing body of scientific evidence that pulsed magnetic fields of the type emitted by VDTs can have teratological effects on rat and chick embryos. Although the results were not directly applicable to humans, they indicated the need for federally sponsored research on the health effects of ELF and VLF fields. In addition, epidemiological evidence of the need to study VDT reproductive hazards was supplied in 1988. Conducted by the Kaiser Permanente Medical Care Program of California, the study of 1,583 pregnant women found that those who worked more than twenty hours a week on VDTs during the first three months of pregnancy had statistically significant increases (80 percent) of miscarriages.[47]

In 1987, IBM quietly applied for a patent on a method of reducing VLF magnetic fields in VDTs and had a low emission monitor on the market by the fall of 1989. Although IBM's action was welcome, it came four years after organized labor recommended it and it applied only to the company's InfoWindow terminals, which were primarily used with mainframe computers and work stations, not in offices. Plus, it did not shield against ELF magnetic emissions.[48] As David Eisen, the Newspaper Guild's director of safety and health said: "It would have been far better if IBM were shielding the ELF frequencies as well. There is no reason they should not be shielding against both."[49] With the exception of the Digital Equipment Company (DEC), which also marketed a terminal that reduced VLF emissions, the rest of the computer industry showed no interest in shielding against EMFs. The feasibility of creating a metal shield that reduced both VLF and ELF emissions was not in doubt, because a shield was being marketed in 1988 for between $400 and $450.[50] But only the computer industry (which could incorporate metal shields in the manufacturing process) had the required capital, market access, distribution networks, and economy of scale to make shielding an affordable reality for all.

IBM's limited action also drew criticism from Paul Brodeur, who charged:

> IBM's move is a half measure because it does not deal with the 60
> Hertz (HZ) fields that are emitted by VDTs. The studies of 60 Hz
> radiation done in the last 10 years clearly show that the fields sup-
> press the immune system, affect cells and promote cancer, particu-
> larly leukemia, lymphoma and brain cancer. Since it is known that
> 60 Hz fields are the dominant radiation emitted by computer termi-
> nals, IBM's failure to acknowledge this hazard seems irresponsible.[51]

Since IBM had always insisted that the nonionizing fields emitted by its terminals posed no harm, formal admission to the contrary might leave the
company open to product liability lawsuits. IBM insisted that the introduction
of its terminal was a response to market demand, not an admission that VLF
emissions were harmful.[52] But this was evading the point: the market
demand for low emission VDTs was from those who were concerned that
unshielded terminals might be harmful. IBM's reaction to the release of a 1989
report by Johns Hopkins University linking higher than normal incidences
of cancer with telephone cable splicers, whose work regularly exposed
them to the same sixty-Hertz EMF fields as emitted by VDTs, is a case in
point. As the *Wall Street Journal* reported: "Reacting to the public outcry, last
week International Business Machines Corp. pledged to reduce the amount
of radiation emitted by all of its future-model computer terminals."[53]

By 1988, research developments had convinced the Swedish government that all computer terminals be shielded to block VLF magnetic fields.
U.S. computer manufacturers adapted by marketing a shielded terminal for
Sweden and the rest of the European market and an unshielded model
for the United States and other markets. The Swedish developments had
virtually no policy-making impact on the U.S. government. It still had not
commissioned research on VLF and ELF fields emitted by VDTs, nor were
there any plans to do so. Nor had it conducted a complete test of computer
monitors' field strengths. The resulting policy-making vacuum led *VDT News*
editor Louis Slesin to write in 1990: "With the growing public concern over
radiation from VDTs, it is amazing that no one in the U.S. has ever done a
comprehensive survey of the electromagnetic emissions from different
models. For instance, would one expect higher electromagnetic fields from
a Compaq or from a Macintosh? We don't really know."[54]

Slesin's question was soon answered by a trade magazine devoted to
the computer industry, not the federal government. The July issue of *Mac-
World* magazine carried a cover story by the investigative writer, Paul

Brodeur, detailing the case that sixty-Hertz extremely low frequency EMFs emitted by VDTs might be linked to health hazards. The magnetic field emissions of ten top-selling monochrome and color monitors were measured four inches from the screen with a gaussmeter, which recorded levels ranging from two to ten times as high (from 4.79 to 22.79 milligauss) as the strength linked to higher than normal incidences of cancer in children (two to three milligauss). Magnetic field strengths were even higher at the sides and back of the tested monitors.[55]

With a circulation well over 325,000, *MacWorld's* "special report" represented an unprecedented breakthrough in media coverage of the VDT EMF debate. It was the first time that a major computer magazine, which usually make their living promoting the computer industry's products, had been willing to challenge industry's claims that VDTs were safe. As a result, stories appeared in *Time,* the *Columbia Journalism Review,* the *Nation,* and the *New York Times,* which reported that "the article has touched off a heated debate in the computer industry and has angered some important advertisers." *MacWorld's* story was discussed four times in a twelve-day span on Cable News Network's "Moneyline" program, and spurred the computer industry—which feared that more bad publicity might hurt its lucrative $6.6 billion monitor market—to retake the initiative.[56] Apple Computer, one of the companies whose color monitors registered potentially dangerous ELF emissions in *MacWorld's* test, announced that it would support medical research on the biological effects of EMFs. Sigma Designs, IBM, and DEC quickly announced plans to introduce shielded monitors that reduced ELF emissions to levels suggested by the proposed Swedish standards.[57]

Fortunately for the computer industry, the federal agencies responsible for public health and safety regarding VDTs expressed no interest in taking action to set protective standards governing their products. An OSHA spokesman said he couldn't comment, "because unfortunately we don't have a subscription to *MacWorld* magazine." The BRH added: "There isn't any scientific consensus on the issue, so there is no present need for the Center to do any testing." On July 24, *MacWorld* and Supermac Technology invited twelve computer companies to meet in San Jose, California, to discuss the nonionizing radiation issue. *MacWorld* editor Jerry Borrell declared that the "goal is a federal standard for EMF emissions." However, this did not fit with the computer industry's plans to retain control over the issue. As a result, the meeting turned out to be more for public relations than substantive purposes. IBM, the industry leader, refused to attend. Fearing erosion of industry autonomy over such decisions, it preferred to formulate a response within established industry forums. Industry representatives at the San Jose meeting concurred with IBM: "The sense of the meeting was that the most effective forum for addressing the [EMF] issue is an established industry group or technical society, such as AEA [American Electronics Association], CBEMA . . . and EIA [Electronic Industries Association]," which are more amenable to the industry's influence.[58] Rebuffed by the computer industry, Borrell used the December 1990 issue to mount a campaign to persuade the federal government to investigate the EMF controversy. As a result, Senator Albert Gore Jr., chairman of the Senate Science Committee, received approximately one thousand postcards, and Congressman Robert Roe (D, N.J.), chair of the House Science Committee, received five thousand postcards. Roe's replacement, Representative George Brown (D, Calif.) also supported the idea of an investigation.[59] But the EMF issue was soon sidetracked by the Persian Gulf crisis, which occupied much of Congress's time and attention in early 1991.

Another, and more important, impetus to industry action on reducing nonionizing radiation emissions came from Europe. In May 1990, the European Community mandated that its members reduce nonionizing radiation emitted by VDTs "to negligible levels from the point of view of the protection of workers' safety and health" by 1993.[60] The question of what "negligible levels" meant became clear in October, when Sweden—which was not then a European Union member—announced the world's first VDT guidelines for ELF fields.[61] CBEMA officials quickly realized that if they didn't develop an alternative (i.e, weaker) standard, the Swedish standard would most likely become the norm for Europe's growing computer market. With economic union planned for 1992, that could threaten the U.S. computer industry's dominance of its most profitable market.[62] "We need to develop a U.S. position to counter Sweden in the European Economic Community," said DEC's Dr. Charles Abernathy. Furthermore, the Swedish standard was on the verge of "becoming the de facto standard in the U.S.," said Apple's John Chubb, because they are "the only thing that customers can quote."[63]

CBEMA worked to head off the stricter Swedish standard at home and abroad. The magnetic field standard would be the same as Sweden's, but the electric field standard would be weaker.[64] Further pressure came from the City of New York's Board of Education, which was preparing purchasing guidelines mandating nonionizing radiation restrictions even stricter than Sweden's. Apple's John Chubb put it bluntly: "If we don't come up with something soon, we're going to pay the consequences." Despite the chain reaction of activity set off by Sweden's announcement of ELF standards, the federal government remained content to defer to the computer industry's leadership. The BRH said that it would only consider action if the computer industry was unable to agree on its own standard.[65] Given the tremendous economic risks at stake for CBEMA, this possibility seemed unlikely.

Playing Politics with EMFs at the EPA

With NIOSH and the BRH mired in a continued state of policy-making inertia, an important development in the VDT nonionizing radiation debate came from the Environmental Protection Agency (EPA). In 1989, an EPA literature review found a pattern linking sixty-Hertz electromagnetic fields, emitted by VDTs and electric power lines, and cancer, leukemia, and lymphoma in children and electrical workers. Consequently, EPA staff scientists proposed that ELF fields be classified as "probable human carcinogens," the second highest category of toxicity in the EPA's five-tier system of classification. Their recommendation, which put ELF fields on a par with such known carcinogens as dioxin, formaldehyde, and polychlorinated biphenals, created an intense political controversy within the Bush administration during the winter of 1990.[66]

On March 6, 1990, William Farland and other EPA officials were called to the White House to discuss the classification controversy. From this point on, decisions would be made by the White House. About a week after the White House meeting, Farland downgraded the ELF field recommendation to "possible human carcinogen." However, even Farland's watered-down recommendation was not enough for the White House, which ordered that the draft report make no recommendation.[67] The Bush administration justified its intervention, saying that classifying extremely low frequency EMFs as "probable human carcinogens" might alarm the public. But the computer industry also had reason for concern. *VDT News* editor Louis Slesin, who felt the original classification was justified by the evidence, recognized the political stakes involved in this debate. "Of course, such a move would have wide-ranging implications, particularly for VDT workers, who are exposed to weak EMFs from their terminals throughout the working day," he wrote. The conflict further intensified when word spread during the summer that the EPA's Science Advisory Board (SAB) might recommend that the original classification be restored. The SAB co-chairpersons had told EPA administrator William Reilly in May that sufficient evidence existed to warrant research into ELF fields.[68] During the summer and fall, the White House turned up the pressure on the EPA to water down the draft report. In August, President Bush's science advisor, Dr. D. Allan Bromley, wrote to Reilly: "This is a very difficult area that, I am sure you agree, requires careful treatment if we are able to serve the public well." He also tried to influence the makeup of the external review panel, a key step in the process when a group of outside scientists review and comment on the draft report. Bromley sent the EPA a list of scientists who believed, in the words of SAB's Donald Barnes, that the connection between ELF fields and health hazards "doesn't make any sense."[69] But his effort to politicize the process was rebuffed by the EPA.

Because electric utility lines, VDTs, and electronic appliances used in millions of homes (such as hair dryers and electric blankets) also emit ELF fields, classifying them as "probable human carcinogens" would have had tremendous ramifications for industry. As a result, the issue of what the draft report should recommend continued to concern the White House. On November 26, the day before the draft report was scheduled to be made public—and more than a month after it had been printed, Bromley pressured Reilly to withhold its release. Fearing that SAB's panel of outside scientists would support the original recommendation that ELF fields be classified as "probable human carcinogens," the White House decided that its own Committee on Interagency Radiation Research and Policy Coordination (CIRRPC)—a liaison group reporting to Bromley's Office of Science and Technology Policy—would conduct the assessment. The next day, Bush's chief of staff John Sununu ordered that the draft report be withheld from the public.[70]

The White House's actions engendered angry responses on Capitol Hill. On December 11, Congressmen George E. Brown, chairman of the House Committee on Science, Space, and Technology, and fellow committee members Frank Pallone (D, N.J.) and James Scheuer (D, N.Y.), sent Bromley a letter accusing him of censoring the EPA report. They stated that his "unprecedented decision" was "more likely to fan public concern than to allay it." Saying, "I want to know what the EPA found in its study," Representative

George Miller (D, Calif.) announced that his Subcommittee on Water, Power, and Offshore Energy Resources would hold hearings in January 1991 to determine "if Bush Administration officials in fact sought to manipulate the report's scientific findings for political purposes."[71] But the Persian Gulf War forced Miller to cancel the hearing. The three congressmen also criticized the Bush administration for permitting the law firm Crowell and Moring, which specialized in lobbying for electric power companies, to be the only speakers at the SAB's external review panel's open meeting.[72] They called upon Reilly, who was now operating under orders from the White House, to "put an immediate halt to the practice of granting to interested parties the right to control who appears before the SAB." If not, they charged, "the 'stacked deck' appearance of the presentations will destroy the very credibility of the SAB review process."[73]

Evaluation of the Potential Carcinogenicity of Electromagnetic Fields was not released until December 14, when the EPA finally agreed to Sununu's condition that it distance itself from the draft report's initial findings.[74] As a result, it included an extraordinary "Note To Reviewers," saying in bold-faced type that *"there are insufficient data to determine whether or not a cause and effect relationship exists"* between ELF fields and cancer. It concluded with the following proviso, also in boldfaced type: *"Given the controversial and uncertain nature of the scientific findings of this report and other reviews of this subject, this review draft should not be construed as representing Agency policy or position."*[75] However, it was difficult to downplay the report's significance when, just three days before its release, the *New York Times* ran a story on the dramatic increase in brain cancer among those under forty-five. The story discussed the possibility of a link with electromagnetic fields.[76]

Despite the disclaimer, and the White House's efforts to delay and weaken its conclusions, the draft report's initial findings could not be ignored. It said in part that "several studies showing leukemia, lymphoma, and cancer of the nervous system in children exposed to magnetic fields from residential 60-Hz electrical power distribution systems, supported by similar findings in adults in several occupational studies . . . show a consistent pattern of response which suggests a causal link."[77] Commenting on the report, the EPA's Farland said: "Over the past few years, more and more people have begun to say there does seem to be something there, that we need to do more work, whereas before we were saying that it was not worth pursuing. This is an important step in getting more research done."[78]

But Farland's optimism was shrouded by the White House's efforts to put a different spin on the EPA report. By insisting that CIRRPC conduct another time-consuming literature review, the White House bought ample time to defuse the controversy and weaken the EPA report's findings.[79] Sununu and Bromley appointed their colleague, Dr. Alvin Young, director of the Office of Agricultural Biotechnology at the Department of Agriculture, to chair the panel. The CIRRPC literature review lasted until June 1992. Not surprisingly, it echoed the Bush administration's view that there is "no convincing evidence in the published literature" to support the claim that ELF fields present "demonstrable health hazards." But there was no disclaimer attached to the CIRRPC's report indicating that it was not the EPA's view.[80] Moreover, the CIRRPC report's politically imposed conclusion was not supported by its scientific content. *Nature* quoted critics as saying that the CIRRPC's conclusion "seems to run counter to [the report's] individual chapters, which urge dozen of new studies." The White House's interference in the EPA's study, was mirrored by the FDA refusal to let BRH staffers test VDT EMF emissions.[81]

Despite the White House's efforts to suppress the EPA's initial findings, four more studies from abroad supported the evidence for further research. In the first study, Australian epidemiologists found that female VDT workers developed brain tumors at five times the rate of nonusers.[82] Then came news from Sweden that occupational exposure to EMFs "can increase the risk of developing cancer—both leukemia and brain tumors." Another Swedish study found that children living within fifty meters of EMF-emitting, high-tension power lines developed leukemia at nearly three times the expected rate of those who lived farther away. As a result, Sweden became the first country to recognize the link between exposure to EMFs and cancer.[83] Finally, a Finnish study, published as the lead story in the *American Journal of Epidemiology*, reported that female VDT workers who were exposed to ELF fields greater than three milligauss had 3.5 times the risk of miscarriage of women who used terminals with acceptable ELF levels (one milligauss). The researchers concluded: "There is a clear need for further studies on the effects of low frequency magnetic fields on the outcome of pregnancy using precise assessment of exposure in the actual working environment. In addition to the effects on users of [VDTs], effects on female workers in industrial and other electrical environments should be investigated."[84]

Despite the EPA's conclusion that "we can identify 60-Hz magnetic fields from power lines, and perhaps other sources in the home as a possible, but not proven, cause of cancer in humans," the federal government has not authorized further research on EMFs.[85] Congress, NIOSH, and the BRH also continued their policy of inaction. The federal government—which usually takes a crisis management approach to occupational safety and health problems—is unlikely to fund scientific research unless it receives absolute medical proof of a link between EMFs and health hazards.[86] This, of course, is the Catch 22 of the nonionizing radiation debate. Holding up absolute proof as the standard to meet, rather than the weight of evidence, the tobacco and asbestos industries long held regulators at bay by sponsoring studies claiming that their products were safe.

The lack of research and testing by federal agencies, such as NIOSH and the BRH, into nonionizing radiation emitted by VDTs may be explained by four key factors. First, the corporate community controls much of the scientific research into EMFs. Second, the scientific establishment tends to dismiss conclusions that don't support the prevailing research paradigm. Third, the major U.S. media refuse to seriously report on research developments (especially foreign) that point to the need for further study. Finally, the federal government prefers funding research that stimulates economic development, and this seriously constrains research into occupational safety and health problems. The federal government's decision not to act has enabled the computer industry to, in effect, make public policy on this important issue.

Chapter 7

The Office of Management and Budget:
Ombudsman to Business

If you're the toughest kid on the block, most kids won't pick a fight with you. The executive order establishes things quite clearly. —James C. Miller III, Reagan's director of OIRA and OMB

[OMB is] "the big kid on the block" to whom all the agencies must kowtow. —David C. Vladeck, Public Interest Research Group attorney

People are not likely to start a fight if they are certain that they are going to be severely penalized for their efforts. —E. E. Schattschneider

In 1980, Congress passed the Paperwork Reduction Act to monitor and reduce the growing burden of regulatory paperwork. The act established the Office of Information and Regulatory Affairs (OIRA) as a "single control point" in OMB to review all pending regulations and studies with the goal of reducing unnecessary paperwork burdens imposed on the public.[1] The Reagan administration, however, envisioned it as the means to ensure that OSHA and NIOSH's policies conformed to its agenda of "regulatory relief" for business.

Congress, the Presidency, and Conflict over the Bureaucracy

Using executive orders, Reagan empowered OIRA to review pending rules and studies in terms of cost/benefit analysis and to consider regulatory alternatives (such as privatization of government functions).[2] The Reagan administration further expanded OMB's powers in January 1985, giving it the authority to review proposed regulations and studies from their inception. With these two executive orders, OMB controlled the social regulatory process from start to finish. As the final arbiter over all pending rules and regulations, OMB became, in James C. Miller III's words, "the toughest kid on the block." Consequently, few agencies were willing or able to fight it. In effect, OMB became an ombudsman for business, cutting through the tangle of administrative procedures to help solve the regulatory problems of corporate America.

There is a fine line between the discretionary power administrators need to respond to unanticipated problems and the subversion of congressional intent.[3] What happens when a president and powerful group interests cross that fine line to subvert an agency's congressional mandate? OMB's interference in NIOSH's epidemiological study of the reproductive problems of female VDT workers on behalf of the BellSouth Corporation illustrates the problem.

The Reagan administration's approach toward the social regulatory process presented a paradox: it strengthened the executive branch's control over safety and health, environmental, and food and drug agencies in the name of deregulating business.[4] Executive order 12291, which consolidated regulatory power in OMB, was the product of the Reagan's Task Force on Regulatory Relief. It was headed by Vice President George Bush and included OMB's James C. Miller III, the director of the newly created OIRA.[5] On April 18, 1981, C. Boyden Gray, counsel to both Bush and the task force, told members of the U.S. Chamber of Commerce that the task force's mission was to intercede on behalf of corporations that felt overburdened by regulations. As Gray put it:

> If you go to the agency first, don't be too pessimistic if they can't solve the problem there. . . . That's what the task force is for. Not too long ago. . . . we told the lawyers representing the individual companies and the trade associations involved to come back to us if they had a problem. Two weeks later they showed up and . . . said they did, and we made a couple of phone calls and straightened it out. We alerted the top people at the agency that there was a little hanky-panky going on at the bottom of the agency, and it was cleared up very rapidly. The system does work if you use it as sort of an appeal. You can act as a double check on the agency that you might encounter problems with.[6]

Likewise, the Reagan administration was very accommodating to BellSouth in the fall of 1985 when it objected to important aspects of NIOSH's VDT study protocol: the only difference was that the task force's ad hoc role of ombudsman to business had been institutionalized in OIRA since 1983.

OMB's Politicization of NIOSH's VDT Study

Since the late 1970s speculation had increased that the higher than normal incidences of miscarriages, birth defects, and infertility among female VDT operators was due to the low level, nonionizing radiation emitted by the terminal's flyback transformer. NIOSH's original plan was to contract out a VDT survey to a California-based group retained to conduct a pesticide and pregnancy study, but, in practice, this proved too unwieldy to execute and was abandoned in early 1983. However, the discovery of three more clusters of miscarriages and birth defects among VDT workers during the next year prompted health and safety groups to ask Congress in 1984 to apply pressure on NIOSH to fulfil its two-year-old promise "to resolve this issue once and for all."[7] In November 1984, after two years of false starts, rumors, delays, and planning, NIOSH began to solicit public comment for its proposed draft of the VDT study protocol from science, industry, and labor. The number of reported adverse reproductive health clusters among VDT workers had now risen to twelve.

Originally, BellSouth agreed to participate in NIOSH's project, assuming that it would be part of a multi-industry study.[8] The reports of miscarriage clusters had heightened fears among women of reproductive age, such as many of BellSouth's operators, that VDTs were unsafe to use. NIOSH's study was an opportunity, as Roy B. Howard, BellSouth's assistant vice president for Industrial Relations, put it, "to allay public and employee concern over the possible effects of VDT's." The computer industry was also confident that VDTs would be exonerated. The Computer and Business Equipment Manufacturers Association's Charlotte LeGates stated: "We have no doubt what the results will be."[9]

However, two unforeseen events changed the situation. First, after an unsuccessful search for suitable populations to take part in a multi-industry study, NIOSH focused on BellSouth's South Central Bell and Southern Bell, and AT&T because they had both VDT users and non-users who did the same job and had similar socioeconomic backgrounds.[10] The study protocol called for four thousand women between the ages of eighteen and thirty-five: two thousand directory assistance operators who used VDTs would serve as the study group; another two thousand operators who were still using the older light emitting diode (LED) technology would constitute the control group.[11] The study would have both retrospective and prospective portions. The retrospective portion, involving the use of questionnaires and the analysis of VDT operators' medical histories and work conditions, would take the first two years. The prospective portion would monitor the operators' health for the next two years.

BellSouth and AT&T were reportedly not pleased that they were the only companies chosen by NIOSH. According to study director Dr. Philip J. Landrigan, "The companies came out and said they didn't really like it. They said they didn't see why it had to be done in their establishment and not some place else." The companies agreed to participate but took NIOSH officials by surprise when they announced that the long-distance operators would be using VDTs by 1986.[12] NIOSH was then forced to cancel the prospective portion of its study, which was most important and had attracted the most interest. It was hoped that the prospective portion of the study would give NIOSH investigators some clues as to why the clusters were occurring among VDT users in unusually high numbers. Without it, NIOSH was unable to track the work and reproductive conditions of non-VDT operators, thereby depriving them of the information necessary to control for deviations in the data of the group using VDTs.

Second, in January 1985, University of North Carolina researchers announced that a study of telephone workers, including employees of Southern Bell, found that VDT workers suffered from angina at rates ten times higher than the national average. They also found that those who used VDTs regularly were twice as likely to suffer from eyestrain, musculoskeletal aches and pains, and stress-induced problems (i.e., headaches, nausea, tension, insomnia, and fatigue) than workers who didn't work on the terminals.[13] In July, NIOSH verified the initial research, finding that nearly 20 percent of female telephone workers who used VDTs for more than half a day suffered from angina. It also added an important new finding: chest pain became more frequent as VDT workers' control over the job decreased.[14]

The angina study cast the proposed VDT study in a new light. As the first study to demonstrate a connection between angina and VDT use, it received nationwide attention. Also, the researchers' finding that management practices at Southern Bell (as well as other companies)—including pressure to increase production, isolation from co-workers, and continuous work without rest breaks—contributed to increased stress and chest pain experienced by VDT workers could be bad publicity for BellSouth. The news of the angina link put NIOSH's inability to find additional companies to take part in the study in a new perspective. The implications were clear; if NIOSH was permitted to ask BellSouth's employees questions regarding stress and fertility, they might find a correlation between VDT use and stress, and/or VDT use and reproductive problems.

In response to BellSouth's inquiries, OMB recommended that it hire Dr. Brian MacMahon, a Harvard University epidemiologist with a long record as an industry consultant, to critique NIOSH's study protocol.[15] Moreover, he also served on the advisory council of the power industry's Electric Power Research Institute, which disputed the possibility that EMFs were linked to reproductive hazards and cancer and had represented industry against NIOSH. In 1978, he had taken part in an industry-orchestrated campaign to persuade Joseph Califano, secretary of Health, Education and Welfare, to overturn NIOSH's recommendation that OSHA tighten the permissible level of exposure to beryllium, a carcinogenic metal.[16]

MacMahon and his collaborator, Dr. Sally Zierler of Brown University, wrote to BellSouth that "it is in our view inconceivable that the study would yield results that are definitive, unequivocal or credible and, even with the modifications that we will propose, such results cannot be assured."[17] Armed with their critique, BellSouth's Howard wrote to Wendy Lee Gramm, OMB's administrator for Information and Regulatory Affairs, on November 20, 1985, stating that "the proposed study, as currently designed, will not provide reliable and scientific information." He also wrote to NIOSH director Dr. J. Donald Millar, objecting that the very presence of the fertility questions in NIOSH's study protocol lent credence to charges that a VDT reproductive/radiation problem existed. Howard cited the recently released House Education and Labor Subcommittee staff report as exonerating VDTs of any nonionizing radiation hazard. But the staff report was a literature review, not a scientific study. It didn't conclusively exonerate VDTs.[18]

The fact that NIOSH first learned of objections to the study protocol from BellSouth, not OMB, amply illustrates the extent to which the research process had become politicized under the Reagan administration. As David LeGrande, the Communications Workers of America's director of Occupational Safety and Health, observed: "BellSouth has done everything they can to prevent the study from being done."[19] Moreover, OMB's objections —inadequate sample size, incorrectly defined sample frame, poorly defined major variables, and the inclusion of too many irrelevant questions regarding stress and fertility—closely echoed those of BellSouth's hired consultants. OMB said that the inclusion of irrelevant stress and fertility questions violated the Paperwork Reduction Act's prohibition against burdening the public with unnecessary paperwork. OMB's rejection of the study protocol was surprising for several reasons. First, it had passed both government and outside peer review panels of scientists. Second, rejection of the protocol was based on a summary of the study. It could have asked NIOSH to see the full study protocol, which, project director Dr. Teresa M. Schnorr noted, would have "answered their questions."[20]

The collusion between BellSouth and OMB raised charges that the integrity and independence of NIOSH's VDT study had been undermined. Landrigan, director of environmental and occupational medicine at the Mount Sinai Medical Center in New York City and former director of NIOSH's VDT study, called OMB's action an "unwarranted intrusion into the scientific authority of NIOSH." "In my opinion, it was a pretty overtly political move," he said. "The companies were just trying to get the government off their backs."[21] Karen Nussbaum, executive director of 9 to 5, accurately foresaw that we'd "be set up with a bad study, one that's flawed in the first place, and doesn't give us any real answers in the end." Congressman Ted Weiss (D, N.Y.), a member of the Government Operations Committee, criticized OMB's "end run" around NIOSH and announced that his Subcommittee on Intergovernmental Affairs would hold hearings to investigate the situation.[22]

Denying charges that it colluded with BellSouth, OMB maintained that it alone made the decision on scientific grounds. Responding to inquiries from Senator Carl Levin's (D, Mich.) office, the OMB's Gramm said, "While we are interested in comments from affected parties, our original conditions were not based upon the comments of the BellSouth consultants and we see no reason to change our position." OMB spokesman Edwin Dale said, "The work by the Harvard guy, Brian MacMahon, was received, but it was not a major influence. We were already moving in the same direction."[23] However, given the fact that OMB has no scientists or epidemiologists on staff, from where was it getting its information? The evidence points to OMB's collusion with BellSouth and its consultants. OMB actively orchestrating the critique of NIOSH's study protocol with BellSouth. An OMB official contradicted Dale's comment that MacMahon's work was insignificant to its decision: "Part of what made BellSouth's comments cogent was the inclusion of a critique by a well-respected epidemiologist."[24] Moreover, it was OMB that recommended MacMahon to BellSouth in the first place.

Statements by the other parties involved also belied OMB's claim to independent and impartial decision making. In his letter to OMB's Gramm, BellSouth's Howard said that his company had a "large investment in these terminals" and was planning to increase it.[25] Shortly after OMB rejected the VDT study protocol, NIOSH's Millar told Congressman Weiss's subcommittee investigation that BellSouth's going to OMB was a common practice for corporations upset with his agency's work. Millar said:

> I am not very fond of it. I accept the fact that the work NIOSH does clearly has implications that are perhaps not true of research done by other agencies. . . . Our findings can have clear-cut economic ramifications for industry, particularly if they result in a recommendation to OSHA for a new workplace standard, as many of our studies do. One just has to expect that major corporations that anticipate some effects growing out of this, will go to whomever they can go to see that these studies are as well done as possible or not done at all, if that can be arranged.[26]

Unionists suspected that BellSouth's complaint to OMB was motivated by fear of legal liability if a link between management-induced stress among VDT operators and adverse pregnancy outcomes was substantiated by NIOSH. "It was the goal of BellSouth to damage the credibility" of the VDT study, the CWA's David LeGrande charged. "They may not want to supply information that may work against them," he added. BellSouth denied that fear of legal liability motivated its insistence that fertility and stress questions be omitted from the study. BellSouth spokeswoman Kathleen Hughes said that OMB's stipulations "have nothing to do with [our] liability."[27] However, Congressman Weiss maintained that there was reason to believe that BellSouth was concerned about legal liability. It was public knowledge that the angina studies called for further study of work-induced stress and fertility as factors that might be causing health problems for VDT workers several months before BellSouth contacted OMB about the removal of the stress and fertility questions from NIOSH's study. "This finding suggests that BellSouth had substantial financial incentives to prevent or delay NIOSH research on stress among VDT workers," Congressman Weiss said.[28]

The Reagan administration's OMB was more accessible to business than to either NIOSH or the public. As Millar, NIOSH's director, told

Congressman Weiss's subcommittee: "We usually are not involved in the discussions that OMB has with the people who are raising questions." To which Weiss replied:

> That is precisely the point . . . The problem is that when OMB gets involved, it is not held accountable, whereas you have to argue out your position with people from the affected industry and other scientists and so on. OMB is reached out to by the affected industry. They have a nice, private discussion about it. They don't bring you into the process at all. They tell you that in fact the protocol has been rejected, to go back to the drawing board, we don't like what you are doing.[29]

OMB told NIOSH officials to meet privately with BellSouth "to hear their concerns." This was a highly irregular move because as Director Millar said, NIOSH does not "have a lot of contact with people except in scientific settings, which are, generally speaking, very open to the public."[30]

On June 5, 1986, OMB extracted its price for granting NIOSH permission to conduct the VDT study—the removal of the stress and fertility questions. OMB said that the stress questions had "no practical utility" because "there is insufficient evidence relating these items to hypotheses concerning VDT exposure and adverse reproductive outcomes." Dr. Irving J. Selikoff, of the Mt. Sinai School of Medicine in New York—the nation's premier epidemiologist, noted that this was true, but only "because the subject has not been studied." He added, "We badly need information about this." Dr. William J. Butler of the University of Michigan, who was conducting a reproductive study of VDT workers that included questions about stress, said that "occupational stress is one of the leading suspected causes of the reported association between VDT exposure and pregnancy outcome. Therefore, collecting information on stress is crucial for the thorough investigation of this occupational health issue."[31] Moreover, OMB ordered the stress questions removal knowing that, as Schnorr, the study's director, said, the stress "questions were important to the study and without them the study will be less credible."[32]

Like BellSouth's consultants, OMB criticized the inclusion of fertility questions on the grounds that "measuring the effect of VDT exposure on fertility is not the purpose of the study." OMB's objection illustrated its lack of epidemiological expertise.[33] Technically, the study's primary purpose was to investigate reproductive outcomes, not the fertility, of women VDT workers. But determining the number of adverse reproductive outcomes related to working with VDTs could not be adequately assessed without determining the degree of fertility. Furthermore, OMB's rejection of the fertility questions disregarded the fact that the study was being done in response to widespread fear that reproductive hazards were linked to VDT use.

Ironically, OMB's demand that fertility questions be deleted undermined NIOSH's efforts to meet another of OMB's objections to the study design: recall bias. Recall bias, which is a recurring problem in epidemiological studies, refers to the fact that interviewee's responses to questions may be subject to memory lapse. NIOSH intended the fertility questions to serve in part as an "indirect method of assessing recall bias" on questions relating to spontaneous abortions.[34] There was an Orwellian-like irony in OMB's decision to forbid NIOSH from asking female respondents questions regarding fertility in a study about the reproductive problems of women who work with VDTs. Selikoff wrote that "NIOSH cannot conduct a meaningful study of reproductive outcome in relation to work if NIOSH is prohibited from asking women (a) whether they were working, and (b) whether they have a uterus." As Selikoff implied, OMB was not capable of making complex epidemiological decisions. Again, OMB's conditions for approval of the VDT study paralleled BellSouth's complaints, reinforcing charges that it was business' ombudsman. The CWA's LeGrande described the process as one in which BellSouth had the ideas for the revisions and "OMB happened to have the letterhead paper."[35]

Following OMB's denial of NIOSH's appeal to maintain the integrity of the VDT study, the conflict shifted to the congressional arena. An analysis of the study protocol commissioned by Congressman Weiss was released by the OTA in August. It was critical of OMB's deletion of the fertility and stress questions, concluding:

> Due to the high visibility of this study and the likely use of the conclusions by a wide variety of individuals, organizations and governments, it is important that its conclusions be as clear as possible. The questions deleted by OMB were intended to provide important and useful information that would reduce the potential for alternative explanations of study results. While the wording of specific questions and the order of the questionnaire might be reexamined and improved, complete deletion of questions on fertility and stress will limit the conclusions that can be drawn from this study.[36]

Weiss concluded that the executive order granting OMB the power to review regulations infringed on the powers given to the regulatory agencies by Congress. On September 3, with time and alternatives running out, he sent HHS secretary Otis R. Bowen a copy of OTA's evaluation that the fertility and stress questions should be reinstated and urged him "to override the Office of Management and Budget's inappropriate demands."[37] Weiss reminded Bowen that he had the statutory power to reinstate the questions in the study, but Bowen's aide replied that it was OMB's decision to make. During the fall of 1986, the effort to reinstate the fertility and stress questions gained momentum both in and outside of Congress. Weiss—joined by Augustus F. Hawkins (D, Calif.) and Mary Rose Oakar (D, Ohio)—wrote to Secretary Bowen urging him to reinstate the questions. They were joined by the leaders of the CWA, the Service Employees International Union, and 9 to 5.[38]

In October, a surprising development added a compelling new dimension to efforts to convince OMB to reinstate the stress and fertility questions. One of BellSouth's consultants, Dr. Sally Zierler, announced that she had serious reservations regarding OMB's politicization of the scientific review process. She added that the fertility and stress questions should be reinstated in NIOSH's study. Her turnaround resulted from discussions with Dr. Diana Zuckerman, one of Congressman Weiss's staff members, who supplied Zierler with the OTA's analysis of the deleted questions and the Health Hazard Evaluation conducted by NIOSH on BellSouth VDT workers in North Carolina. After seeing this information, Zierler wrote to Weiss, expressing her misgivings about OMB's role:

> I have become increasingly aware of the role of the Office of Management and Budget in setting up barriers to governmental scientific activity. Inadvertently, I feel that I participated in a process that served to undermine the spirit of peer review. . . . The adversarial undertone of the exchange between NIOSH and the industry-initiated review created a climate of mistrust and led to accusations of being bought by industry. Regardless of the intention of the review from the reviewers perspective (and that intention was solely in the interest of scientific integrity), the effect of the review was to delay the study's implementation (at the cost of increased publicity, thus increasing the potential for recall bias—ironically, the major problem the industry reviewers were addressing) and to confer to OMB (a nonscientific agency) the power to act as scientists without the benefit of scientific expertise.[39]

Referring to BellSouth's interference in NIOSH's VDT study, Zierler added that "if the study findings could lead to policies that affect private industries, then these industries should have no participation in the review process."[40] Zierler's reevaluation of the need for the stress and fertility questions highlights the dangers of OMB's collusion with industry. As the Government Operations Committee reported: "The use of consultants paid by the industry presents an obvious conflict of interest. . . . Although the consultants were described by BellSouth as independent, their interest in the study apparently resulted from their consulting relationship with the industry; they had not taken advantage of earlier opportunities to express concerns about the study, when scientists from across the country were asked to comment on the study in December 1984."[41]

Zierler's reversal forced BellSouth to announce that it had no further objection to the inclusion of the stress and fertility questions in the study. BellSouth said that Zierler's reevaluation was "based on new scientific evidence and information that was not available" when she last reviewed the study questionnaire in April.[42] However, BellSouth, its consultants, and OMB could have obtained answers to their questions from NIOSH's Dr. Teresa M. Schnorr, the project director, in April. Zierler's and BellSouth's turnaround was vindication of NIOSH's plan to include the stress and fertility questions. However, OMB refused to reinstate them.

In light of Zierler's and BellSouth's reconsideration, the battle shifted to Congress. Congressman Hawkins wrote to Bowen on October 20, asking him to reinstate the stress and fertility questions. Bowen responded on November 12, saying that HHS "has reached accord with OMB on the design, procedures, and content of the study," and that "NIOSH is proceeding with the study as directed."[43] Hawkins replied to Bowen, stating that "it would seem that OMB does not have a leg to stand on in opposing the reinsertion of the [stress and fertility] questions." On December 23, Bowen sent his final reply to Hawkins, stating that "the Department cannot reinsert questions into a study without prior approval by OMB as required by the Paperwork Reduction Act."[44] It was clear that OMB was making the decisions, and Bowen had no intention of challenging its authority. Then, Senator Levin wrote to OMB director Miller, stating that "the deletion of the questions on stress and fertility throws the value of the VDT study into question" and urging him to reinstate them.[45] Ignoring BellSouth's and Zierler's reversal, Gramm repeated the same objections to Levin in December that OMB had given to NIOSH in June.[46]

When the study finally got under way in May 1987, Schnorr reiterated her concern that the OMB-ordered "changes may hurt the ultimate value of the study."[47] The lost opportunity to investigate whether there was a correlation between reproductive outcomes and VDT use was accentuated in August by news of a Swedish study, which found that a higher number of miscarriages occurred in mice exposed to EMFs similar to that emitted by VDTs. This further illustrated the need to ask female computer users questions about fertility and stress. Congressman Weiss stressed: "These findings are extremely important and reaffirm the need for a definitive study assessing the dangers of VDTs for pregnant women." He estimated that "OMB's interference with NIOSH's study has set back efforts by at least two years."[48]

NIOSH's VDT study was published in the *New England Journal of Medicine* on March 14, 1991, nine years after NIOSH first proposed it. It found that "the use of VDTs and exposure to the accompanying electromagnetic fields were not associated with an increased risk of spontaneous abortion."[49] The removal from the study protocol of plans to measure EMFs and ask respondents stress and fertility questions destroyed the study's ability to explain whether EMFs were a factor in miscarriages.[50] The fact that both the control and study groups were exposed to extremely low frequency fields made it impossible for NIOSH to compare the effects of EMF exposure on VDT users.[51] Nevertheless, the study's shortcomings were overlooked while the press reported that VDT use was not linked to miscarriages.[52]

OMB Interference in the VDT Study

OMB intervention in NIOSH's VDT study on BellSouth's behalf was indicative of a larger pattern of political interference in scientific research. In a study of the fifty-one Centers for Disease Control research projects between January 1984 and March 1986, the Harvard School of Public Health and the Mt. Sinai School of Medicine found that OMB was seven times more likely to reject or limit the scope of occupational safety and health and environmental studies than those that focused on other subjects, such as infectious diseases.[53] Unlike infectious disease research, occupational and environmental studies have been especially vulnerable to OMB interference because their results can have economic ramifications for affected industries. The researchers also found that OMB was more likely to reject or limit the scope of reproductive health studies than other types of studies. Reproductive studies of workers, which, like the VDT study, might reveal a correlation between computer use and adverse reproductive outcomes, were also more likely than other studies to have economic implications for business interests. Add to this the federal government's research bias against women's health studies (as documented in the previous chapter) and it is not surprising that OMB was more likely to reject reproductive studies than other studies. As both an investigation of occupational safety and health and women's reproductive health, the VDT study was more vulnerable than other studies to OMB's interference.

The pattern of OMB's interference in the VDT study was strikingly similar to its pattern of intervention in the other studies. Harvard/Mt. Sinai researchers found that OMB's review, "which was superimposed on the peer review process, generally relied on single consultants rather than a panel of experts. The process was poorly documented and often demonstrated a dismaying ignorance of the fundamentals of science and public decision making."[54] They concluded that Reagan's OMB had politicized the process of medical research to a degree unequaled by previous administrations:

> The health policy implications are serious; OMB is clearly interfering with the substance of CDC research. OMB has delayed, impeded, and thwarted governmental research efforts designed to answer public demands for information on serious public health questions. Rather than minimize the cost of information collection, the paperwork review process has resulted in a diversion of tax dollars from productive health research into paperwork clearance activities and unnecessary contracting costs.[55]

In effect, the Reagan administration placed private economic interests before the public's interest in health and science. OMB's interference in the VDT study was part of a larger and more pervasive pattern of the Reagan administration's collusion with industries that were affected by pending regulations and studies. Disregarding a 1980 congressional law requiring the regulation of infant formula, Reagan's OMB vetoed pending Food and Drug Administration regulations. As a result, contaminated infant formula soon began to circulate in an unregulated market.[56] In 1982, the FDA proposed banning six carcinogenic color additives and dyes in accordance with the

Delaney amendment's prohibition against the use of cancer-causing agents. Alerted by a friend who represented the industry's trade association, Vice President Bush had OMB kill the proposal. Reagan's OMB went so far as to strip the FDA commissioner of the power to order carcinogenic agents off the market. Not even twenty-one deaths and more than eight hundred injuries caused by allergic reaction to sulfites was sufficient to move OMB to permit the FDA to require warning labels. A public outcry and the threat of congressional action ensued before the Reagan administration approved the warning labels.[57] When the FDA proposed regulations stipulating a mandatory warning that aspirin use by children who have influenza or chicken pox could cause Reyes syndrome, a potentially fatal disease, lobbyists for the industry's Aspirin Foundation of America asked Bush for assistance. He contacted OMB, which forced the FDA to agree to voluntary warnings—which proved to be ineffectual.[58] OMB rejected NIOSH's peer reviewed and approved dioxin/Agent Orange study protocol on behalf of the Dow and Monsanto Chemical Companies.[59] After OMB rejected the Environmental Protection Agency's asbestos guidelines, Congressman John Dingell (D, Mich.) noted that "OMB's arguments against EPA's guidelines were virtually identical to arguments presented—in secret and outside of the regular procedures—to OMB by industry officials."[60]

A major expansion of OMB's power to intervene in agency rule making on industry's behalf occurred under the tenure of Douglas H. Ginsburg, who is best remembered as the Reagan Supreme Court nominee who withdrew his name from consideration when it was revealed that he had smoked marijuana. Less well known, but more lasting in its impact, was his role in undermining occupational safety and health regulation as OMB's director of OIRA (1984–85).[61] Complaining that OMB's final "review comes too late" in the regulatory process, Ginsburg oversaw the development and implementation of executive order 12498. Signed by President Reagan in January 1985, it gave OMB's OIRA the power to review proposed regulations from the start of the process. Just as agencies were required to submit annual fiscal budget requests to OMB, they were now required to submit annual "regulatory budgets," listing high priority regulations in the making.[62] In effect, executive order 12498 gave OIRA greater power over the regulatory agencies by permitting it to secretly squelch regulations and studies before the public was even aware of their existence. Supporters said it would enable the president to control the burgeoning social regulatory bureaucracy.

In practice, however, it enhanced OMB's power to interfere in the regulatory process on industry's behalf. As the U.S. Chamber of Commerce noted, business stood to "benefit from OMB's efforts to coordinate and provide a preview of the regulatory actions of the executive branch."[63] As a result, the Department of Labor, which houses OSHA, became "Number One" on OIRA's "hit list," with one hundred pending regulations under OMB review. The Department of Health and Human Services, which includes NIOSH, was number two on OIRA's hit list, with eighty-eight pending regulations.[64]

Increased OMB interference, combined with severe budget and staff cuts, crippled NIOSH's ability to study the health hazards confronting America's workers. That NIOSH was singled out by Reagan's OMB for special treatment is illustrated by the fact that between 1980 and 1986 its budget was cut 19 percent—42 percent when adjusted for inflation—at the same time its parent agency, the CDC, received a 28 percent increase. NIOSH's staff fell from 1,019 in 1980 to 806 in 1986, a 21 percent decrease.[65] In 1986, the House Committee on Government Operations reported that occupational safety and health data collection was seventy-two years behind that for communicable diseases and that increasing spending for preventive research would have a greater payoff in terms of reduced occupational illness than spending for medical care after the diagnosis of illness.

The Administrative Procedures Act requires that the regulatory process be conducted in an open manner, but the Reagan administration's OMB closed it to the public. "One of the most troubling aspects of OMB's review of regulations," Congressman Weiss said, "is the secrecy in which it takes place. Behind closed doors, nameless and faceless OMB employees—using the powers granted them not by statute, but by executive order—have forced expert agencies like the Food and Drug Administration to alter regulations. Often these orders are issued over the phone, with no documentation of the communication."[66] This practice became so common at OIRA that some members of Congress remarked that Miller's "office served as a back-room 'conduit' for industries anxious to escape federal regulations, but less anxious to have their advocacy appear in a public docket." In fact, Miller became notorious for refusing "to publicly log his meetings with outside parties." He defiantly told Congressman Dingell's subcommittee in 1981, "We will not maintain a file and a record" of contacts with business interests seeking regulatory relief. Miller's deputy, Jim Tozzi, put it bluntly: "I don't leave fingerprints."[67]

The trend toward institutionalizing secrecy was further accelerated in Reagan's second term with the help of executive order 12498. It forbade the social regulatory agencies from publicly discussing or soliciting comment on proposed regulations without OMB's permission. OMB claimed that limiting the public's access would open up the regulatory review process. However, there was nothing open about OMB's ability to squelch pending regulations without the public's knowledge. As Alan B. Morrison observed: "What makes matters worse is the fact that OMB is under no similar injunction of secrecy. Given the predilections of OMB desk officers, industry will know perfectly well what is being proposed and will surely have its input into OMB's decision whether to permit an agency to begin to consider a problem in earnest."[68] This is precisely what happened in the case of the VDT study, and numerous others that were rejected or substantially revised.

Reviewing OMB's pattern of interference in scientific research, the House Committee on Government Operations concluded that OMB was "not qualified to make health policy decisions, or research of any kind."[69] Senator William Proxmire (D, Wisc.) remarked that "there has been increasing political pressure to place economic consideration above considerations of public health and the three Commissioners to serve during the Reagan administration have been kept on increasingly short leashes. The result has been a triumph of politics over science and has led to criticism from both sides of the aisle."[70]

Although every president since Nixon has expanded OMB's powers over the social regulatory process, none did so as dramatically as Reagan. The effect of the Reagan administration's OMB policy was to undermine the primacy of the rule of law, and to elevate administrative discretion based on the preferences of powerful groups affected by regulation. The Reagan administration's redefinition of the agencies' congressionally mandated missions upset the equilibrium that existed between the two branches, which provoked Congress to attempt to restore the balance. In 1986, Congress required that future directors of OIRA be confirmed by the Senate, but politically fragmented and distracted, it was unable to muster majorities to rein in OMB.[71] Even if it had, veto-proof majorities would have been next to impossible to mobilize. Most of the limited success in holding OMB accountable to the law came as a result of suits filed in the courts.[72]

The Reagan administration made two arguments to justify its grant of expanded powers to OMB. First, it argued that OMB played only an advisory role, final decisions were made at the departmental level. The Reagan administration admitted that, in practice, this was a hollow distinction when it said that "the agency head remains free *to risk presidential discipline* and take the action he believes appropriate."[73] This was the Reagan administration's way of saying it would not tolerate department heads who made decisions that were not in accord with OMB. HHS secretary Bowen understood this when he told Congressman Weiss that the final say over the fate of the stress and fertility questions rested with OMB. OMB made it clear that it had final authority, too, telling Bowen, "Our approval [of the VDT study] is conditioned on HHS agreeing to all provisions."[74] OMB has a simple check on recalcitrant agency heads; the Paperwork Reduction Act requires that all forms submitted to the public (e.g., rules and studies) carry a control number assigned by OMB upon its approval. Any government regulation that does not carry the control number is "bootleg," and the public (i.e., business) is free to ignore it.[75] OMB can simply refuse to assign a control number until an agency head complies with its wishes.

Second, the Reagan administration maintained that the expansion of OMB's powers to oversee the social regulatory process was implied by the president's constitutional duty to "take care that the laws be faithfully executed."[76] But this argument is contradictory at its core. If the president is free to ignore the will of Congress, then how is he *faithfully* executing the laws they pass? The resulting abuse of administrative power created the environment which led to OMB's interference in scientific research.

The Reagan administration went well beyond Congress' intent in passing the Paperwork Reduction Act. Congress intended that "the Government-wide management system created should . . . help solve information management problems."[77] As the act's legislative history indicates, Congress did not intend for OMB to control the content of biomedical and epidemiological research. Fearing that OMB might be tempted to meddle, the Association of American Colleges and the Association of Schools of Public Health, among others, asked Congress to exempt biomedical and epidemiological research from the law's requirements. The Senate Committee on Governmental Affairs sympathized with their request but did not think the exemption was necessary for three reasons. First, most research was conducted by nongovernmental parties through "assistance grants," which

were exempt from the law's provisions. Second, they believed that congressional oversight would be sufficient to maintain the independence of
government sponsored biomedical and epidemiological research. Finally,
because it had not been a major problem during the previous thirty-eight
years of budget agency review, the committee thought that the OMB director would continue to be the defender of the integrity of biomedical and epidemiological research. As the committee said, the OMB "director has
sufficient flexibility in the administration of this Act to ensure that our nation's
health research effort is not impaired."[78]

The Reagan administration's deregulatory policies resulted in the
paralysis of the occupational safety and health policy-making process, the
politicization of scientific research, and the insulation of corporate interests
from public accountability. Isolated, demoralized, and deprived of much of
their decision-making power, the social regulatory agencies soon realized
it was easier to comply with than fight OMB. OMB intervention in regulatory issues that affect business interests followed the same pattern in the Bush
administration. As head of the Council on Competitiveness, Vice President
Dan Quayle played the same role that Bush had played in the Reagan
administration. As with Reagan's Task Force on Regulatory Relief, Bush's OMB
director was a council member and played the key role in seeing that the
regulatory agencies conformed to its priorities. Like its predecessor, the Council on Competitiveness was a high-powered and secretive conduit for corporations seeking regulatory relief. The council described itself as being in
the business of "reducing regulatory burdens on the free enterprise system."[79]
President Bush's three-month moratorium on proposed new regulations was
recommended by the Council on Competitiveness, just as President Reagan's sixty-day suspension of pending regulations in 1981 came from the
Task Force on Regulatory Relief.[80] President Clinton abolished the Council on Competitiveness in 1993, but as long as pressures on the White House
to maximize conditions for economic growth continue, OMB will play an
important role managing the social regulatory process.

It is ironic that, in the name of preventing wasteful paperwork burdens from being imposed on the public, OMB's interference in scientific
research imposed a greater paperwork burden on government administrators. OMB forced NIOSH to go through three revisions of the study, which
generated additional paperwork. Also ironic was OMB's disregard for the
cost of the VDT study despite its order that agencies should be cost effec-

tive. NIOSH spent $53,451 just to comply with OMB-ordered paperwork reduction revisions—more than 13 percent of the study's $400,000 cost.[81] Also, OMB's exclusion of the stress and fertility questions made it virtually certain that another study would be needed, which would require additional funds. In 1984, NIOSH estimated that the study would cost $100,000 and take three years to complete.[82] In the final analysis, OMB's interference was the main reason the study's cost increased fourfold, why it took twice as long to complete, and why its findings were of limited value.

Chapter 8

State and Local Arenas:
Laboratories of Democracy or Labyrinths of Frustration?

*I*n discouraging organized labor from approaching the Occupational Safety and Health Administration by its intensely anti-union, deregulatory stance, the Reagan administration had, in effect, made a non-decision that kept the video display terminal issue out of the federal arena. Blocked at the federal level, advocates of safety and health regulations governing the workplace use of VDTs focused their efforts on the state and local levels of government, which have been called "laboratories of democracy" for their willingness to experiment with new solutions to social and political problems. In all, VDT regulatory proposals were considered in thirty states, and in numerous counties and cities. But failure to overcome intense business and governmental opposition to VDT regulations resulted in the states becoming labyrinths of frustration for organized labor. Obstacles included a well-organized corporate coalition of manufacturers and users who backed up their opposition to VDT regulations with threats of economic blackmail and state and local government officials who feared that controls on the market would undermine their ability to attract high-tech business investment.[1]

The Response to Reagan's New Federalism

The Reagan administration's health and safety policies were both a blessing and a curse for the business community. Cutbacks in federal health and safety regulation were a boon to businesses seeking regulatory relief but also created a Pandora's Box of problems, as unions sought compensating remedies at the state and local levels. As Stephen A. Bokat, the U.S. Chamber of Commerce's general counsel, put it: "It's an incredible hassle for companies that do business in all 50 states to cope with 50 different laws."[2] The devolution of occupational safety and health policy making to the state and local level was encouraged by the Reagan administration's "New Federalism" policy, the companion to its "regulatory relief" campaign. A counterattack against the transferral of the primary responsibility for health and safety policy making from the states to the federal government during the 1960s and 1970s, it called for giving back to the states much of the power over health, education, and welfare issues.

However, organized labor viewed Reagan's New Federalism as an opportunity born of necessity. Believing that VDT safety and health regulations should be OSHA's responsibility, unions and their supporters hoped to achieve a regulatory breakthrough at the state and local level that would generate public support for a renewed assault on the national level. Maine state representative Edith S. Beaulieu (D), who introduced the nation's first VDT bill in March 1981, said her goal was to draw the nation's attention to the VDT problem and prod OSHA into setting national standards. "It makes a lot more sense to have one standard rather than a collection of incompatible state rules," she explained.[3] But it was futile for organized labor to approach OSHA regarding VDT regulations in the intensely anti-union deregulatory atmosphere created by the Reagan administration. As Geri D. Palast, the Service Employees International Union's legislative director, explained:

> The Occupational Safety and Health Administration has faced one cutback after another and are [sic] in no position to either take on new programs as a matter of philosophy or as a matter of funding. Therefore we feel that once we begin to focus the attention of the states on this problem, we can make a breakthrough which we can then expand throughout the states and raise to an issue of national dimension.[4]

New England was an early hotbed of VDT legislative activity. Bills were passed in Maine, Connecticut, Rhode Island, and Massachusetts to study the VDT safety and health problem during the early to mid 1980s, but none enacted mandatory regulations. But corporate pressure on state legislators not to be the first to enact mandatory regulations governing the private sector was an effective tactic for defeating VDT bills. Harry Harris, the vice president of the Southwestern Area Commerce and Industry Association of Connecticut, warned state legislators that if Connecticut became the first state to enact mandatory VDT regulations, it would be "less attractive economically."[5]

The early passage of study bills fueled subsequent legislative efforts to secure mandatory safety and health regulations in other states. The specific contents varied from state to state (some called for metal shields to reduce the level of nonionizing radiation emitted by the terminals' flyback transformer), but the typical VDT bill called for ergonomically designed work stations with adjustable chairs, detachable keyboards, reduction of screen glare from bright lights and sunlight, periodic rest breaks, daily work limits, shields to reduce printer noise, the outlawing of keystroke monitoring, and alternative work provisions for pregnant VDT workers. Many of these provisions had been adopted in Europe, Australia, New Zealand, and Canada.[6]

These events prompted the Computer and Business Equipment Manufacturer's Association to form the Coalition for Workplace Technology to prevent VDT regulations from becoming law in the United States. The CWT was backed by a formidable lobbying alliance of twenty-two trade associations representing the full spectrum of corporate VDT users. Corporate interests viewed the VDT legislative campaign as a cover for labor's attempt to organize office workers. The Massachusetts Newspaper Publishers Association's *Bulletin* remarked that the VDT safety and health issue was "organized labor's subtle way of expanding operations to unorganized businesses, especially Hi-Tech where it has made little progress."[7] CBEMA president Vico E. Henriques warned Congress that organized labor's legislative campaign would impose onerous burdens on employees and employers alike:

> They would force people to sit in special chairs, even if they were satisfied and comfortable in the present model; mandate covering windows with blinds even if there were no glare problem, or even if the glare problem came from another source. They would force low light levels in all working places using visual displays. . . . They would reduce the number of hours people could work on displays to a maximum of four or five. . . . They would force employers to pay for meaningless devices and activities, such as metal shielding for terminals and radiation inspections.[8]

CBEMA was ever vigilant against the slightest suggestion that a state law had mandated workplace VDT regulations. It even criticized the Office of Technology Assessment's report, *Automation of America's Offices,* for giving the impression that some states had passed laws regulating VDTs in the workplace. Although a few states had passed study bills, "no states have laws defining VDT-related ergonomics or mandating VDT rest breaks," Oliver Smoot, CBEMA's executive vice president declared.[9]

Corporate interests used both carrots and sticks to persuade state legislators to oppose VDT legislation. Southern New England Telephone's provision of free lunch for legislators and Digital Equipment Corporation's placement of a new plant—and eight hundred new jobs—in the district of the labor committee's chairman helped corporate interests defeat VDT legislation in Connecticut.[10] After Suffolk County (NY) executive Patrick Halpin did an about-face and vetoed the VDT bill, he was rewarded with business supporters eager to buy tickets to his three-hundred-dollars-a-plate reelection fundraiser.[11]

However, the use of the stick in the form of economic blackmail was more common. In 1983, Oregon's VDT bill was defeated after Consolidated Freightways, Inc. threatened to cancel its $8 million expansion plans and move all of its thirteen hundred–plus jobs out of Oregon.[12] In a letter to Governor Victor G. Atiyeh (R), Vice President N. R. Benke said that Consolidated Freightways "felt that it is not desirable to expand operations in states where oppressive legislation causes unnecessary and costly restrictions." Consolidated Freightways denied that it was attempting to blackmail the legislature, but the state's choice was clear. "If the Senate bill passes, they (the board of directors) won't build the building in Portland. If it fails, they will," said Phillip Seeley, another Consolidated vice president. Consolidated Freightways' threat received widespread publicity and solidified opposition to the VDT bill in the legislative and executive branches. Governor Atiyeh opposed the bill, saying its passage would have a "chilling effect" on the state's economy. "I hope this signal goes out loud and clear to some of the dreamers in the Oregon Legislature," he said.[13] Fear of a chilling effect, and the opposition of other employers, such as AT&T, Hewlett-Packard, and Textronix, Inc., the state's largest private employer, convinced the Oregon Senate Labor Committee to strip all the bill's requirement's except the annual eye exam. Legislative leaders then effectively killed the bill by establishing an interim committee to study the VDT issue.[14]

In New York, home to IBM, the world's largest computer company, and other industry giants, such as Eastman-Kodak and Xerox Corporation, "the computer industry has pulled out all the stops," said District Council 37's legislative council Fred Jacobs in 1984. "Many computer companies are headquartered in New York, and they have made defeating any and all VDT legislation their number one priority."[15]

Despite their initial success in defeating organized labor's efforts to secure passage of mandatory VDT regulations in fifteen states from 1982 to 1984, CBEMA and CWT were not claiming victory. The American Newspaper Publisher's Association's legal counsel, Claudia James, warned the group's members that VDT bills were "not going to go away."[16] Indeed, in December 1984, the SEIU and 9 to 5 launched an ambitious national "Campaign for VDT Safety" with the introduction of a new VDT bill in the Massachusetts legislature. In announcing the campaign, SEIU president John Sweeney said the safety and health problems facing office workers in the 1980s were "no less serious than the problems faced by industrial workers in the 1930's and they are even more insidious because of their subtlety."[17] Labor's strategy was to focus lobbying, organizing, and educational campaigns in the eighteen states where its support was strongest. The campaign sponsored two types of VDT bills: those mandating ergonomics standards and those that promoted an employee's right to know about hazards related to the technology.[18]

The Campaign for VDT Safety got an early boost in March 1985 when New Mexico governor Toney Anaya signed an executive order mandating ergonomic and purchasing guidelines for state employees. 9 to 5 hailed New Mexico's regulations as "better than anything that exists somewhere else," but the Campaign for VDT Safety was unable to overcome the chilling effect that corporate threats of economic blackmail had on politicians.[19] Three months after the breakthrough in New Mexico, the Oregon legislature became the first to pass a VDT bill. Although it did not apply to the private sector, Atiyeh vetoed the bill, claiming that it would inhibit the state's growing computer industry.[20] The *Los Angeles Times* reported that "Atiyeh . . . thought such a law would be harmful to the state's business climate. Oregon has been making a big push to cultivate high-tech industries and has succeeded to such a degree that the area around Beaverton, a town just west of Portland, is now called 'Silicon Forest.'"[21]

By 1987, bills addressing the workplace use of VDTs had been introduced in twenty-five states and the District of Columbia. Up to that point, four states had passed study bills, five had established purchasing guidelines for state employees, and three had established ergonomic guidelines, but none had succeeded in mandating VDT protection in the private sector workplace (where most VDT operators work). The fate of Pennsylvania state senator Buzz Andrezeski's VDT bill in 1986 was typical of the vast majority of legislative efforts: it was "buried 'deeper than you could dig with a shovel.'"[22]

The War between the States

Corporate opponents of VDT regulation had an ally in the economic war between the states for high-tech investment. Luring high-technology industries, such as computers, was seen by many states as the answer to their loss of smokestack industries during the 1970s and 1980s. In 1984, *Chemical Week* reported that "an enthusiasm for high technology, bordering on a mania . . . has been sweeping through state development offices around the country."[23] Virtually every state, and many cities, established high-technology councils to ensure that it not be left behind in the race to win high-technology investments. April Young, executive director of the Fairfax, Virginia, Economic Development Agency told *Business Week,* "There are 4,500 economic development agencies in this country, and it's fair to say that every one of them is after high tech."[24] These high-technology councils, composed of businessmen, educators, and labor leaders but dominated by corporate executives, served as boosters of their state's economic virtues and planners for future development policy. Along with state economic development officials, many of them made pilgrimages to the nation's three meccas of high technology—California's Silicon Valley, Massachusetts' Route 128, and North Carolina's Research Triangle—in the hopes of learning the secrets of their success, and to lure firms to their states. According to the OTA, seventeen states had programs to teach workers' high-technology skills by 1983, and the idea was under consideration in four more. Many states established venture capital funds to nurse and promote emergent high-technology development, and tax credits to attract new investments.[25] President Reagan made high-tech computer development an important part of his 1983 State of the Union address, and followed it up the next day with a visit to a computer keyboard manufacturing site in inner-city Boston. Ironically, Reagan had cut federal funds from the program that made the factory he visited a viable enterprise. Cuts in federal aid increased the pressure on states to find new sources of income. As a result, many states were locked in a game of competitive bidding to see who could offer the most attractive incentive packages to companies looking to get the best deal.[26]

However, the states' demand for high-tech jobs and capital investments was growing faster than the supply. High-technology firms could not replace all the jobs that were lost in manufacturing. As a result, pressure on the states to lure new high-tech investment from other states increased. Connecticut's

High Technology Council and the state Department of Economic Development (DED) worked together to keep high-tech industries happy. "We have to make sure they feel comfortable here and do not search for greener pastures. Midwestern states are going crazy recruiting" our companies, said the DED's David Driver.[27] By 1984, the competition to attract high-tech investment was growing so fierce that Trygve Vigmostad, deputy director of Michigan's Office of Economic Development, described the situation as a "war between the states" that "is heating up."[28]

This dynamic aided corporate efforts to defeat VDT regulations that might add to high-tech firms' cost of doing business. "In most state capitols today, seldom is heard a discouraging word about high technology. States are trying to attract the high-flying high tech industries, which promise jobs and taxes for the future, with every thing from tax incentives to promotion of research institutes," said CBEMA president Henriques. "But a small, highly vocal group is introducing legislation into several states that could put a roadblock in front of these efforts," he warned.[29]

This economic pressure made state economic development officials and most politicians soldiers for CBEMA's cause. Even where there was strong legislative support for VDT regulations (as in Connecticut, Oregon, New York City, and Suffolk County), corporate opponents had only to convince the head of the executive branch—whose position includes the promotion of business development—to use his veto. Similarly, California's Occupational Safety and Health Board rejected the advice of its Expert Advisory Committee on VDTs that mandatory standards be adopted. It did so based on the objections of CalOSHA's director, R. W. Stranberg, a political protégé of Governor George Deukmejian (R).[30] Wavering legislators were pressured to consider the argument that if their state became the first in the nation to enact mandatory VDT regulations, the other forty-nine would quickly be touted as superior locales for high-tech investment. As a Connecticut state legislative supporter of VDT regulations put it: "VDT use is high in Connecticut industries—we have all the major insurance companies in the world headquartered here. So state legislators are scared to death that the more we make this a public issue, the more women who work in these industries will realize they need to be organized—and this will jeopardize the state's economy."[31] Pleased with the defeat of VDT bills, CBEMA's Charlotte LeGates said, "Legislators have been highly responsible and will allow themselves to be persuaded by the facts."[32]

The Power Not to Tax

The lengths to which the states are willing to go to court big business is illustrated by their use of the investment tax credit (ITC). ITCs give major corporations the right to deduct a percentage (e.g., in New York it's 5 percent) of their annual investment in manufacturing plant and equipment from their tax bill. States engaged in the competitive chase offer ITCs to lure new businesses and keep the one's they have from leaving. However, there is no convincing evidence that corporations view the ITC as the decisive factor in their multifaceted decision to stay put or leave. Fifteen of sixteen corporations doing business in New York surveyed by District Council 37 agreed that the ITC had no impact on their investment decisions. The decision to reinvest in New York is made "whether you have an ITC or not," said an IBM spokesman. "We probably would have made the investment anyway without the credit," he added. "We think New York is a great place to work."[33] Indeed, IBM received an estimated $75 million in investment tax credits between 1982 and 1987. Fellow CBEMA member Xerox Corporation received an estimated $8.2 million during the 1987–89 period. These massive subsidies were given to IBM and Xerox during a time when they made $58,402,000,000 and $3,682,800,000 in profits, respectively. The investment tax credits given to IBM and Xerox during this period virtually wiped out their state tax bills. Moreover, New York state officials pursued this costly policy at a time when they were experiencing revenue shortfalls that forced legislators to limit and cut expenditures for underfunded social welfare and education programs.[34]

The lobbying clout of corporate giants such as IBM and Xerox, combined with Albany's desire to placate business interests, keeps this subsidy in place despite a 1985 state report's conclusion that "the ITC has probably not been a significant factor in the locational decisions of business [and] is inherently wasteful because a corporation receives a credit for all of its qualified investment, including that which would have occurred in any event."[35] The ITC's ineffectiveness as an instrument of fiscal policy was even recognized by Congress, which eliminated it from the federal tax code in the Tax Reform Act of 1986.[36] The exact amounts of the ITC each corporation gets is an official state secret that is not released until two or three years after the fact, leaving the public in the dark on the appropriateness of these decisions. Moreover, it is a tax policy that favors giant corporations over their smaller, and more economically vulnerable, competitors. Only about 3 percent of the corporations in New York have investments large enough to qualify for the tax credit. In 1982, IBM and Eastman Kodak alone accounted for 43 percent of all the credits given by New York.[37]

The Power of the Publishers

As one of the first industries to use VDTs, the publishing industry was a staunch opponent of VDT regulations. The Newspaper Guild, which represents many reporters, was the first union to raise the VDT safety and health issue in collective bargaining talks. As a result, many publishers charged that the VDT safety and health issue was a cover for labor's attempts to organize new workers and gain benefits. Faced with five VDT bills introduced in the state legislature in 1984 alone, the Massachusetts Newspaper Publishers Association (MNPA) became concerned that reporters might report the VDT issue to their own advantage. The MNPA also told the editors of its member papers to "carefully screen" all VDT stories for anti-employer and anticomputer industry bias. Having invested millions of dollars in converting from typewriters to VDTs, newspaper publishers had an economic interest in opposing VDT legislation. The MNPA told its editors and publishers that labors' "misinterpretation of facts and statements is . . . dangerous, especially to business interests."[38] But the MNPA's policy was damaging to the public interest. Its efforts to slant the coverage of the VDT story deprived the public of the full account of the controversy. The ability to shape the content of VDT news that reached the public greatly aided MNPA and its allies in their successful quest to kill VDT legislation in the Massachusetts state house.

The Illinois Press Association (IPA) took a leading role in opposing the VDT bill in the Illinois legislature. At the bill's hearing in 1984, the IPA's Dale Barker criticized workers' depiction of VDT work as monotonous, repetitive, and contributing to high levels of stress, vision, and musculoskeletal problems: "Unfortunately many jobs are tedious. What this bill plainly attempts to do is simply legislate work out of the workplace. Is the next step a law to say that no worker can go home more tired than when he arrived?" Barker charged that the Newspaper Guild was "using fear and ignorance to create something of a panic." The only reason they had "turned to the legislative arena," she surmised, was because of their failure to get "these grossly featherbedding [VDT] provisions into local contracts."[39] Like its counterparts in Massachusetts and Illinois, the Ohio Publishers Association used its power of the press to turn public opinion against the VDT bill. In its campaign to discredit supporters of VDT regulations, *Columbus Dispatch* depicted VDT proponents as irrational and antiprogress:

> It's a good thing that some of the present members of the Ohio General Assembly weren't around when the pencil was invented. Had they been, the world's most basic writing instrument might today come equipped with a tip safety shield with see-through visor, work gloves, protective eyeglasses, ear shields, and an anti-chew guard. And it would, of course, contain no lead and be made of splinter-free material. All of this would have been done in the name of 'operator safety.' Well, the doodlers and scribblers were spared this nonsense, but the users of the world's current basic writing instrument—the video display terminal—may not be so lucky.[40]

The point of view of the *Columbus Dispatch* and other opponents of the VDT bill prevailed. Pringle's bill was referred to committee, where it died at the end of the 1984 legislative session.[41] When it came to VDT safety and health legislation, the usually liberal *New York Times* decried "the heavy hand of governmental regulation." A major VDT user, it criticized Suffolk County's ill-fated VDT bill as being "bizarre" and "picky" and charged that its passage "would set a reckless precedent for other jurisdictions."[42] By 1991, however, the heavy hand of the market resulted in many of its newsroom employees wearing protective wrist splints, fifteen out of work on CTD disability, and ten more on reduced duty.[43] The role of the newspaper industry in opposing VDT safety and health legislation illustrates the point that the power of the press is superseded only by the power of the publishers.

The Shift to Suffolk County

Rebuffed at the state level, VDT proponents had better success at the county and local levels of government, where support was better concentrated. In 1987, state legislator John J. Foley (D) introduced a VDT bill that made Suffolk County, New York, the focal point of the national conflict over VDT safety and health for the next two years. Foley's bill (similar in content to those introduced in many states) applied only to employees who worked at a VDT for more than twenty-six hours a week in businesses that had five or more machines.

For Foley, a self-described New Deal Democrat, the VDT bill was an outgrowth of his interest in labor issues. Foley's attention was drawn to the issue by his wife, a CWA member, and his son, a professor of public health who was a specialist on the effects of stress.[44] The Foley bill was supported by unions and affiliated groups, such as the CWA (representing four thousand VDT workers in the county) and the Civil Service Employees Association (representing twenty-six thousand government workers in the county). Opposing the measure were many of the county's corporate VDT users, including AT&T, New York Telephone (which employed two thousand VDT operators in the county), Grumman Corporation (Long Island's largest private employer), and Newsday, Inc. (a major user of VDTs). Local high-technology firms and trade associations—including the Long Island Association (the region's chamber of commerce and largest business group with thirty-six hundred members), the New York State Bankers Association, the Business Council of New York State, the Long Island Forum for Technology (LIFT), and the Association for a Better Long Island (ABLI), a group representing forty real estate developers—also opposed Foley's bill.

Pressure against the Foley bill also came from the public sector. Concerned about the flight of corporate neighbors, such as Grumman Electronics Systems, Islip town supervisor Frank R. Jones testified against the bill. Acting county executive William A. LoGrande (R) complained that the bill would regulate small firms. Foley responded to LoGrande's objection by limiting his bill's jurisdiction to companies that used more than twenty VDTs.[45] Given that the worst safety and health problems among VDT operators were in smaller firms, Foley's concession weakened the bill's effectiveness considerably. However, Foley's modification helped get the bill passed on June 23, 1987, by a vote of thirteen to two, with three abstentions. Then, LoGrande vetoed the VDT bill, calling the measure "unconstitutional" because it applied only to large employers. The override attempt fell one vote short when two county legislators who had supported Foley's bill were persuaded by opponents to vote against it.[46] Organized labor responded by targeting LoGrande for defeat and threw their support in the 1987 race for county executive behind Assemblyman Patrick G. Halpin (D). A cosponsor of Assemblyman Frank Barbaro's VDT bill in the state assembly, Halpin promised to sign the VDT bill into law if elected.[47] Labor's campaign efforts were rewarded when Halpin defeated LoGrande, making him Suffolk County's first Democratic county executive, and the Democrats won control of the county legislature.

When Foley reintroduced his bill in March 1988, it contained two new features aimed at addressing the business community's concerns. First, employers would be required to pay only 80, not 100, percent of the cost of eye exams and prescriptions. Second, to meet opponents criticism that regulations would freeze the technology in place when it was still evolving, Foley added a provision to create a five-member board that would suggest state-of-the-art updates in the law's ergonomic standards every two years.[48] Despite these modifications, the business community continued to oppose the Foley bill. The LIA proposed a voluntary plan in a last ditch effort to stave off mandatory VDT regulations, but on May 10, 1988, the county legislature, known for its independence, passed the Foley bill by the same margin as it did the year before.[49]

Business pressure on Halpin to veto the measure was intense, and he waited for the full thirty-day period allowed under county law before vetoing the VDT bill on June 10. Ultimately, the business community's threats of economic and job loss were decisive. "More than one business leader has told me bluntly they would move from Suffolk County . . . or not relocate here" if the VDT bill became law, he said. In return for his veto, Halpin said that Suffolk County's leading businessmen had given him their "personal commitment" that they would maintain adequate VDT standards. James Larocca, the LIA's president, called the veto "an extraordinary act of courage by a guy who has matured very quickly in the job."[50]

Despite intense pressure from the bill's opponents the Legislature overrode Halpin's veto by a thirteen-to-five vote on June 14, establishing Suffolk County as the first governmental body in the nation to regulate the workplace use of VDTs in the private sector.[51] The business community's reaction was immediate and unfavorable. Northwest Airlines announced it was canceling plans to move 180 jobs into the county, and the Metropolitan Life Insurance Company said it would not hire an additional 200 employees. Real estate developers complained that clients, such as the Chubb Insurance Company, canceled deals when they learned of the proposed VDT law. The news stirred interest as far away as Wyoming, where Cheyenne proclaimed its willingness to provide a home for the corporate exodus.[52]

New York Telephone announced a hiring freeze in Suffolk County and said that it would close a directory assistance office in Babylon at the end of 1989. The Babylon office employed 125 people with an annual payroll of $3 million. Thomas J. Calabrese, general manager for the company's Long Island operations, said: "We regret having to take these steps. But as we testified at various hearings this bill imposes unnecessary costs on our company, which ultimately will be borne by our customers."[53] The same message was carried on nationwide television by the *ABC Evening News*, which quoted New York Telephone executive Steve Marcus as saying that "it's going to stifle business development in our view and its going to have an impact on our revenues."[54]

Organized labor's victory did not bring an end to the battle over VDTs in Suffolk County. Instead, it continued in the executive and judicial arenas. Despite their legislative victory, proponents of VDT regulations were now confronted with the dilemma of enforcement. In light of Halpin's promise to "do my best to implement this law so that it has the minimal impact on our business community," how vigorously would he enforce it?[55] Halpin gave the VDT bill a low priority—only one person, who also handled housing and sanitation problems, to oversee the implementation of the VDT law.

Nevertheless, opponents preferred no regulations to weakly enforced ones. Moreover, Suffolk's law was a dangerous precedent that the rest of the nation might follow. On June 23, four local businesses challenged the legality of the law in court. They charged that the county overstepped its constitutional bounds by mandating that employers pay for 80 percent of VDT workers eye exams and prescriptions, a function reserved to federal and state governments. "We want to give the Suffolk County Legislature a message that they shouldn't tread in areas where they have no jurisdiction, especially when their acts create unnecessary negative impacts of [sic] the Long Island economy," said Gary Neil Sazer, the LIA's counsel.[56] On October 5, state supreme court judge John Copertino issued a preliminary injunction stopping Suffolk County from implementing the eye care provision (the day before it was to go into effect) of its VDT law. The judge stated that the VDT law may interfere with state and federal rules regarding workers compensation, interfere with interstate commerce, and impose "financial hardship" on employers by making them pay 80 percent of employee eye care costs.[57] Judge Copertino officially overturned the VDT law's eye care provision on December 27, 1989. His decision turned on the technical question of state and local jurisdictions, not on the substance of law's concerns. In a decision that was upheld on appeal, Judge Copertino said that "though the legislation is well-intentioned and ultimately may be proved an important first step in bringing the worker health concerns addressed in the law to the attention of the public, the Suffolk County Legislature lacked the authority" to pass it.[58] He added that "in an era of almost daily revelations about workplace health and safety, it would be better to allow the state to continue its traditional oversight and control."[59]

As James O'Connor notes, and the county executive's vetoes demonstrate, public dependence on corporate-generated jobs and tax revenue tends to create a community of interests between elements of the business sector and government. In an era of tightening budgets, the Islip town supervisor didn't need to be lobbied by Grumman executives to understand that he, too, should oppose the VDT bill. Rather, the Islip town supervisor's concern that Grumman might leave the region was sufficient to ensure his opposition to the bill. The loss of Grumman's considerable contribution (i.e., $616,000 in school, town, and county taxes; $403,000 in sales and use taxes; $66 million paid annually to eighteen hundred employees; and $10 million worth of contracts it gives to other local businesses) would have a devastating impact on the area's economy.[60] Halpin's position on the VDT issue changed under the pressure of similar arguments made by business lobbyists.

The flexibility of computer and communications technology (which makes it possible to transmit work across political boundaries) makes corporate flight a more potent threat than ever before. As New York Telephone spokesman Bruce W. Reisman said after Suffolk County passed its VDT law: "It is easy for us to put VDT jobs in an adjacent location . . . artificial geographic boundaries mean little."[61] Despite the threats, few, if any, firms actually moved out of Suffolk County when the VDT law was enacted. The decisions by New York Telephone and Metropolitan Life to curtail new employment in the county were actually made before the VDT bill's passage. Claiming that the VDT law would deter business investment was an effective lobbying tactic for pressuring legislators, but it alone was not enough for companies to leave. Hewlett-Packard went ahead with its plans to build a new facilities in the county, as did Computer Associates, Inc. The county legislature's legal counsel, Paul Sabatino, reported that many firms asked his office for advice on how to comply with the law, and that a survey by the county found that the vast majority of firms were complying with its requirements.[62] This is not surprising given that business decisions to leave are usually due more to a multitude of factors such as the rising cost of supplies, labor, real estate, and traffic congestion, than the estimated costs of complying with a single regulation.

Suffolk County's Ripple Effect

The passage of a VDT law in Suffolk County created a legislative ripple effect that spread as far as the West Coast. Bills were introduced in thirteen states, and in localities such as New York City and San Francisco. Although New York City's bill did not apply to the private sector, both the business community and Mayor Edward Koch (D) eyed it with suspicion. Paul Magarill, the New York Chamber of Commerce and Industry's legislative counsel, called the VDT bill "extremely dangerous. There's no question that they'd try to extend it to the private sector."[63] In reply to industry complaints that a VDT law would stifle business, Diane Stein, the VDT Coalition's spokesperson, told the city council that the bill "does nothing more than adopt the recommendations of companies like IBM and Bell Laboratories and codify them."[64] Koch pocket vetoed New York City's bill just before leaving office, claiming that the cost of compliance, $10–$30 million, would create a less hospitable business climate. However, the city council responded that the cost would be only $3 million and that would be made up by savings from improved worker productivity and health.[65] That the cost of compliance was not an insurmountable obstacle for the city to meet was shown in June 1990, when the Dinkins administration reached a collective bargaining agreement with District Council 37 with virtually the same provisions.[66]

The passage of Suffolk County's VDT law also inspired California activists, who had been lobbying unsuccessfully at the state level, to shift their energies to the local level. Mayor Art Agnos (D) signed a VDT bill regulating both the public and private sectors into law on December 27, 1989.[67] Business opponents warned that compliance with the VDT law would cost tens of millions of dollars and worsen San Francisco's antibusiness image.[68] San Francisco's law was challenged by two local firms in court. Their legal fees were paid by IBM and other VDT manufacturers who preferred to remain anonymous. Like Suffolk County's law, San Francisco's law was struck down on the grounds that it interfered with the state's power to set occupational safety and health regulations.[69] Given that all the major cities in California were considering bills modeled on San Francisco's law, the court's ruling was an important victory for the corporate VDT coalition. It meant they didn't have to deal with the potential nightmare of complying with different regulations on a city by city basis. Moreover, San Francisco's VDT law had generated tremendous interest nationwide with more than four hundred cities requesting copies of the legislation.[70] Having to lobby against hundreds of VDT bills and comply with a myriad of enacted laws had the potential to turn the state and local arena into a labyrinth of frustration for corporate interests.[71]

Ultimately, advocates for VDT safety and health legislation did not meet with success at the state and local levels of government. Only two states enacted laws dealing with VDTs, but neither included mandatory regulations. In 1986, Rhode Island directed its Department of Labor to develop an informational brochure on VDT work hazards, and in 1989, Maine required employers to provide education and training for their VDT workers. However, Rhode Island's brochure was never written, and Maine's law was "whittled down" to the point where it cost business an "insignificant amount of money to implement," said a spokesman for the Maine Chamber of Commerce and Industry.[72] Eight states have voluntary training and/or purchasing guidelines for state employees, and New York City has a collective bargaining agreement with its employees covering ergonomic factors, but none have regulations governing the private sector where the vast majority of VDT operators work.[73]

The VDT safety and health issue illustrates the difficulties inherent in trying to achieve policy with nationwide implications at the state and local level. The business community could easily exploit its most important weapon—the threat to boycott or withdraw its business from the first state to seriously consider enacting mandatory VDT regulations. The war between the states for the high-tech investment dollar in an era of tight budgets and slow growth also gives the corporate community a tremendous advantage in shaping the safety and health debate. These factors increase government officials fears that imposing VDT regulations on business will result in a loss of economic investment, jobs, and tax revenue. The failure of state and local governments to protect the occupational safety and health of VDT workers illustrates the need for national standards and a strong OSHA to regulate the harmful effects of VDTs.

Chapter 9

Workers' Safety and Health in Postindustrial Society

The VDT safety and health issue is compelling because it illuminates the contradictions between democracy and capitalism as the United States makes the transition from the industrial to the postindustrial era. How long will workers in the postindustrial economy continue to be forced to forego the protection of the Occupational Safety and Health Act? Will the United States become a more stratified, less democratic society as present trends indicate?[1] Can organized labor meet the challenge of defending workers' rights and reverse this antidemocratic trend? These are social problems that all Americans, not just VDT workers, will have to grapple with in the future.

Although much has been said and written about the wonders of the office of the future and the information superhighway, little attention has been paid to the social costs of computing. Illnesses related to the use of video display terminals are the major occupational safety and health problem of postindustrial society. Many of the safety and health problems can be traced to poorly designed work practices that force VDT users to contort themselves to the dictates of the system of production. Misguided efforts to use the VDT to emulate assembly-line type methods creates problems of increased health hazards and worker alienation for office workers similar to those faced for many years by their industrial counterparts.

Recommendations

Many of the ailments suffered by VDT users can be prevented or alleviated by the application of ergonomic knowledge. NIOSH's recommendations, which follow, should serve as the starting point for correcting the ergonomic problems that afflict VDT workers. Regular office lighting is too bright for the performance of many VDT tasks. VDTs should not be placed so that the screen faces windows (if they are not covered) or lights. Intensive screen viewing requires the use of lower levels of illumination. Preferably, employees should be able to adjust the lighting to their particular work needs. Glare shields can also be used to reduce screen glare. Employees should have an eye examination when first assigned to VDT work and follow-up exams on an annual basis. Chairs should have adjustable seat height, backrest supports, and tension, and tables should also be adjustable. Computers should have detachable keyboards. At the very least, VDT workers should be given a fifteen-minute rest break after two hours of work, or after one hour of intensive work. However, VDT workers who feel the first signs of health problems may need to take more frequent breaks or be given appropriate non-VDT work to perform.[2] In addition, total daily work time at the VDT should not exceed four hours, and workers' keystroke counts should not be used to pit workers against one another. The Occupational Safety and Health Administration should be allowed to complete its work on the much needed and long overdue ergonomics standard.

Voice recognition computer systems, which allow the user to dictate information to the VDT, may help those suffering from crippling cumulative trauma disorders. However, voice recognition systems are no substitute for measures to redesign work stations and the work process to prevent CTDs from occurring. Less reliance on computer use is suggested as a way to reduce repetitive strain. This is not intended as an exhaustive list of recommendations. New safety and health innovations are being devised as more is learned about ergonomic problems of working with VDTs.

As this book has indicated, research and laboratory studies have linked nonionizing radiation to health problems. As a result, Sweden now requires the use of low electromagnetic emission monitors. The National Board for Measurement and Testing's guidelines were developed as a result of combined influence of the Swedish labor movement and the Social Democratic Party. They have become the de facto standard for the European Union and the world, and MPRIII standards are in the works. The Swedish Confederation of Professional Employees developed stricter guidelines in 1992, including an energy-saving feature that reduces the computer's power when it is not in use. This saves money and reduces electromagnetic fields while the VDT is dormant. However, relatively few low emission monitors are available in the U.S. market. U.S. manufacturers, who steadfastly refused for many years to make low EMF monitors for the domestic market, now face pressure to meet the MPRII and TCO standards. TCO's guidelines prompted President Clinton to issue an executive order in 1993 to encourage the computer industry to sell monitors that meet its energy-saving "Energy Star" guidelines. As a market incentive to the industry, President Clinton directed the executive branch, the world's largest computer buyer, to purchase power-down computers.[3] The resolution of flat panel, liquid crystal displays has improved to the point where they are now used in laptop computers and, with further improvements, may approximate the resolution found in desktop terminals. Using liquid crystals in place of cathode ray tubes eliminates the problem of nonionizing radiation's threat to human health.

As this book has indicated, research into the effects of extremely low frequency EMFs on human health is highly politicized and dominated by the computer industry. The Scandinavians, especially the Swedish government, have pioneered research in this field and their findings point to a connection between health problems and extremely low frequency EMFs—the same type emitted by VDTs. The U.S. government, which has much greater economic and scientific resources at its disposal, should fund independent research into the nonionizing radiation problem.

The scope and severity of the safety and health hazards associated with video display terminals presents a serious public health problem for children as well. Young children are actively encouraged by parents and educators to use computers to do school work, play games, and cruise the Internet. Moreover, children may sit too close to the VDT and not maintain correct posture. Virtually all the public health studies deal with adults, but children using computers face the same risks. Because their bodies are still growing, children may be even more vulnerable than adults to CTDs and extremely low frequency nonionizing radiation. Will eye strain create more severe and chronic vision problems for computer-using children? These questions need to be investigated by public health officials. The generation of computer-using children growing up in the 1980s and 1990s may provide our first epidemiological answers to these questions. Parents, however, needn't wait for the answers to take basic precautions.

Market Failure and the Need for Worker Participation

The growing volume of safety and health problems related to VDT use in the workplace testifies to the fact that the unregulated market approach has not worked. Although some computer manufacturers and employers have made efforts to alleviate these ergonomically related ailments, many have not taken sufficient steps to educate themselves and their workers. Over the long run, employers who take protective measures can reap productivity benefits in terms of healthier workers and higher morale. But the competitive pressures of the market, and the unwillingness of many employers to address safety and health problems, put employers who do take preventive measures at a competitive disadvantage. The long-term benefits to be gained by health hazards' prevention conflicts with and is subordinated to the market's ultimate goal: short-term maximization of profit. This lesson has been learned many times, most recently when organized labor fought for and secured the passage of the Occupational Safety and Health Act in 1970.[4] Now it needs to be learned again.

Giving workers a greater voice in the work process contributes to a healthier, more productive work force. OSHA's chief ergonomist, Roger Stephens, found that VDT workers are more likely to follow ergonomic instructions if they are included in their preparation.[5] As Shoshana Zuboff indicates, information-based computer work in postindustrial society requires that management take a new approach to the organization of work. Rather than emulating the assembly-line model of industrial work, which regiments, alienates, and contributes to health problems among workers, companies should use the creative talents of their employees by restructuring the work process to give them more responsibility.[6] Harley Shaiken stated it best: "It's the way the system is structured that's the real problem. . . . at stake is really a profound new way of ordering work. Now, the computer technology gives us a choice. We can have more autonomy or more authority in the workplace. And these systems when they're used to monitor and control and ultimately pace and discipline workers, are using computer technology to extend authority."[7]

NIOSH recommends that jobs be redesigned to make them more interesting and intellectually stimulating. This involves restructuring the work process to encourage cooperation and interaction, rather than competition and alienation, among workers. It should also be restructured to give employees some say over the pacing of the work process, to integrate other tasks with VDT work, and to make sure that the demands of work schedules do not place undue burdens on employees personal lives. As Dr. Gabriele Bammer, an expert on the problem of repetitive strain injuries at the Australian National University, explains: "There is overwhelming evidence that improving work organization is crucial to preventing work-related

Repetitive Strain Injury. . . . This means reducing work pressure, increasing worker control over the job, designing the job so that workers can help each other out and increasing the variety of tasks to be done, particularly limiting the time spent in repetitive work like keyboarding."[8]

The recommendations for restructuring work and giving employees a stronger voice in decision making have implications that go beyond the prevention of occupational safety and health hazards to the very relationship between capitalism and democracy. Taken as a whole, they pose a challenge to traditional, hierarchical assumptions about the organization of work and, in effect, recommend greater workers' participation in the postindustrial workplace. Larry Hirschhorn argues that workers must be given greater responsibility in the postindustrial workplace. Workplace participation is vital if workers are to learn from their mistakes. These "control system failures," as Hirschhorn calls them, not only create more productive and stimulated workers but also "may help to bring out in the culture a developmental concept of the self, a concept that leads people to seek out learning opportunities throughout their lives."[9] Carole Pateman asserts that "it is possible for the authority structure in industry to be considerably modified, for workers to exercise almost complete control over their jobs and to participate in a wide range of decision making, without any loss in productive efficiency."[10] She adds that giving employees a voice in workplace decision making contributes to a greater feeling of political efficacy. This point is reinforced by Benjamin Barber, who notes that a strong civic democracy depends on the development of workplace democracy: "The sharing of decision-making by workers and management . . . not only serve economic egalitarianism but foster civic spirit."[11]

The Role of Unions

Organized labor must play a leading role if the United States is to become a more democratic society in the postindustrial era. Unions have historically championed the interests of the average worker/citizen, fighting for a more equitable distribution of society's costs and benefits, and for the democratization of political rights. As the battle for VDT safety and health protection shows, unions are willing to fight for protective rights for all workers, not just those they represent. Organized labor, and most workers, have been battered by both the state and capital, which have worked to undermine the Wagner Act framework of labor relations. OSHA and the National Labor Relations Board have been of little help to workers trying to defend their rights in the postindustrial era.[12]

Democratic Party leaders, political allies since the New Deal, have distanced themselves from the labor movement with the growth of the postindustrial, global economy. Whereas the AFL-CIO hoped that President Clinton's Commission on the Future of Worker-Management Relations would restore the eroding balance of power between capital and labor, Commerce Secretary Ron Brown said its mission was to devise "an entirely new way for American firms to compete and win in global marketplaces." Contemplating whether the Wagner Act framework should be weakened to permit the reinstitution of company unions, President Clinton's labor secretary, Robert Reich, said, "The jury is still out on whether the traditional union is necessary for the new workplace." Secretary Brown added that "unions are okay where they are. And where they are not, it is not clear yet what sort of organization should represent workers."[13] Statements like these from high-ranking officials indicate the extent to which Democratic Party thinking on the role of unions has changed.

But organized labor also had internal, organizational problems of its own. Organized labor's preoccupation with defending the rights of its declining membership in its predominantly male, blue-collar industrial unions hindered its ability to focus on the opportunity presented by the VDT safety and health issue to organize the predominantly female office work force. Although many unions have made great strides in organizing women and opening leadership opportunities, the AFL-CIO's failure to mount a strong campaign to organize women office workers limited its ability to mobilize popular support for the VDT issue in the political arena.[14]

Given the problems that unions labor face in organizing the white-collar work force, they might make greater use of associational unionism. Generally, associational unionism provides services, benefits, and professional support for its members, encourages more flexible work rules and greater workers' participation in the labor process, but doesn't collectively bargain for workers.[15] Associational unionism might be better suited to the unique characteristics of white-collar VDT workers, who are less likely to be receptive to the concept of unions than blue-collar workers. As Charles Heckscher writes, "The problem of worker representation extends far beyond . . . [the domain of traditional unionism to] . . . issues faced by all levels of employees

—and especially by the white collar and professional employees who are increasingly seen as the leading edge of economic growth."[16] Moreover, as Casey Ichniowski and Jeffrey S. Zax have shown, employee associations often prove to be staging grounds for the development of unions. Similarly, Deborah Bell has found that the presence of employee associations in state and local governments helped unions organize workers.[17]

Organizing drives often fail because they are too narrowly focused on signing up workers who do not have much of a social connection to one another or to a union. To broaden the scope of its support in the community, labor might establish closer links with local "workers centers." They usually serve as support groups and local clearinghouses for poor, immigrant, or minority workers, helping them deal with language and cultural barriers. Workers centers often combine efforts to organize workers with efforts to help the broader community deal with its social and political problems.[18] Historically, labor's greatest strength has been its community support. Although many white-collar workers do not live near their workplace, and VDT work can be transmitted to other workplaces, unions should examine where and how workers centers might benefit organizing drives. For example, many VDT data-entry workers are minority women. Unions might focus on an organizing campaign that uses the support of local churches and neighborhood groups. Labor's greatest strength comes when it is transformed from an interest group into a social movement.[19] Workers centers could be a catalyst in that transformation.

Labor, Capital, and Power

The power inequities between labor and capital need to be addressed if the reforms and recommendations are to become a reality for all VDT workers. Pluralists assert that capital's economic power is dissipated in the political arena by intrabusiness strife and the countervailing power of opposing interest groups.[20] However, there was little intrabusiness strife to erode the corporate coalition's unity on political goals in this case. United, the computer manufacturers and corporate users were able to convert their economic resources into political influence to defeat organized labor's regulatory initiatives. Second, whereas pluralists maintain that policy issues arise separately in the political arena, both federal and state government officials considered the issues of VDT safety and health regulation and economic growth to be two sides of the same coin.[21] In this zero-sum game, public officials rejected VDT regulations because they were considered to be a drag on economic growth.

Although pluralists maintain that American politics is played on a level playing field, structural factors give corporate interests a decisive advantage over organized labor. Occupational safety and health policy making for VDT workers is dominated by a corporate coalition of computer manufacturers and corporate users of office automation systems in conjunction with a network of insurance companies, voluntary safety groups (the National Safety Council), professional associations (the Human Factors Society and the Institute of Electrical and Electronics Engineers), and private, standard-setting organizations (the American National Standards Institute). This policy network, which Daniel M. Berman calls the "compensation-safety apparatus," has been the dominating factor in occupational safety and health policy making since the Progressive era.[22] Although its policy influence over industrial health and safety has been somewhat abated by the OSH Act, the corporate-controlled policy network's dominance over the information sector remains unchecked.

The mobilization of bias supporting the compensation-safety apparatus was sustained by both governmental and corporate uses of nondecision-making tactics. The corporate coalition's effectiveness was greatest when its interests were most threatened. The computer industry's establishment of a voluntary VDT ergonomics standard in cooperation with ANSI and HFS deflated organized labor's calls for, and OSHA's work on, an ergonomics standard. Despite the fact that research indicated the need for further study, the computer industry and corporate users promoted the conventional scientific view that nonionizing radiation was harmless to humans. This stance was effective in persuading public officials that publicly funded research was unnecessary because most of the U.S. research in this little-explored area was sponsored by the computer and electronics industries, and because of corporate efforts to censor, ignore, and refute news of studies that pointed to the need for further research. In the wake of governmental inaction, the corporate coalition, ANSI, HFS, and the IEEE became quasi-governmental policy makers with a de facto veto over the final shape of voluntary VDT guidelines. This structural bias made it easier for capital to defend the policy status quo against organized labor's challenge.

The Role of the State

Corporate dominance of the VDT issue was also made possible by the state's dependence on capital as the generator of economic growth and tax revenues. This dependence made the state susceptible to pressure from the corporate coalition. The state's responsiveness to corporate pressure was accentuated by the importance it placed on fostering unfettered high-technology/computer development as the engine of economic recovery in the globally competitive, postindustrial era.

The anticipated negative economic impact of safety and health regulations on the manufacture and widespread use of VDTs, and the ripple effect it would have on the economy, gave public officials an incentive to oppose organized labor's attempts to secure VDT regulations. The Reagan and Bush administrations used the Office of Management and Budget to undermine NIOSH research studies and to prevent OSHA regulations from coming through the administrative pipeline. Interfering in NIOSH's study of reproductive hazards on BellSouth's behalf, OMB forbade NIOSH from asking female VDT workers questions regarding stress and fertility. This made it virtually impossible for NIOSH to determine if there was a connection between VDT use and reproductive disorders. The Reagan administration's anti-union, deregulatory stance discouraged organized labor from asking OSHA to promulgate a VDT standard. Despite evidence of an epidemic of CTDs among VDT workers, the Bureau of Labor Statistics does not keep detailed statistics on the number who were afflicted. Although cumulative trauma disorders are a major problem for VDT workers, and CTDs have been among the fastest growing occupational illnesses during the 1980s and 1990s, the federal government refused to allocate adequate monies to fund positions for an ergonomics program in OSHA and NIOSH. These nondecisions masked the true magnitude of the problem and made it more difficult for organized labor to attract public attention to its case for regulation.

In Congress, both political action and inaction were used to defeat protective policies for VDT workers. Under the Democrats, organized labor was not able to advance its case for VDT regulations beyond the hearings' stage in the House of Representatives. The corporate coalition's public relations campaign to redefine the VDT safety and health issue as a question of employee comfort that was best handled on a voluntary basis by employers persuaded most congressmen that federal action was unnecessary.

With few exceptions there was little interest in pushing the VDT issue in Congress. When the Republicans gained control of Congress in 1995, one of the first orders of business was to cut OSHA's funding, thus forcing the Clinton administration to stop work on its ergonomics standard.

The futile efforts of regulatory advocates to achieve a breakthrough at the state and local levels shows the difficulties inherent in trying to make national policy at the state and local level. The ease with which VDT work can be transmitted beyond local, state, and national boundary lines, combined with states' fierce competition for the high-tech investment dollar, gives the corporate community a tremendous advantage in shaping of occupational safety and health policy in the postindustrial era. As a result, state government officials rejected organized labor's calls for VDT regulations in order to avoid losing much needed economic investment, jobs, and tax revenue to other states or countries.

As the case of VDT workers seeking occupational safety and health protection makes clear, the fragmented framework of the American political system makes it relatively easy for opponents to frustrate needed policy-making reforms. However, the chances for policy reform increase during times of economic and social change. Presently, the United States is going through a transformation from a largely national, industrial economy to the global, postindustrial economy. As it did during the 1930s, organized labor will need to transform itself from an interest group into a social movement in order to generate the massive grass-roots support needed to help effectuate democratic reforms.

Notes

INTRODUCTION

1. A selected list follows: Barbara Hilkert Andolsen, *Good Work at the Video Display Terminal* (Knoxville: University of Tennessee Press, 1989); Barbara Baran and Suzanne Teegarden, "Women's Labor in the Office of the Future" (paper presented at the conference on "Women and Structural Transformation," Rutgers University, New Brunswick, N.J., November 18–19, 1983); *The Technological Woman,* ed. Jan Zimmerman (New York: Praeger, 1983); Rosemary Crompton and Gareth Jones, *White-Collar Proletariat: Deskilling and Gender in Clerical Work* (Philadelphia: Temple University Press, 1984); Roselyn L. Feldberg and Evelyn N. Glenn, "Proletarianizing Clerical Work," in *Case Studies on the Labor Process,* ed. Andrew Zimbalist (New York: Monthly Review Press, 1979), 51–72 and "Technology and Work Degradation: Effects of Office Automation on Women Clerical Workers," in *Machina Ex Dea: Feminist Perspectives on Technology,* ed. Joan Rothschild, (Elmsford, N.Y.: Pergamon Press, 1983), 59–78; Robert Howard, *Brave New Workplace* (New York: Viking Books, 1986); Karen Sacks and Dorothy Remy, eds., *My Troubles Are Going to Have Trouble with Me: Everyday Trials and Triumphs of Women Workers* (New Brunswick, N.J.: Rutgers University Press, 1984); and Jackie West, "New Technology and Women's Office Work," in *Work, Women and the Labour Market,* by Jackie West (London: Routledge and Kegan Paul, 1982), 61–79.

2. The literature is voluminous; a selected sample follows: International Labour Office, *Working with Visual Display Units,* Occupational Safety and Health Series, No. 61 (Geneva: ILO, 1989); American Medical Association, Council on Scientific Affairs, "Council Report: Health Effects of Video Display Terminals," *JAMA* 257 (March 20, 1987): 1508–1512 and "Health Effects of Video Display Terminals: An Update" (paper presented by George H. Bohigian, M.D., April 1989); Paul Brodeur, "Annals of Radiation: Part III—Video Display Terminals," *New Yorker,* June 20, 1989, 39–68; Mary Sue Henifin, "The Particular Problems of Video Display Terminals," in *Double Exposure: Women's Health Hazards on the Job and at Home,* ed. Wendy Chavkin (New York: Monthly Review Press, 1984), 69–80; Joel Makower, *Office Hazards* (Washington, D.C.: Tilden Press, 1981); Karel Marha, Barry Spinner, and Jim Purdham, *The Case for Concern about Very Low Frequency*

Fields from Visual Display Terminals: The Need for Further Research and Shielding of VDTs (Hamilton, Ontario: Canadian Centre for Occupational Health and Safety, 1983); National Academy of Sciences, National Research Council, Committee on Vision, Panel on Impact of Video Viewing on Vision of Workers (hereafter cited as NAS), *Video Displays, Work, and Vision,* (Washington, D.C.: National Academy Press, 1983); *Potential Health Hazards of Video Display Terminals* (Cincinnati, Ohio: NIOSH, 1980); Jeanne M. Stellman and Mary Sue Henifin, *Office Work Can Be Dangerous to Your Health* (New York: Pantheon Books, 1983); and *The VDT Book: A Computer User's Guide to Health and Safety* (New York: New York Committee for Occupational Safety and Health, 1987).

3. A few law articles have dealt with the issue of VDT workers' rights. See Sheryl Gordon McCloud, "VDTs in the Workplace," *Southern California Law Review* 58 (1985): 1493–1499; Sara Rapport, "Health Rights of Video Display Terminal Operators," *Harvard Women's Law Journal* 8 (1985): 247–264; and Charles Wallach, "Employer Liability in Video Display Operators' Health Complaints," *Glendale Law Review* 6 (1985): 1–14.

4. Shari Roan, "When It's a Blur: New Developments in Equipment, Lighting and Prescriptions May Help Ease Strain of Staring at VDTs," *Los Angeles Times,* January 19, 1993, p. E1.

5. U.S. Department of Human Services, National Institute for Occupational Safety and Health (hereafter cited as NIOSH), *An Investigation of Health Complaints and Job Stress in Video Display Operations,* by Michael J. Smith, Barbara G. F. Cohen, Lambert W. Stammerjohn, and Alan Happ (Cincinnati: Public Health Service, 1981).

6. Quoted in Marvin J. Dainoff, "The Illness of the Decade," *Computerworld,* April 13, 1992, 27.

7. Doug Bartholomew, "RSI: Is it Your Problem?" *Information Week,* November 9, 1992, 33.

8. Bob DeMatteo, *Terminal Shock: The Health Hazards of Video Display Terminal Workers,* 2d ed. (Toronto: NC Press, 1986); Environmental Protection Agency, Office of Research and Development (hereafter cited as EPA), *Evaluation of Potential Carcinogenicity of Electromagnetic Fields,* review draft (Washington, D.C.: GPO, 1990).

9. From a national survey of 1,008 full-time office workers by Louis Harris and Associates, for "Office Environment Index: Summary Report: United States," in Steelcase, Inc., 1991 *Steelcase Worldwide Office Environment Index* (Grand Rapids, Mich.: Steelcase, 1991), 13.

10. Ibid., 5.

11. Barbara Garson, *The Electronic Sweatshop: How Computers are Transforming the Office of the Future into the Factory of the Past* (New York: Simon and Schuster, 1988); "VDTs: Sweatshops of the Future?" *Public Sector,* July 12, 1985, 10–11. Employers have even farmed out VDT work on a piecework basis to those working at home. See Dennis Chamot and John L. Zalusky, "The Electronic Sweat-

shop: The Use and Misuse of Work Stations in the Home" (presented at a National Executive Forum: Office Work Stations in the Home, National Academy of Sciences, Washington, D.C., November 9–10, 1983); Philip Mattera, "High-Tech Cottage Industry: Home Computer Sweatshops," *Nation,* April 2, 1983, 390–392; Richard Moore and Elizabeth Marsis, "Telecommuting: Sweatshop at Home Sweet Home?" *In These Times,* April 18–24, 1984.

12. On the two-tier economy, see AFL-CIO, *Future of Work.* For the postindustrial economy's dependence on low-paid women workers, see Aaron Bernstein, "What's Dragging Productivity Down? Women's Low Wages," *Business Week,* November 27, 1989, 171.

13. U.S. Department of Labor, Bureau of Labor Statistics (hereafter cited as BLS), *Employment and Earnings,* January 1995, table 39.

14. BLS, *Employment and Earnings,* table 39; percentage calculated by the author.

15. U.S. Department of Labor, Women's Bureau, "Women and Workforce 2000," Fact Sheet No. 88-1, January 1988, 4.

16. Wendy Chavkin, ed. *Double Exposure: Women's Health Hazards on the Job and at Home* (New York: Monthly Review Press, 1984).

17. For example, see Robert Stewart Smith, The Occupational Safety and Health Act: Its Goals and Achievements (Washington, DC: American Enterprise Institute, 1976); Steven Kelman, Regulating America, Regulating Sweden (Cambridge, MIT Press, 1981); David P. McCaffrey, OSHA and the Politics of Health Regulation (New York: Plenum Press, 1982); and Graham K. Wilson, The Politics of Safety and Health (New York: Oxford University Press, 1985)

18. E. E. Schattschneider, *The Semisovereign People: A Realist's View of Democracy* (Hinsdale, Ill.: Dryden Press, 1975), 108.

19. Peter Bachrach and Morton S. Baratz, *Power and Poverty: Theory and Practice* (New York: Oxford University Press, 1970), 43.

20. Peter Bachrach and Morton S. Baratz, "Two Faces of Power," *American Political Science Review* 56 (December 1962): 947–952.

21. Bachrach and Baratz, *Power and Poverty,* 44. See also "Decisions and Nondecisions: An Analytical Framework," *American Political Science Review* 57 (1963): 641–651.

22. "Is Your Computer Making You Sick?" *Open Computing,* February 1995, 20.

23. For 1994 sales, see Alan Cane, "Survey of the Computer; Battle for the Desktop," *Financial Times,* May 31, 1994, 1.

24. George Taninecz, "Technology Booming," *Industry Week,* May 15, 1995, 23.

25. Norman C. Remich Jr., "Growth Continues; Appliance Industry," *Appliance Manufacturer,* January 1994, 22.

Chapter 1   THE HAZARDS OF WORKING WITH VIDEO DISPLAY TERMINALS

CRT (cathode ray tube) is an older term for video display terminal. The term *visual display unit* (VDU) is commonly used in Europe. Although *visual* is more accurate than *video,* the latter term—which is widely used in the United States—is used to avoid confusion.

1. What follows is a sampler of sources on VDT-related safety and hazards. House Committee on Education and Labor, *OSHA Oversight: Video Display Terminals in the Workplace: Hearings before the Subcommittee on Health and Safety,* 98th Cong., 2d sess., 1984, 59. See also *Potential Health Hazards of Video Display Terminals;* Bob DeMatteo, *Terminal Shock: The Health Hazards of Video Display Terminal Workers,* 2d ed. (Toronto: NC Press, 1986).

2. NAS, *Video Displays, Work, and Vision,* 1.

3. NIOSH, *An Investigation of Health Complaints and Job Stress in Video Display Operations,* by Michael J. Smith et al. (Cincinnati: Public Health Service, 1981), 11.

4. Cathy Trost, "The Price of Progress: Computers, While Increasing Productivity, Have Spawned New Occupational Ailments," *Wall Street Journal,* September 16, 1985, p. 34C.

5. Office of Technology Assessment, *Biological Effects of Power Frequency Electric and Magnetic Fields,* background paper by Indira Nair, M. Granger Morgan, and H. Keith Florig (Washington, D.C.: GPO, 1989). See also "Very Weak Magnetic Fields Cause Chick Abnormalities," *VDT News,* March/April 1988, 1.

6. Paul Brodeur, *Currents of Death: Power Lines, Computer Terminals, and the Attempt to Cover Up Their Threat to Your Health* (New York: Simon and Schuster, 1989), chaps. 33–45; Bill Paul, "Radiation Study Finds High Incidence of Cancer Among Phone Cable Splicers," *Wall Street Journal,* November 29, 1989, p. B4. "IBM Shielding Move Prompts New Conflicts," *VDT News,* January/February 1990, 5; "CRT Use Linked to Cancer: Australian Study Finds Brain Tumor Risk for Women, Not Men," *VDT News,* July/August 1992, 1; and "Alzheimer's Linked to EMF Exposure," *VDT News,* September/October 1994, 1.

7. Marja-Liisa Lindbohm, Maila Hietanen, Pentti Kyyrönen, Markku Sallmén, Patrick von Nandelstadh, and Helena Taskinen, "Magnetic Fields of Video Display Terminals and Spontaneous Abortion," *American Journal of Epidemiology* 136 (November 1, 1992): 1041–1051. In a follow-up analysis of their data, the authors found a stronger relationship between miscarriages and magnetic EMFs than originally reported. See *American Journal of Epidemiology* 138 (November 15, 1993): 902–905. "EMF-Miscarriage Link Supported," *VDT News,* January/February 1994, 1.

8. Ionizing radiation is also emitted, but (except for some poorly manufactured terminals in the 1970s and early 1980s) it is contained by the backside of the phosphor-coated screen. See "Allergies to VDTs," *VDT News,* May/June 1987, 1; "Hypersensitivities to VDTs," *VDT News,* July/August 1989, 4–5. Gunnar Swanbeck and Thor Bleeker, "Skin Problems from Visual Display Units," *Acta Derm Venereol* 69 (1989): 46–51; "Face Rashes Linked with Use of VDTs," *Science News* 120 (September 5, 1981): 150; "Skin Rash Debate," *VDT News,* November/December 1986, 17–18; "Skin Problems in Sweden," *VDT News,* May/June 1987, 10; "North Carolina Study Finds VDT Heart Illness Link," *VDT News,* May/June 1985,

4–5; "NIOSH Investigations: Non-Ionizing Radiation and Angina Rates," *VDT News,* November/December 1985, 10–11; EPA, *Evaluation of Potential Carcinogenicity of Electromagnetic Fields,* review draft (Washington, D.C.: GPO, 1990).

9. Marilyn K. Goldhaber, Michael R. Polen, and Robert A. Hiatt, "The Risk of Miscarriage and Birth Defects among Women Who Use Visual Display Terminals During Pregnancy," *American Journal of Industrial Medicine* 13 (June 1988). See also Tamar Lewin, "Pregnant Women Increasingly Fearful of VDT's," *New York Times,* July 10, 1988, p. 19 and "Protecting the Baby: Work in Pregnancy Poses Legal Frontier," *New York Times,* August 2, 1988, p. A1; Laura Stock, "Kaiser Study Finds High Miscarriage Rate in VDT Workers," *Monitor,* Summer 1988, 13; Philip Shabecoff, "U.S. Sees Possible Cancer Tie to Electromagnetism," *New York Times,* May 23, 1990, p. A22; and William K. Stevens, "Scientists Debate Health Hazards of Electromagnetic Fields," *New York Times,* July 11, 1989, p. C1; "VDT Use Linked to Increased Miscarriage Risk," *VDT News,* July/August 1988, 1; and "Study Adds to Pattern of Pregnancy Risk, *VDT News,* January/February 1991, 1.

10. Gregg LaBar, "Bent Out of Shape; Musculoskeletal Injuries as a Workplace Epidemic," *Occupational Hazards,* June 1991, 37.

11. Craig Brod, *Technostress: The Human Cost of the Computer Revolution* (Reading, Mass.: Addison-Wesley, 1984).

12. André Piche and Jacques Piche, "Health Problems of Data Entry Clerks and Related Job Stressors," *Journal of Occupational Medicine* 29 (December 1987): 942–948.

13. Steelcase, Inc., *Office Environment Index: 1989 Detailed Findings* (Grand Rapids, Mich.: Steelcase, 1989), 65. The survey included 1,041 full-time office workers.

14. Lawrence M. Scheifer, *Effects of VDT/Computer System Response Delays and Incentive Pay on Mood Disturbances and Somatic Discomfort* (Cincinnati: NIOSH, 1986) and NIOSH, *Investigation of Health Complaints,* abstract page.

15. Peter L. Schnall, Carl Pieper, Joseph E. Schwartz, Robert A. Karasek, Yvette Schlussel, Richard B. Devereux, Antonello Genau, Michael Alderman, Katherine Warren, and Thomas J. Pickering, "The Relationship Between 'Job Strain,' Workplace Diastolic Blood Pressure and Left Ventricular Mass Index," *Journal of the American Medical Association* 263, no. 14 (April 11, 1990): 1929–1935; International Labour Office, *Working with Visual Display Units,* Occupational Safety and Health Series, No. 61 (Geneva: ILO, 1989), 8–9.

16. Researchers at the University of Bologna reported an increase of hormones called catecholamines, a known sign of stress, in VDT operators who worked for more than four hours a day. See "Vision, RSIs & Stress Issues Dominate WWDU 89," *VDT News* (November/December 1989): 2–5.

17. "Survey of Secretaries Finds Greater Stress with VDT's than Memory Typewriters," *Secretary,* March 1986.

18. NIOSH, *Investigation of Health Complaints;* Ann Dooley, "Stress, Health Hazards Linked to CRT Use," *Computerworld,* February 16, 1981, 1; and David Moberg,

"Terminal Boredom and Higher Stress," *In These Times*, November 10–16, 1982, 2.

19. NIOSH, *Investigation of Health Complaints*, 12.

20. Library of Congress, Office of Technology Assessment (hereafter cited as OTA), *The Electronic Supervisor: New Technology, New Tensions* (Washington, D.C.: GPO, 1987); Michael J. Smith, Pascale Sainfort, Katherine Rogers, and David LeGrande, *Electronic Performance Monitoring and Job Stress in Telecommunications Jobs* (Madison: University of Wisconsin, Department of Industrial Engineering and the Communications Workers of America, 1990); 9 to 5, National Association of Working Women, *Computer Monitoring and Other Dirty Tricks* (Cleveland: 9 to 5, 1986); Frank Swoboda, "Study Links Electronic Monitoring, Stress," *Washington Post*, October 14, 1990; "Survey of VDT Users Indicates Link Between Health Problems, Monitoring," *Occupational Safety & Health Reporter*, December 5, 1985, 560. "Monitoring Compounds Worker Stress from VDT Units, Researcher Tells Meeting," *Occupational Safety & Health Reporter*, April 8, 1987.

21. They conclude that workers performing repetitive, assembly-line tasks suffer more job-related stress than the peasant of preindustrial era. "Relationship Between Stress, Degree of Job Control Seen in Research Findings," *Occupational Safety & Health Reporter*, May 27, 1987, 1461; "Worker Stress Linked to High Blood Pressure in Medical Journal Study by New York Doctor," *Occupational Safety & Health Reporter*, April 18, 1990, 2054–2055.

22. Shari Roan, "When It's a Blur: New Developments in Equipment, Lighting and Prescriptions May Help Ease Strain of Staring at VDTs," *Los Angeles Times*, January 19, 1993, p. E1.

23. See *VDT User's Guide to Better Vision* and *The Effects of Video Display Terminal Use on Eye Health and Vision*, both from the American Optometric Association (St. Louis: American Optometric Association, 1994); "Optometric Association Urges VDT Workers to get Annual Eye Exams to Protect Vision," *Occupational Safety & Health Reporter*, October 27, 1983; NAS, *Video Displays, Work, and Vision*, 1; and California, Assembly Committee on Labor and Employment and the Senate Committee on Industrial Relations, *Video Display Terminal Safety: Problems Relating to Vision*, A Joint Interim Hearing, December 17, 1985.

24. Anne-Marie Schiro, "Secretaries' Poll on Computers," *New York Times*, March 14, 1983, p. 18.

25. "Vision and VDTs Discussed at Optometrists' Meeting," *VDT News*, May/June 1985, 5; "Data Entry Operators Report Eye Problems," *VDT News*, July/August 1989, 3–4.

26. "Who Gets RSIs?" *VDT News*, July/August 1989, 4.

27. Dr. Vern Putz-Anderson, ed., *Cumulative Trauma Disorders* (Philadelphia: Taylor and Francis, 1988), quoted in Peter T. Kilborn, "Automation: Pain Replaces the Old Drudgery," *New York Times*, June 24, 1990, sec. 1, p. 1.

28. For example, see Mitch Betts, "Repetitive Stress Claims Soar," *Computerworld*, November 11, 1990, 1, and "Repetitive Motion Disorders Lead Increase in Job

Illnesses," *New York Times,* November 16, 1990, p. A26.

29. BLS, *Workplace Injuries and Illnesses in 1993* (Washington, D.C., 1994), 2.

30. For more on the lack of VDT-related CTD statistics, see the testimony of Lawrence J. Fine, M.D., director, Division of Surveillance, Hazard Evaluations, and Field Studies, NIOSH, in House Committee on Government Operations, *Dramatic Rise in Repetitive Motion Injuries and OSHA's Response: Hearings before the Employment and Housing Subcommittee,* 101st Cong., 1st sess., June 6, 1989, 116. Also, the BLS verified that they do not keep data on VDT-related CTDs; telephone interview with Larry Drake, July 19, 1990. Scannel cited in Peter T. Kilborn, "Rise in Worker Injuries Is Laid to the Computer," *New York Times,* November 16, 1989, p. A24. Habes quoted in Trost, "Price of Progress," 34C.

31. For the newspaper and telecommunications industries, see "Vision, RSIs & Stress Issues," 2–5; for the Minolta study, see Schiro, "Secretaries' Poll," 18.

32. "Study Spots High RSIs at NYNEX," *VDT News,* January/February 1990, 4.

33. NIOSH, *Health Hazard Evaluation Report: Newsday, Inc., Melville, New York,* HETA 89-250-2046 (Cincinnati: NIOSH, 1990), 1; Ronald E. Roel, "Study Ties Computer Typing, Injuries," *Newsday,* June 6, 1990, 19.

34. "Adapt Work Stations to Workers' Needs, Experts Encourage Industrial Hygienists," *Occupational Safety & Health Reporter,* November 5, 1986, 599–600.

35. Quoted in Ellen Cassedy and Karen Nussbaum, *9 to 5: The Working Women's Guide to Office Survival* (New York: Penguin Books, 1983), 68.

Chapter 2   THE OFFICE OF THE FUTURE MEETS THE FACTORY OF THE PAST

1. Some of the material in this chapter appears in different form in my essay, "Video Display Terminals and the Deskilling of Work in the 'Office of the Future,'" in *Beyond Survival: Wage Labor in the Late Twentieth Century,* ed. Cyrus Bina, Laurie Clements, and Chuck Davis (Armonk, N.Y.: M. E. Sharpe, 1996).

2. "The Office of the Future," *Business Week,* June 30, 1975, 48.

3. Adia Personnel Services, *The Impact of Office Automation: 84/85 International Survey* (Menlo Park, Calif.: Adia Personnel Services [c. 1985]), 22.

4. Michael D. Zisman, "Office Automation: Revolution or Evolution?" *Sloan Management Review* (Spring 1978): 9.

5. "Office 'Miracles' that Electronics Is Bringing," *U.S. News & World Report,* September 18, 1978, 76–78.

6. IBM, *1987 Annual Report* (Armonk, N.Y.: IBM, 1988), 17.

7. Adia Personnel Services, *Impact of Office Automation,* 12.

8. Harley Shaiken, "Choices in the Development of Office Automation," in *Office Automation: Jekyll or Hyde?* ed. Daniel Marschall and Judith Gregory (Cleveland: Working Women Education Fund, 1983), 10.

9. "Consultants Question Computer's Impact on Workplace," *Computerworld,* May 28, 1984, 18.

10. "Office of the Future," 50, 53.

11. Foreword to William H. Leffingwell, *Office Management: Principles and Practice* (New York: McGraw-Hill, 1925), vi.

12. Ibid., 35, 36.

13. OTA, *Automation of America's Offices* (Washington, D.C.: GPO, 1985), 9; Margaret Lowe Benston, "For Women, the Chips Are Down," in *The Technological Woman,* ed. Jan Zimmerman (New York: Praeger, 1983), 46–47.

14. Mills, *White Collar,* 226–227.

15. Harry Braverman, *Labor and Monopoly Capital: The Degradation of Work in the Twentieth Century* (New York: Monthly Review Press, 1974), 347.

16. John Dewey, *Democracy and Education* (New York: Free Press, 1966), 85.

17. "Office of the Future," 49; "The 'Automated Office' Is Thriving," *Office Management,* May 1983, 13.

18. SRI International, "Office Automation Consulting and Research" (Palo Alto, Calif.: SRI International, n.d.), 2; Wassily Leontief and Faye Duchin, *The Impacts of Automation on Employment, 1963–2000: Final Report* (New York: Institute for Economic Analysis, New York University, 1984), 5:7.

19. SRI International, "Office Automation," 2; Marvin Kornbluth, "The Electronic Office: How It Will Change the Way You Work," *Futurist,* June 1982, 37.

20. Vincent E. Giuliano, "The Mechanization of Office Work," *Scientific American,* September 1982, 164.

21. "Information Processing and Tomorrow's Office," *Fortune,* October 8, 1979, 32. An advertising supplement prepared by International Data Corporation, a market research company.

22. Quoted in Craig Brod, *Technostress: The Human Cost of the Computer Revolution* (Reading, Mass.: Addison-Wesley, 1984), 45–46.

23. John Naisbitt, *Megatrends* (New York: Warner Books, 1982), 16.

24. Richard J. Matteis, "The New Back Office Focuses on Customer Service," *Harvard Business Review* (March–April 1979): 146–159.

25. Ibid., 150.

26. NIOSH, *Investigation of Health Complaints,* 13; emphasis added.

27. "Study of New Jobs Since '79 Says Half Pay Poverty Wage," *New York Times, Sept. 27, 1988,* p. A22; AFL-CIO, *The Future of Work* (Washington, D.C.: AFL-CIO, 1983), 8; William Serrin, "A Great American Job Machine? The Myth of the 'New Work,'" *Nation,* Sept. 18, 1989, 269–271.

28. Philip Kraft, "Mid-Level Managers: Will They Fade Out as Automation Changes the Office?" *Computerworld,* September 28, 1981, SR 29; Sally Cusack, "Is Automation Turning Managers into Clerks?" *Computerworld,* October 15, 1990, 83; Trish Hall, "A Changing World for Secretaries," *New York Times,* April 27, 1988, p. D1. For clerical worker trends, see OTA, *Automation of America's Offices,* 33, 55; U.S. Department of Labor, Women's Bureau, *1993 Handbook on Women Workers: Trends & Issues* (Washington, D.C., 1994), 235.

29. Paraphrased and quoted in "Monitoring Workers by Computer," *Business Week,* August 9, 1982, 62F.

30. *Stories of Mistrust and Manipulation: The Electronic Monitoring of the American Workforce* (Cleveland: Working Women Education Fund, 1990), 1. This figure is in keeping with the OTA's 1987 estimate of six million workers in OTA, *Electronic Supervisor,* 32; and the American Civil Liberties Union's (hereafter cited as ACLU) estimate of ten million workers in Karen B. Ringen, "Electronic Monitoring," in *Liberty at Work: Expanding the Rights of Employees in America,* ed. ACLU (New York: ACLU, 1988), 9.

31. "Remarks at the White House Conference on Productivity," September 22, 1983, in *Public Papers of the Presidents of the United States: Ronald Reagan* (Washington, D.C.: GPO, 1985), 2:1329; Meese quoted in Gary T. Marx, "The Company is Watching You Everywhere," *New York Times,* February 15, 1987, p. 21. For management's response, see the comments of James O'Brien, executive director of the MTM Association, a business consulting group, 9–13, in "The MacNeil/Lehrer News Hour," PBS telecast, "Big Brother in the Workplace," December 28, 1983 (New York: Journal Graphics Transcripts, 1983).

32. Ronald Rice, Bonnie Johnson, Deborah Kowal, and Charles Feltman, "The Survival of the Fittest: Organizational Design and the Structuring of Word Processing," cited in *Computer Chips and Paper Clips: Technology and Women's Employment,* ed. Heidi I. Hartmann, Robert E. Kraut, and Louise A. Tilly (Washington, D.C.: National Academy Press, 1986), 1:143.

33. 9 to 5, National Association of Working Women, *Computer Monitoring and Other Dirty Tricks* (Cleveland: 9 to 5, 1986); Karen Nussbaum, "Outlaw Monitoring; It Abuses the Worker," *USA Today,* July 11, 1986; Gary T. Marx and Sanford Sherizen, "Monitoring on the Job: How to Protect Privacy as Well as Property," *Technology Review,* November/December 1986, 63–72; Marx, "Company is Watching," 21; Jesse Wing, "Subliminal Messages," in ACLU, *Liberty at Work,* 40–43; Chuck Fogel, "The Electronic Boss: How Management is Using the Latest Technology to Control Employees in the Workplace," *Solidarity,* July 1987, 11–14.

34. OTA, *Electronic Supervisor,* 29.

35. "VDTs and Productivity," *Guild Reporter,* March 23, 1984, 8.

36. "The MacNeil/Lehrer News Hour"; see James O'Brien's remarks, 9–13.

37. Ibid., 9; OTA, *Electronic Supervisor,* 1; "Statistical Compensation Survey," *DEMA,* 2. For Equitable officials, see "The MacNeil/Lehrer News Hour," 9.

38. Danann quoted in "Monitoring Compounds Worker Stress from VDT Units," *Occupational Safety & Health Reporter;* ACLU, *Liberty at Work,* 9–11.

39. "Statistical Compensation Survey," *DEMA,* 2.

40. Michael J. Smith, Pascale Sainfort, Katherine Rogers, and David LeGrande, *Electronic Performance Monitoring and Job Stress in Telecommunications Jobs* (Madison: University of Wisconsin, Department of Industrial Engineering and the Communications Workers of America, 1990); "Occupational Stress Insurance Claims Grow as Workers Confront More Office Technology," *Occupational Safety & Health Reporter,* October 26, 1988, 1071; "Survey of VDT Users Indicates Link Between

Health Problems, Monitoring," *Occupational Safety & Health,* 560; Brod, *Technostress.*

41. For Connecticut telephone workers, see Fogel, "Electronic Boss," 13; "Bell Canada Counts Group, Not Individual, Keystrokes," *VDT News,* November/December 1989, 8.

42. Margery W. Davies, *Women's Place Is at the Typewriter* (Philadelphia: Temple University Press, 1982), 51–53, 102.

43. BLS, *Employment and Earnings,* tables 9 and 39; percentage calculated by the author. See also Women's Bureau, *1993 Handbook on Women Workers,* 34–35, 235.

44. *Indoor Air Quality: A National Survey of Office Worker Attitudes,* public opinion poll for Honeywell, Inc., 1985, cited in "Numbers Worth Knowing," *VDT News,* May/June 1987, 2. Despite the computer's widespread use throughout American society, the BLS does not maintain statistics on the number of women who use VDTs. This point was verified in telephone conversations with two Department of Labor officials: Mary Murphree, New York office of the Women's Bureau; and Larry Drake, Occupational Outlook section, BLS, Washington, D.C., July 19, 1990.

45. 1994 national median earnings, ibid., 209; women's clerical workers' earnings as a percentage of men's, ibid., 210; both figures calculated by the author.

46. House Committee on Government Operations, *Dramatic Rise in Repetitive Motion Injuries and OSHA's Response: Hearings before the Employment and Housing Subcommittee,* 101st Cong., 1st sess., June 6, 1989, 36; OTA, Electronic Supervisor, 55.

47. Peter T. Kilborn, "Rise in Worker Injuries Is Laid to the Computer," *New York Times,* November 16, 1989, p. A24.

48. Louis Uchitelle, "Surplus of College Graduates Dims Job Outlook for Others," *New York Times,* June 18, 1990, p. A1; Elizabeth M. Fowler, "Graduates Find Tighter Job Market," *New York Times,* July 10, 1990, p. D19.

49. Anne-Marie Schiro, "Secretaries' Poll on Computers," *New York Times,* March 14, 1983, p. 18.

50. Kelly Services, "Poll Says Secretaries Think Automation Makes Work Less Stressful," press release (Troy, Mich.: Kelly Services, 1984), 2.

51. 9 to 5, National Association of Working Women, *The 9 to 5 National Survey on Women and Stress* (Cleveland: 9 to 5, 1984).

52. Steelcase, Inc., *Office Environment Index: 1989 Detailed Findings* (Grand Rapids, Mich.: Steelcase, 1989), 65.

53. Kelly Services, "Tomorrow's Secretary," 1; and "Romance Growing Between Secretaries and Word Processing, but Love Does Not Necessarily Bring More Money," press release (Troy, Mich.: Kelly Services, 1984), 3.

54. Quoted in Brod, *Technostress,* 45–46.

55. Steelcase, Inc., *Office Environment Index: 1989 Detailed Findings* (Grand Rapids, Mich.: Steelcase, 1989), 63.

56. Schiro, "Secretaries' Poll," 18.

57. Kelly Services, "American Secretaries Say They Are Satisfied with Current Jobs: Yet Less than Half Would Advise Daughter to Pursue Secretarial Career," press release (Troy, Mich.: Kelly Services, 1984), 2, 3.

58. For stress in secretaries under age twenty-five in Kelly Services, see "Tomorrow's Secretary: Computer-Wise and Ambitious," press release (Troy, Mich.: Kelly Services, 1984), 2; Kelly Services, "Poll Says Secretaries," 1.

59. Hall, "Changing World for Secretaries," D1.

60. Kelly Services, "Romance Growing," 2; BLS, *Employment and Earnings,* table 39.

61. Kelly Services, "American Secretaries," 1–2.

62. John Maxwell Hamilton, "A Bit Player Buys into the Computer Age," *New York Times, Business World,* December 3, 1989, 24. Duchin quoted in Hall, "Changing World for Secretaries," D1.

63. Vary T. Coates, OTA, "Office Automation Technology and Contingent Work Modes," in U.S. Department of Labor, Women's Bureau, *Flexible Workstyles: A Look at Contingent Labor,* Conference Summary (Washington, D.C.: GPO, 1988), 31. Part-time workers are those who are on the company payroll but work for only a portion of the week. Temporary workers are outsiders who are provided by an agency to fill a company's particular need for a specific period of time.

64. Ibid., 30. Also, Barnaby J. Feder, "Bigger Roles for Suppliers of Temporary Workers," *New York Times,* April 1, 1995, p. 37.

65. For part-time workers, see BLS, *Employment and Earnings,* table 23. For the figure on temporary workers, Mary Murphree, U.S. Department of Labor, Women's Bureau, telephone interview, July 16, 1990.

66. Coates, "Office Automation," 30; Levine and Olsten quoted in "Time for Temps," *New York Times,* November 22, 1987, sec. 3, p. 1.

67. Robert E. Calem, "Working at Home, for Better or Worse," *New York Times,* April 18, 1993, sec. 3, p. 1; *Pros and Cons of Home-based Clerical Work: Hearings before the Employment and Housing Committee,* 99th Cong., 2d sess., February 26, 1986, 22; Giuliano, "Mechanization of Office Work," 163; Mattera, "High-Tech Cottage Industry," 390–392.

68. OTA, *Automation of America's Offices,* chap. 8, "Off-Shore Office Work"; "U.S. Clerical Work Sent Overseas," *Monitor,* October–December 1988, 5.

69. Hamilton, "Bit Player," 22–25; Coates, "Office Automation," 32.

70. Steve Lohr, "The Growth of the Global Office," *New York Times,* October 18, 1988, p. D1.

71. Kevin P. Power, "Now We Can Move Office Work Offshore to Enhance Output," *Wall Street Journal,* June 9, 1983, p. 32.

72. "The Instant Offshore Office," *Business Week,* March 15, 1982, 136E.

73. "Work Sent Overseas," *Monitor,* 5.

74. Hamilton, "Bit Player," 24.

75. Power, "Now We Can Move Office Work Offshore," 32. The computer industry is exporting manufacturing jobs to low-wage locales like the Philippines and Malaysia. Workers, who toil for long hours under harsh conditions, have been

denied their rights to organize unions. The U.S. government is required by law to monitor workers' rights, but has not done so in the case of these two allies. See Denis MacShane, "Dreaming of the Forty-Hour Week," *Nation,* May 15, 1989.

76. NIOSH, *Investigation of Health Complaints,* 13; emphasis added.

Chapter 3   ORGANIZING OFFICE WORKERS FOR OCCUPATIONAL SAFETY AND HEALTH

1. Adolf Sturmthal, "Comparative Essay," in *White-Collar Trade Unions: Contemporary Developments in Industrialized Societies* (Urbana: University of Illinois Press, 1966), 365–398.

2. "Choices in Development of Office Automation," in *Office Automation: Jekyll or Hyde?* ed. Daniel Marschall and Judith Gregory (Cleveland: Working Women Education Fund, 1983), 5–14.

3. Olov Ostberg, "CRTs Pose Health Problems for Operators," *Journal of Occupational Health and Safety,* November/December 1975; Gunnar Swanbeck and Thor Bleeker, "Skin Problems from Visual Display Units," *Acta Derm Venereol* 69 (1989): 46–51; "Face Rashes Linked with Use of VDTs," 150; "Skin Problems in Sweden," *VDT News,* May/June 1987, 10; Swedish law quoted in "Few VDT Rules Around the World: Despite Massive Use Sweden Alone Has Broad Law," *Women's Occupational Health Resource Center Newsletter,* April/July 1986, 1; also see Campaign for VDT Safety, *Summary of Regulatory Activity on VDTs in Other Countries* (Cleveland: 9 to 5, n.d.). TCO plans to release stricter MPRII standards in the near future.

4. "Council Directive of 29 May 1990 on the Minimum Safety and Health Requirements for Work with Display Screen Equipment," *Official Journal of the European Communities,* June 21, 1990, 14–18; Clare Newsome, "Are You Sitting Uncomfortably? Britain is Stubbornly Resisting Measures to Reduce Computer Injury, Risky Health and Output," *Independent,* February 13, 1995, 23.

5. National Labour Inspection of Norway, *Regulations for Working with Display Screen Equipment,* 1995.

6. Gwenda Blair, "Through a Glass, Dimly: Why 75 Secretaries at the UN Walked off Their Ultra-Modern Jobs," *In These Times,* February 28–March 6, 1979, 24; Ann Dooley, "CRTs at UN Prompt Workers to Walk off Jobs," *Computerworld,* March 26, 1979, 9.

7. Olov Ostberg, "The Health Debate," *Reprographics Quarterly* 12 (1979): 80–82.

8. "Few VDT Rules Around World," *WOHRC News,* 6; Campaign for VDT Safety, *Summary of Regulatory Activity.*

9. VDU Workers' Rights Campaign, *Conference Report: Time for Action on VDU Hazards* (London: City Centre, 1986), 3.

10. Letter to author from Gill Kirton, member of the ad hoc committee, VDU Workers' Rights Campaign, London, June 20, 1986.

11. "Few VDT Rules Around World," 6.
12. "NZ Journalists Win Benefits," *VDT News*, May/June 1988, 8.
13. John G. Kilgour, "Office Unions: Keeping the Threat Small," *Administrative Management*, November 1982, 23.
14. Cited in Steelcase, Inc., "Office Environment Index: Summary Report: United States," in *Steelcase Worldwide Office Environment Index, 1991* (Grand Rapids, Mich.: 1991), 14.
15. BLS, *Employment and Earnings*, January 1995, table 9; percentages calculated by the author. For BLS projection of new entrants in the work force, see "Needed: Human Capital," *Business Week*, September 19, 1988, 102–103.
16. U.S. Department of Labor, Women's Bureau, "Women and Workforce 2000," Fact Sheet No. 88-1, January 1988, 4.
17. Margery W. Davies, *Women's Place Is at the Typewriter* (Philadelphia: Temple University Press, 1982) and "Women's Place is at the Typewriter: The Feminization of the Clerical Labor Force," *Radical America*, July/August 1974, 1–28.
18. Linda Valli, *Becoming Clerical Workers* (Boston: Routledge and Kegan Paul, 1986), 197ff.
19. Alice Kessler-Harris, "Where Are the Organized Workers?" in *A Heritage of Her Own: Toward a New Social History of American Women,* ed. Nancy F. Cott and Elizabeth H. Pleck (New York: Simon and Schuster, 1979), 347–348. Also, see her *Out to Work: A History of Wage-Earning Women in the United States* (New York: Oxford University Press, 1982), 148; Barbara Mayer Wertheimer, *We Were There: The Story of Working Women in America* (New York: Pantheon, 1977), 235; Martin Oppenheimer, *White Collar Politics* (New York: Monthly Review Press, 1985), especially chap. 6, "The Hidden Proletariat: Women Office Workers."
20. Various researchers have uncovered employee feelings of resentment and insecurity beneath the veneer of identification with management. See, for example, C. Wright Mills, *White Collar* (New York: Oxford University Press, 1951), 305; and Roselyn L. Feldberg and Evelyn N. Glenn, "Clerical Work: The Female Occupation," in *Women: A Feminist Perspective,* 3d ed., ed. Jo Freeman (Palo Alto, Calif.: Mayfield Publishing, 1984), 330–331.
21. See Sharon Hartman Strom, "'We're No Kitty Foyles': Organizing Office Workers for the Congress of Industrial Organizations, 1937–1950," in *Women, Work and Protest: A Century of Women's Labor History,* ed. Ruth Milkman (New York: Routledge and Kegan Paul, 1985), 206–234; Kessler-Harris, "Where Are the Organized Workers?" 348–349.
22. Ibid. and Everett M. Kassalow, "White-Collar Unionism in the United States," in Sturmthal, *White-Collar Trade Unions,* 339, 356.
23. Deborah Bell, "Unionized Women in State and Local Government," in Milkman, *Women, Work and Protest,* 287–288; Dale Melcher, Jennifer L. Eichstedt, Shelley Eriksen, and Dan Clawson, "Women's Participation in Local Union Leadership: The Massachusetts Experience," *Industrial and Labor Relations Review* 45 (January 1992): 267–280.

24. Many railroad clerical workers were organized by the brotherhoods, and the United Auto Workers had some success at organizing the Big Three's office workers. See Mills, *White Collar,* 303–304; Kassalow, "White Collar Unionism in the United States," 305–364; and "Unleashing the White Collar: How UAW White-Collar Workers Have Been Making Their Own History for Nearly 50 Years," *Solidarity,* January 1985, 22. Exceptions to this rule include entertainment workers (including musicians, actors, and stagehands) and postal and other government workers.

25. Kenneth Noble, "Decline in Industrial Unions Cited," *New York Times,* October 25, 1985, p. A18; BLS, *Employment and Earnings,* table 40.

26. BLS, *Employment and Earnings,* table 42; "Public Sector Unions Fare Better in Their Less-Hostile Arena," *Wall Street Journal,* February 26, 1991, p. A1.

27. See Thomas Byrne Edsall, *The New Politics of Inequality* (New York: W. W. Norton, 1984) and Frances Fox Piven, "Structural Constraints and Party Development: The Case of the American Democratic Party," in *Labor Parties in Postindustrial Societies,* ed. Frances Fox Piven (New York: Oxford University Press, 1992), 235–264.

28. "Conference Told Union Organizing Must Focus on Women's Issues," *White Collar Reporter,* July 18, 1984, 77–78; American Federation of Labor–Congress of Industrial Organizations, *The Changing Situation of Workers and Their Unions* (Washington, D.C., 1985), 9.

29. BLS, *Employment and Earnings,* table 42.

30. President's Kennedy's Executive Order 10988, "Employee-Management Cooperation in the Federal Service" (27 F.R. 550, 551), January 17, 1962.

31. Bell, "Unionized Women in State and Local Government," 296.

32. National District 925 is an outgrowth of Boston local District 925 established in 1977 by 9 to 5 and the SEIU. See Ellen Cassedy and Karen Nussbaum's *9 to 5: The Working Women's Guide to Office Survival* (New York: Penguin Books, 1983) for a summary of its policies on office work.

33. NIOSH, *A Report on Electromagnetic Radiation Surveys of Video Display Terminals* (Washington, D.C.: GPO, 1977), 19.

34. "Display Unit Problem Brings Issue of Health and Safety to Industry's Attention," *Occupational Safety & Health Reporter* 9 (January 31, 1980): 810; Joann S. Lublin, "Health Fears on VDTs Spur Union Action," *Wall Street Journal,* October 27, 1980, p. 31.

35. July 6, 1984 issue, quoted in "Free Exams, Glasses Said 'In' for VDTs," *Guild Reporter,* August 10, 1984, 3.

36. "Effects of Video Display Terminals Examined in Two NIOSH-Funded Efforts," *Occupational Safety & Health Reporter,* December 20, 1979, 685; Cole quoted in Gail Bronson, "Video Display Units Blamed for Anxiety, Pains and Strains," *Wall Street Journal,* June 16, 1980, p. 18; Ann Dooley, "CRT Operators Strike at Blue Shield of Calif.," *Computerworld,* February 16, 1981, 4.

37. "Union Coalition Seeks Government Study of Video Display Terminals' Effects

on Users," *White Collar Reporter,* November 30, 1979, pp. A9–10.

38. See Jean Tepperman, *Not Servants, Not Machines: Office Workers Speak Out* (Boston: Beacon Press, 1976) and *60 Words A Minute and What Do You Get? Clerical Workers Today* (Somerville, Mass.: New England Free Press, 1976).

39. See Joann S. Lublin, "Secretaries' Revolt: Female Office Workers Form Groups to Fight Sex Bias, Petty Chores," *Wall Street Journal,* February 23, 1978, p. 1; Women's Work Project, *Women Organizing the Office* (New York: Women in Distribution, Union for Radical Political Economics), 1978; Elyse Glassberg, Naomi Baden, and Karin Gerstel, *Absent from the Agenda: A Report on the Role of Women in American Unions* (New York: Coalition of Labor Union Women, 1980); "CLUW Task Force," *VDT News,* September/October 1984, 15. For an overview, see Ruth Milkman, "Women Workers, Feminism and the labor Movement Since the 1960s," in Milkman, *Women, Work and Protest,* 299–322.

40. Cassedy and Nussbaum, *9 to 5.* Its reports include: *Race Against Time: Automation of the Office,* 1980; *Warning: Health Hazards for Office Workers,* 1981; *The Human Factor: 9 to 5's Consumer Guide to Word Processors,* 1982; *Nine to Five Campaign on VDT Risks: Analysis of VDT Operator Questionnaires of VDT Hotline Callers,* 1984; *Hidden Victims: Clerical Workers, Automation, and the Changing Economy,* 1985; and *Computer Monitoring and Other Dirty Tricks,* 1986.

41. On National Secretaries' Day strategy, see "How to Use the 9 to 5 Working Women's Agenda," flyer in *9 to 5 Newsletter,* March/April 1985. "9 to 5 Bill of Rights for the Safe Use of VDTs," in *Nine to Five Campaign on VDT Risks Hotline* (1983).

42. "Dynamic Trio: Three Labor Activists Lead a Growing Drive to Sign Up Women," *Wall Street Journal,* January 29, 1985, p. 1. Nussbaum now heads the Women's Bureau in the U.S. Department of Labor.

43. Jane Fonda, *Jane Fonda's Workout Book* (New York: Simon and Schuster, 1981), 244–248.

44. House Committee on Education and Labor, *OSHA Oversight: Video Display Terminals in the Workplace: Hearings before the Subcommittee on Health and Safety,* 98th Cong., 2d sess., 1984, 63.

45. Ibid., 65; William Serrin, "Computers in the Office Change Labor Relations," *New York Times,* May 22, 1984, p. B2.

46. House Committee on Education and Labor, *OSHA Oversight: Video Display Terminals in the Workplace,* 64.

47. Serrin, "Computers in the Office," p. B2. Equitable was also reported to be planning a nationwide reduction in claims staffing from four to three thousand. Canuso is quoted in House Committee on Education and Labor, *OSHA Oversight: Video Display Terminals in the Workplace,* 65–66.

48. "Why Clerical Workers Resist the Unions," *Business Week,* May 2, 1983, 126.

49. Ibid., 64–65; and Ruth Milkman, "Pink-Collar Unions: Breakthrough at 'The Equitable,'" *Nation,* December 3, 1983, 564–566; William Serrin, "Upstate Office Workers Gain a Landmark Pact," *New York Times,* November 10, 1984; Cathy Trost,

"The Price of Progress: Computers, While Increasing Productivity Have Spawned New Occupational Ailments," *Wall Street Journal,* September 16, 1985, p. 34C.

50. "Labor Gets a Little Toe in the Office Door," *Business Week,* December 3, 1984, 38; Peter Perl, "Clerical Workers Organized at Major Insurance Firm," *Washington Post,* November 10, 1984, and "How an Organizing Breakthrough Was Won at Equitable Life," *Public Employee Press,* December 6, 1985, 8–9.

51. Philip J. Jennings, "Organizing Bank and Insurance Workers: The International Experience," *Interface* (Spring 1987): 3–4. For a management perspective, see Keith Wharton, "White Collar Unions, European Style," *Administrative Management,* August 1980, 43ff.

52. For example, in June 1984, the Newspaper Guild sent model collective bargaining language to its locals that focused on VDT workers and their problems, including transfers for pregnant employees, rest breaks, eye exams. See "More Protections for Pregnant Workers, VDT Users Favored in Proposed Guild Program," *Occupational Safety & Health Reporter,* June 20, 1984. The SEIU had some success with the collective bargaining process, winning provisions to establish labor/management committees to study the NIOSH ergonomic guidelines in a Denver and California local. See "SEIU Contract with Kaiser in Denver Calls for HMO to Study Effects of VDTs," *Occupational Safety & Health Reporter,* May 23, 1985. The CWA won a similar arrangement with Pacific Northwest Bell. See "Company VDT Programs, Furniture, Hazard Studies Discussed at Conference," *Occupational Safety & Health Reporter,* March 3, 1986.

53. "Labor Gets a Little Toe in the Office Door," *Business Week,* 38.

54. "Pink-Collar Workers: The Next Rank and File?" *Business Week,* February 24, 1986, 116–118.

55. Michael A. Pollock, "Labor Goes After Its Great White-Collar Hope," *Business Week,* August 19, 1985, 41.

56. Herbert R. Northrup, "The AFL-CIO Blue Cross–Blue Shield Campaign: A Study of Organizational Failure," *Industrial and Labor Relations Review* 43 (July 1990): 525–541; "Unions Still Dividing Territory for Blues Organizing Campaign," *Daily Labor Report,* February 7, 1986, A2. No mention of the failure of this highly publicized organizing drive—which was chaired by the SEIU's John J. Sweeney—is to be found in a book on the white-collar work force that he coauthored with 9 to 5's Karen Nussbaum, *Solutions for the New Workforce: Policies for a New Social Contract* (Cabin John, Md.: Seven Locks Press, 1989).

57. The Newspaper Guild, "Third and Final Report of the Research and Information —Safety & Health—Guild Reporter Committee," 1986 Convention, 2.

Chapter 4   A QUESTION OF BUSINESS

1. Cathy Trost, "The Price of Progress: Computers, While Increasing Productivity, Have Spawned New Occupational Ailments," *Wall Street Journal,* September 16, 1985, p. 34C; Martin F. Payson, "Wooing the Pink Collar Work Force,"

Personnel Journal, 63 (January 1984), 48–53; and Martin Lasden, "Unrest in the Data-Entry Department: Time Running Out?" *Computer Decisions,* May 1983, 167.

2. Bruce Hoard, "Steps Outlined to Forestall Office Unions," *Computerworld,* February 15, 1982, 67; see also John G. Kilgour, "Union Organizing Activity Among White Collar Employees," *Personnel,* March/April 1983, 19.

3. Revenue percentage and quotation cited in a CBEMA membership pamphlet, circa 1986. CBEMA's total membership varies from year to year, but the large manufacturers, such as IBM, Apple, and Compaq, form the permanent nucleus.

4. Edward S. Herman, *Corporate Control, Corporate Power: A Twentieth Century Fund Study* (New York: Cambridge University Press, 1981), 2. Prepared Statement of Dr. Howard R. Brown, M.D., medical director, *New York Times,* and George Cashau, director of Technical Research, American Newspaper Publishers Association, in House Committee on Education and Labor, *OSHA Oversight: Video Display Terminals in the Workplace: Hearings before the Subcommittee on Health and Safety,* 98th Cong., 2d sess., 1984, 299.

5. Loren Stein and Diana Hembree, "VDT Regulation: The Publishers Counterattack," *Columbia Journalism Review* (November/December 1984), 42.

6. Senate Committee on Government Affairs, *Structure of Corporate Concentration: Institutional Shareholders and Interlocking Directorates Among Major U.S. Corporations. A Staff Study,* 96th Cong., 2d sess. 2 vols., December 1980, 26. See also, Jake Kirchner, "Senate Study Points to Corporate Interlocks: Among DP, Commun. Suppliers," *Computerworld,* February 16, 1981, 16.

7. E. E. Schattschneider, *The Semisovereign People: A Realist's View of Democracy* (Hinsdale, Ill.: Dryden Press, 1975); Murray Edelman, *The Symbolic Uses of Politics* (Urbana: University of Illinois Press, 1964).

8. National Council on Compensation Insurance, *VDTs and Office Safety: An Overview, Radiation, Stress, Vision and Ergonomics* (New York: 1986), 20–21; emphasis added.

9. Letter to author from David Durbin, research economist, NCCI, New York, December 15, 1988; "No Significant Increase in VDT Claims Despite Rising Public Concern, NCCI Says," press release (New York: NCCI, August 2, 1988), 3–4. The thirteen states that served as the basis for data collection were not mentioned in the NCCI report, nor press release.

10. "Occupational Stress Insurance Claims Grow as Workers Confront More Office Technology," *Occupational Safety & Health Reporter,* October 26, 1988, 1071; *Washington Post,* May 30, 1985.

11. "Occupational Stress Insurance Claims," 1071. Also, "VDT Operators Winning Disability Awards," *Guild Reporter,* December 14, 1984, 1; Laura Lent, "VDT Operator Wins Worker's Comp," *Ms.,* March 1984, 21.

12. Trost, "Price of Progress," p. 34C.

13. Bureau of National Affairs, *VDTs in the Workplace: A Study of the Effects on Employment* (Washington, D.C.: GPO, 1984), 27.

14. Milt Freudenheim, "Costs Soar for on-the-Job Injuries," *New York Times,* April 11, 1991, p. D1.

15. House Committee on Education and Labor, *OSHA Oversight: Video Display Terminals in the Workplace,* 299.

16. Renee S. Ross, "It's Finally Time to Debunk the Myth That VDTs Are Harmful to Health," *PC Week,* April 15, 1986, 41.

17. See House Committee on Science and Technology, *Potential Health Effects of Video Display Terminals and Radio Frequency Heaters and Sealers: Hearings before the Subcommittee on Science and Technology,* 97th Cong., 1st sess., May 12, 1981, 400–401. When Congressman Gore asked Wolbarsht if he was testifying on behalf of the computer industry, he replied: "just for this particular hearing" (401). But Wolbarsht had conducted a vision and VDT study for IBM the year before. See Myron L. Wolbarsht, F. A. O'Foghludha, D. H. Sliney, A. W. Guy, A. A. Smith Jr., and G. A. Johnson, "Electromagnetic Emission from Visual Display Units: A Non-Hazard," in *Ocular Effects of Non-ionizing Radiation: Proceedings of the Society of Photo-Optical Instrumentation Engineers,* ed. M. L. Wolbarsht and D. H. Sliney (Bellingham, Wash.: Society of Photo-Optical Instrumentation Engineers, 1980), 229:187–195. He later appeared in a CBEMA video asserting that VDTs do not affect vision. Wolbarsht quoted in Paul Hyman, "NIOSH Widens Probe: Checks CRTs for Health Effects," *Electronic Buyers' News,* April 30, 1980, 1.

18. Adia Personnel Services, *The Impact of Office Automation: 84/85 International Survey* (Menlo Park, Calif.: Adia Personnel Services [c. 1985]), 18.

19. For 1994 sales, see Alan Cane, "Survey of the Computer; Battle for the Desktop," *Financial Times,* May 31, 1994, 1. For the number of computers in workplace use, see "Is Your Computer Making You Sick?" *Open Computing,* February 1995, 20.

20. Norman C. Remich Jr., "Growth Continues; Appliance Industry," *Appliance Manufacturer,* January 1994, 22.

21. Ira Sager and Robert Hof, "If it Computes, It's Gonna Sell," *Business Week,* January 9, 1995, 75.

22. Rhett B. Dawson, "Unlimited opportunities; information technology industry," *Appliance,* January 1995, 56.

23. "Troubles with VDUs Could Be in the Job," *New Scientist,* August 27, 1981, 513.

24. Ibid.

25. COT's information brochure does not mention its prior existence as the Center for Workplace Technology. Nor does it mention the role that the rift between manufacturers and users played in COT's creation. Instead, it states that COT was created to "fulfill" the "need" for "a national clearinghouse for authoritative information on issues related to video display terminals and office automation." Still, COT's political function was the same as its predecessor: to coordinate corporate opposition in the effort to preempt the drive for VDT regulations. Center for Office Technology, information brochure, n.d.

26. In his book, *On Bended Knee: The Press and the Reagan Presidency* (New York: Schocken Books, 1989), Mark Hertsgaard described ANPA as being "as conservative a grouping as existed within the journalism business" (220).

27. Stein and Hembree, "VDT Regulation," 42; "Then and Now," *Columbia Journalism Review* (November/December 1986).

28. Stein and Hembree, "VDT Regulation," 43–44.

29. Ibid., 43.

30. Ibid., 43.

31. Ben H. Bagdikian, *The Media Monopoly,* 4th ed. (Boston: Beacon Press, 1989), 45.

32. "The Inside Story: Big Blue Surprise . . . ," *VDT News,* September/October 1986, 2–3.

33. Jeff Sorensen and Jon Swan, "VDT's: The Overlooked Story Right in the Newsroom," *Columbia Journalism Review* (January/February 1981): 32–38.

34. "The VDT Story: Why We Stick with It," *Columbia Journalism Review* (November/December 1984): 19.

35. Both articles were written by Malcolm W. Browne, "Experts Debate the Amount of Microwave Radiation that Can Cause Danger to Health," *New York Times,* December 27, 1977, p. 23; and "'Benign' Radiation Increasingly Cited as Dangerous," *New York Times,* October 21, 1980, p. C1. The closest the *Times* came to mentioning the VDT safety and health controversy during this period was a passing reference in the 1977 article to Paul Brodeur's concern about VDTs and radiation.

36. Gail Bronson, "*New York Times*' Video-Display Devices Ruled Out by Study as Cause of Cataracts," *Wall Street Journal,* February 15, 1978, p. 12.

37. John Noble Wilford, "A Study of Computer Terminals Finds the Radiation Insignificant," *New York Times,* May 29, 1981, p. B6.

38. Sandra Salmons, "The Debate Over the Electronic Office," *New York Times Magazine,* November 14, 1982, 132ff.

39. "Editors' Notebook," *VDT News,* May/June 1990, 2.

40. Don Bacheller, copy editor and Newspaper Guild shop steward, New York, April 26, 1992.

41. Sorensen and Swan, "VDT's," 32–38.

42. The killed story was by William Hines, "VDT's Can Hurt Vision: Expert," *Chicago Sun-Times,* March 11, 1980.

43. "The VDT Problem: Seeing No Evil," *Chicago Reader,* March 20, 1980, 4.

44. See "Computers Are Changing Newsrooms Across Nation," and "The Times is Planning to Install Soon an 'Electronic Newsroom' by Harris," in the *New York Times,* February 19, 1976, p. 50; also Sorensen and Swan, "VDT's," 32–38.

45. "VDTs: The Issue No One Cares About," WBAI radio, November 18, 1987. Pinsky has followed the VDT story as associate editor of *VDT News* and as a staff member for NYCOSH. He is author of *The EMF Book: What You Should Know About Electromagnetic Fields, Electromagnetic Radiation and Your Health* (New York: Warner Books, 1995).

46. The study also noted the close relationship between IBM and the banking

industry. In rank order, the top four institutional shareholders in IBM—with seats on its board of directors—were: J. P. Morgan, Manufacturers Hanover, Bankers Trust, and Citicorp. Senate Committee on Government Affairs, *Structure of Corporate Concentration,* 25.

47. IBM, *Securities and Exchange Commission: Form 10-K Annual Report for the Year Ended December 31, 1994* (Armonk, N.Y., 1995), exhibit 2.

48. During the 1980s, when labor launched its drive for VDT regulations, IBM's economic power was virtually unsurpassed. IBM ranked as the world's most profitable corporation for five years in a row (1985–89) and, it would have been number one again in 1990 if it had not been for Royal Dutch Shell's Persian Gulf War–induced windfall profits. Still, it was the second most profitable corporation ($6 billion) with worldwide sales of $69 billion. See "The Global 1000," *Business Week,* July 15, 1991, 52–53.

49. Robert J. Cole, "Dow Slips 7.18 for Third Consecutive Loss," *New York Times,* February 22, 1991, p. D6.

50. Robert Sobel, *IBM: Colossus in Transition* (New York: Bantam Books, 1983), 84–85, 117, 136. In 1932, the Justice Department charged IBM with monopolizing the tabulating card market; IBM pleaded guilty in 1934. In 1952, IBM was charged with monopolizing the tabulating machine industry; the Justice Department negotiated a consent decree with IBM in 1956. The last and most important suit charged IBM with monopolizing the computer industry; IBM was able to stall the case until the Reagan administration dropped the suit in 1982.

51. *United States Government Manual,* 1936. Cited in David Eakins, "Business Planners and America's Postwar Expansion," in David Horowitz, ed. *Corporations and the Cold War* (New York: Monthly Review Press, 1969), 145–146.

52. For Watson's relationship with Kennedy and Johnson, see Kim McQuaid, *Big Business and Presidential Power: From FDR to Reagan* (New York: William Morrow, 1982), 215, 219–220, 234–235, 254–255. For his ties to Carter, see Philip M. Stern, *The Best Congress Money Can Buy* (New York: Pantheon, 1988), 162.

53. IBM, *1990 Annual Report* (Armonk, N.Y.: IBM, 1991) 63. Former IBM chair and CEO Thomas J. Watson Jr., Carter's ambassador to the USSR, may also be included. For Dam, see IBM, *Form 10-K,* 2–3.

54. Doug Henwood, "Corporate Profile: *The New York Times,*" *Extra!* March/April 1989, 8.

55. Doug Henwood, "Times Mirror: Up from Manliness," *Extra!* January/February 1991, 10.

56. Richard Thomas DeLamarter, *Big Blue: IBM's Use and Abuse of Power* (New York: Dodd, Mead, 1986), 329.

57. Doug Henwood, "The *Washington Post:* The Establishment's Paper," *Extra!* January/February 1990, 11. Dave Moberg, "*Washington Post* Labor Struggles," *Extra!* May/June 1989, 1. For example, "Peter Perl . . . decided to report on a firm which trained companies on how to get rid of unions. When Perl disclosed he was from the *Post,* the firm's founder, Francis T. Coleman Jr., said admiringly,

'You're [the newspaper] considered a leader in this field.' Invited to attend one of Coleman's $325-a-day sessions, Perl discovered that of the 30 people there, four were vice presidents or managers of his own newspaper."

58. For Akers, see Henwood, "The *New York Times*," 9. For Petersen and Jordan, see Doug Henwood, "Dow Jones: Going for the Glitz?" *Extra!* May/June 1990, 10.

59. Ben H. Bagdikian, "The Lords of the Global Village," *Nation*, June 12, 1989, 807–811.

60. IBM, 1990 Annual Report, 62; Doug Henwood, "Capital Cities/ABC: No. 2, and Trying Harder," *Extra!* March/April 1990, 8–9.

61. DeLamarter, *Big Blue*, 329; Herman, *Corporate Control, Corporate Power*, 197–198.

62. Henwood, "Dow Jones," 10.

Chapter 5   THE FEDERAL POLITICS OF ERGONOMIC INACTION

1. *Public Papers of Ronald Reagan: 1983* (Washington, D.C.: GPO, 1984).

2. COT was known as the Center for Workplace Technology until its reorganization in 1985.

3. Quoted in Cathy Trost, "The Price of Progress: Computers, While Increasing Productivity, Have Spawned New Occupational Ailments," *Wall Street Journal*, September 16, 1985, p. 34C. See also Computer and Business Equipment Manufacturers Association, *Fact Sheet 2: Comfort Aspects of Visual Displays* (Washington, D.C., 1984).

4. See House Committee on Science and Technology, *Potential Health Effects of Video Display Terminals and Radio Frequency Heaters and Sealers: Hearings before the Subcommittee on Investigations and Oversight*, 97th Cong., 1st sess., May 12–13, 1981; *The Human Factor in Innovation and Productivity: Hearings before the Subcommittee on Science, Research and Technology*, 97th Cong., 1st sess., September 9–11, 15–17, 1981; and *Job Forecasting: Hearings before the Subcommittee on Investigations and Oversight*, 98th Cong., 1st sess., April 6–7, 1983. House Committee on Education and Labor, *New Technology in the Workplace: Hearings before the Subcommittee on Labor Standards*, 97th Cong., 2d sess., June 23, 1982. House Committee on Education and Labor, *OSHA Oversight: Video Display Terminals in the Workplace*, 98th Cong., 1st sess., 1983; and House Committee on Education and Labor, *OSHA Oversight: Video Display Terminals in the Workplace: Hearings before the Subcommittee on Health and Safety*, 98th Cong., 2d sess., 1984.

5. House Committee on Education and Labor, *OSHA Oversight: Video Display Terminals in the Workplace*, 98th Cong., 2d sess., 1984, 301.

6. House Committee on Government Operations, *Dramatic Rise in Repetitive Motion Injuries and OSHA's Response: Hearings before the Employment and Housing Subcommittee*, 101st Cong., 1st sess., June 6, 1989, 2.

7. Frank Swoboda, "OSHA to Defy House Ban with New Workplace Rules," *Washington Post*, March 20 1995, p. A1.

8. NAS, *Video Displays, Work, and Vision* (Washington, D.C.: National Academy Press, 1983), 213.

9. "Year-old Tubes Vision Hazards?" *Guild Reporter,* March 12, 1982, 1.

10. NAS, *Video Displays, Work, and Vision,* 235, 236.

11. "Newspaper Union Criticizes VDT Study As Understating Employee Health Hazards," *Occupational Safety & Health Reporter,* July 21, 1983, 178.

12. House Committee on Education and Labor, *OSHA Oversight: Video Display Terminals in the Workplace,* 98th Cong., 2d sess., 1884, 1–111. The NIOSH recommendations are on p. 212; for LeGrande's testimony, see p. 86.

13. Ibid., 113–208, 231–366.

14. Ibid., 301.

15. Ibid., 302.

16. Ibid., 301. Also see "Education, Not Legislation, Is Key to Alleviating Fears Concerning VDTs," *Occupational Safety & Health Reporter,* June 14, 1984, 26.

17. Panasonic Industrial Company and Professional Secretaries International, *The Causes of Stress in the Modern Secretary* (Secaucus, N.J.: Panasonic and Professional Secretaries International, 1986), 16.

18. Professional Secretaries International, "Professional Secretaries/Panasonic Conduct Survey on Secretarial Stress," News Release, (Kansas City: Professional Secretaries International, 1986), 1.

19. Steelcase, Inc., *Office Environment Index: 1988 Detailed Findings* (Grand Rapids, Mich.: Steelcase, 1988); cited in Michael R. Kagay, "Workers Want Their Employers to Listen to Them, Survey Shows," *New York Times,* June 14, 1988, p. A25.

20. House Committee on Education and Labor, *OSHA Oversight: Video Display Terminals in the Workplace,* 98th Cong., 2d sess., 1984, 301.

21. "VDT Health," a public service announcement produced by the American Council on Science and Health, n.d.

22. House Committee on Education and Labor, *OSHA Oversight: Video Display Terminals in the Workplace,* 98th Cong., 2d sess., 1984, 301.

23. American Council on Science and Health, *Introducing . . . American Council on Science and Health* (New York: American Council on Science and Health, n.d.). Theodore D. Goldfarb, ed. *Taking Sides: Clashing Views on Environmental Issues,* 4th ed. (Guilford, Conn.: Duskin, 1991), 153. For another example of the ACSH's proindustry, antiregulatory stance, see executive director Dr. Elizabeth M. Whelan's article, "The Charge of the Cancer Brigade," *National Review,* February 6, 1981, in Goldfarb, *Taking Sides,* 164–169. She maintained that the EPA's estimate that 60 to 90 percent of all cancer was caused by environmental factors was wrong and described OSHA's 1980 proposal that the workplace use of a handful of carcinogens be banned or restricted as a policy that "would require industries to invest large sums of money to protect their workers from allegedly harmful chemicals" (165). In the same volume (157–163), see Dr. Samuel S. Epstein's "Losing the War Against Cancer," *Ecologist* 17 (1987), in which he cites

the ACSH's industry ties and quotes a characterization of Dr. Whelan as a practitioner of "voodoo science."

24. American Council on Science and Health, *American Council on Science and Health,* 2.

25. "'People Problems' Must Be Solved Before VDTs Introduced, Study Finds," *Employee Relations Weekly,* December 17, 1984.

26. "Health Risks from VDT's Aren't a Concern to Most Companies that Use Them," *Wall Street Journal,* May 21, 1985, p. 1.

27. Trost, "Price of Progress," p. 34C.

28. "Health Risks from VDT's," p. 1.

29. "Use of Ergonomics 'Buzzword' No Guarantee that Workers Will Benefit, Researcher Says," *Occupational Safety & Health Reporter,* May 1, 1986, 1215.

30. William M. Bulkeley, "Technology: Computer Users' Ills Attract More Attention," *Wall Street Journal,* May 1, 1991, p. B1.

31. Charles Levenstein, "Worksite Health Promotion," *American Journal of Public Health* 79 (January 1989): 11. The editorial was prompted by an article in the same issue by Jonathan E. Fielding and Philip V. Piserchia, "Frequency of Worksite Health Promotion Activities," 16–20. Also see "Wellness Programs Are Promoted by More Firms. But a Critic Asks Why," *Wall Street Journal,* January 17, 1989, p. 1.

32. "Uncovering Health Dangers in VDTs," *Business Week,* June 30, 1980, pp. 52D–52E.

33. "Use of Ergonomic Furniture Grows; Proper Use Seen Key to Worker Health," *Occupational Safety & Health Reporter,* April 5, 1984, 1186; emphasis added. See also Channer's testimony in House Committee on Education and Labor, *OSHA Oversight: Video Display Terminals in the Workplace,* 98th Cong., 2d sess., 1984, 119.

34. Peter H. Lewis, "Paying More Attention to Furniture," *New York Times,* October 9, 1988, sec. 3, p. 11.

35. House Committee on Education and Labor, *OSHA Oversight: Video Display Terminals in the Workplace,* 98th Cong., 2d sess., 1984, 77–78, 80–81.

36. Mitchell Betts, "Opposition to VDT Regulation Continues in House Hearings," *Computerworld,* June 11, 1984, 28.

37. House Committee on Education and Labor, Subcommittee on Health and Safety, *Oversight of OSHA with Respect to Video Display Terminals in the Workplace,* staff report, 99th Cong., 1st sess., August 1985, 28.

38. News release from Congresswoman Mary Rose Oakar, "Oakar to Release OTA Study on Office Health Hazards," Washington, D.C., September 14, 1984, 1.

39. Letter from Congresswoman Oakar to author, October 22, 1984.

40. News release from Congresswoman Oakar, 1.

41. "Office Health Under Study," *9 to 5 Newsletter,* September/October 1986, 2.

42. "Potential Hazards to Office Workers Cited by OTA; More Research Recommended," *Occupational Safety & Health Reporter,* September 20, 1984, 336.

43. "Office Health Under Study," *9 to 5 Newsletter,* 2.

44. General Accounting Office, *Office Health Hazards: Federal Activities Funded in Fiscal Years 1981–1986* (Washington, D.C.: GPO, 1986); "NIOSH VDT Budget," *VDT News,* November/December 1984, 2.

45. LeGrande quoted in "Maryland Chambers of Commerce Opposed to Labor-Supported VDT Legislation," *Occupational Safety & Health Reporter,* August 1, 1985, 210.

46. Harvey J. Hilaski, "Understanding Statistics on Occupational Illnesses," *Monthly Labor Review,* March 1981, 25–29. Hilaski remarks that "after considering the recordkeeping criteria and the factors inhibiting detection and recognition of occupational disease, one can better understand why the BLS estimates of occupational illnesses are suspected of being seriously understated" (29).

47. Surgeon General, *The Surgeon General's Report on Health Promotion and Disease Prevention* (Washington, D.C.: GPO, 1979); OTA, *Preventing Illness and Injury in the Workplace,* (Washington, D.C.: GPO, April 1985), 5.

48. House Committee on Government Operations, *Occupational Health Hazard Surveillance: 72 Years Behind and Counting,* H.R. 99-979, 99th Cong., 2d sess., October 8, 1986, 11.

49. "Selikoff Gives Pessimistic Appraisal of Obstacles to Health Data Utilization," *Occupational Safety & Health Reporter,* May 10, 1984, 1315.

50. Thomas Edsall makes the same point in *The New Politics of Inequality* (New York: W. W. Norton, 1984), 140.

51. Arthur Oleinick and Jeremy V. Gluck, "Faulty Data Play Down Job Injuries," *New York Times,* August 15, 1993, sec. 3, p. 13.

52. For the lack of VDT related CTD statistics, see Lawrence J. Fine, M.D., director, Division of Surveillance, Hazard Evaluations, and Field Studies, NIOSH, in House Committee on Government Operations, *Dramatic Rise in Repetitive Motion Injuries,* 116. Also, in a telephone interview on July 19, 1990, the BLS's Larry Drake verified that they do not keep data on VDT-related CTDs.

53. National Association of Public Health Policy, Council on Occupational and Environmental Health, Women's Committee, *Women's Occupational Health Agenda for the 1990's,* working draft, March 1988, 1–3. Also see "Health Group Study Advocates VDT Standards, Supports Tougher OSHA Indoor Air Quality Rules," *Occupational Safety & Health Reporter,* October 21, 1987, 850–851.

54. House Committee on Energy and Commerce, *NIH Reauthorization and Protection of Health Facilities: Hearings before the Subcommittee on Health and the Environment,* 101st Cong., 2d sess., February 8, June 18, 1990. Also see Jeanne Mager Stellman and Joan Bertin, "Science's Anti-Female Bias," *New York Times,* June 4, 1990, p. A23.

55. Congresswoman Patricia Schroeder cited in Gina Kolata, "N.I.H. Neglects Women, Study Says," *New York Times,* June 19, 1990, p. C6. Also see House Select Committee on Aging, *Women Health Care Consumers: Shortchanged on Medical Research and Treatment: Hearings before the Subcommittee on Housing and Consumer Interests,* 101st Cong., 2d sess., July 24, 1990.

56. Philip J. Hilts, "N.I.H. Starts Women's Health Office," *New York Times*, September 11, 1990, p. C9. The GAO's report and a congressional hearing on the issue in June prompted the NIH to announce the establishment of an Office of Research on Women's Health in September.

57. Kolata, "N.I.H. Neglects Women, Study Says," C6.

58. Human Factors Society, *The American National Standard for Human Factors Engineering of Visual Display Terminal Workstations* (Santa Monica, Calif.: Human Factors Society, 1988).

59. "ANSI/HFS Standard Approval Renews Debate over Use," *VDT News*, March/April 1988, 3.

60. "Labor Applauds, Questions New ANSI Standard on VDT Workstations," *Monitor* (Summer 1988): 13–14; "ANSI/HFS Standard Update," *VDT News*, July/August 1988, 2–3. O'Neill quoted in "ANSI/HFS Standard Approval," *VDT News*, 3.

61. "ANSI/HFS Standard Approval," *VDT News*, 3.

62. "Job Redesign Needed, but Must Be Done by Employers Themselves, OSHA Official Says," *Occupational Safety & Health Reporter*, May 29, 1986.

63. House Committee on Government Operations, *Dramatic Rise in Repetitive Motion Injuries*, 89.

64. Ibid., 93.

65. Ibid., 107.

66. Ibid., 110.

67. Ibid., 130; "Adapt Work Stations to Workers' Needs, Experts Encourage Industrial Hygienists," *Occupational Safety & Health Reporter*, November 5, 1986, 599–600.

68. BLS, *Workplace Injuries and Illnesses in 1993* (Washington, D.C., 1994), 2. Also Peter T. Kilborn, "Automation: Pain Replaces the Old Drudgery," *New York Times*, June 24, 1990, sec. 1, p. 1; Maria Mallory and Hazel Bradford, "An Invisible Workplace Hazard Gets Harder to Ignore," *Business Week*, January 30, 1989, 92–93 and "Workplace Hazards Hit a Nerve," same issue, 104.

69. House Committee on Government Operations, *Dramatic Rise in Repetitive Motion Injuries*, 2.

70. The NIOSH statement is in ibid., 118; OSHA Notice CPL 2, May 12, 1986, quoted in "Musculoskeletal Disorders Addressed by Initiation of OSHA Inspection Program," *Occupational Safety & Health Reporter* 16 (June 12, 1986): 23.

71. Peter T. Kilborn, "Rise in Worker Injuries Is Laid to the Computer," *New York Times*, November 16, 1989, p. A24.

72. Swoboda, "OSHA to Defy House Ban," p. A1.

Chapter 6   THE NONPROBLEM OF NONIONIZING RADIATION

1. See Karel Marha, Barry Spinner, and Jim Purdham, *The Case for Concern about Very Low Frequency Fields from Visual Display Terminals: The Need for Further Research and Shielding of VDTs* (Hamilton, Ontario: Canadian Centre for

Occupational Health and Safety, 1983) and Karel Marha and David Charron, *The Very Low Frequency (VLF) Testing of CCOHS Terminals,* (Hamilton, Ontario, 1983). A unit of measurement of the frequency of electromagnetic fields, one hertz is equal to one cycle, or wavelength, per second.

2. EPA, *Evaluation of the Potential Carcinogenicity of Electromagnetic Fields,* review draft (Washington, D.C.: EPA, 1990); Bob DeMatteo, *Terminal Shock: The Health Hazards of Video Display Terminal Workers,* 2d ed. (Toronto: NC Press, 1986), chap. 2; Paul Brodeur, *Currents of Death: Power Lines, Computer Terminals, and the Attempt to Cover Up Their Threat to Your Health* (New York: Simon and Schuster, 1989), 231–232.

3. Thomas S. Kuhn, *The Structure of Scientific Revolutions,* 2d ed. enl. (Chicago: University of Chicago Press, 1970), viii, 5.

4. David Dickson, *The New Politics of Science* (Chicago: University of Chicago Press, 1988), 47.

5. Bromley quoted in William H. Miller, "Science and Technology Policy: Science Friction," *Industry Week,* May 4, 1992, 54.

6. NIOSH, *A Report on Electromagnetic Radiation: Surveys of Video Display Terminals,* by C. Eugene Moss, William E. Murray, Wordie H. Parr, Jacqueline Messite, and Gerald J. Karches (Washington, D.C.: GPO, 1977), 12–13. Parr quoted in Elliot Pinsley, "Automating the Printed Word," *Bergen Record,* March 11, 1980, p. A1.

7. See Paul Brodeur, *The Zapping of America* (New York: Norton, 1977) and two articles by Stephen J. Lynton in the *Washington Post,* "U.S. Radio-Frequency Radiation High," July 11, 1977, p. A10 and "Microwave Radiation Health Hazard Worries Scientists," July 10, 1977, p. A4.

8. R. B. Plunkett Jr., "VDTs in the Office: Hazardous to Your Health?" *New York Daily News,* May 26, 1981, p. 23. For the FDA report, see Bureau of Radiological Health, *An Evaluation of Radiation Emission from Video Display Terminals,* (Washington, D.C.: GPO), 1981.

9. See U.S. Army Doctor Phillip Winter's testimony, in House Committee on Science and Technology, *Potential Health Effects of Video Display Terminals and Radio Frequency Heaters and Sealers: Hearings before the Subcommittee on Investigations and Oversight,* 97th Cong., 1st sess., May 12–13, 1981, 118ff. Rep. Gore declared: "I think the significance of Col. Winter's testimony is that for the first time a government scientist has acknowledged that radiation in low levels can cause damage to the body." Quoted in Plunkett, "VDTs in the Office," 25.

10. The power density for pulsed rf/mw fields was limited to ten microwatts per square centimeter in the former Czechoslovakia, compared to one milliwatt per square centimeter in the United States. A microwatt is one thousandth of a milliwatt: DeMatteo, *Terminal Shock,* 61–65; and Lynton, "Microwave Radiation," A4 and "U.S. Radio-Frequency Radiation High," A10.

11. Paul Hyman, "NIOSH Widens Probe: Checks CRTs for Health Effects," *Electronics Buyers' News,* April 30, 1980, 1. See Wolbarsht's IBM-sponsored study, "Electro-

magnetic Emission from Visual Display Units: A Non-Hazard," in *Ocular Effects of Non-ionizing Radiation*, ed. M. L. Wolbarsht and D. H. Sliney (Bellingham, Wash.: Society of Photo-Optical Instrumentation Engineers, 1980), 187–195.

12. House Committee on Science and Technology, *Potential Health Effects of Video Display Terminals*, 193.

13. Ibid., 395.

14. "The Story That Never Was . . . ," *VDT News*, September/October 1986, 3.

15. The Gore/Villforth exchange is in House Committee on Science and Technology, *Potential Health Effects of Video Display Terminals*, 90–91. The use of the phrase "Catch-22" is Gore's, p. 11. "Where is the FDA Hiding?" *VDT News*, March/April 1992, 3.

16. NAS, *Video Displays, Work, and Vision* (Washington, D.C.: National Academy Press, 1983), 3, 59–60.

17. Philip M. Boffey, *New York Times*, July 12, 1983, p. B1; John Wilke, *Washington Post*, July 12, 1983, p. A3.

18. Parr quoted in Pinsley, "Automating the Printed Word," A1. Wolbarsht quoted Hyman, "NIOSH Widens Probe," 1; emphasis added.

19. See "Appendix A. Summary of Adverse Pregnancy Clusters Involving VDTs in Canada and U.S.," in 9 to 5, National Association of Working Women, "Technical Memorandum: Campaign on VDT Risks" and "Update" (Cleveland: 9 to 5, 1983); DeMatteo, *Terminal Shock*, 84–85; Brodeur, *Currents of Death*, 27, 243; "Eleventh Problem Pregnancy Cluster Reported," *VDT News*, May/June 1984, 6–7; and Dana Priest, "Miscarriages at *USA Today* Cause Concern," *Washington Post*, December 9, 1988, p. A1.

20. 9 to 5, National Association of Working Women, *Analysis of VDT Operator Questionnaires of VDT Hotline Callers* (Cleveland: 9 to 5, 1984); "Birth Defect and Miscarriage Clusters Stir Up More Fears Over VDTs," *Microwave News*, November 1981, 1.

21. NIOSH, *Health Hazard Evaluation Report: General Telephone Company of Michigan, Alma, MI* (Cincinnati: NIOSH, 1985), 6.

22. *Toronto Star* worker quoted in Joann S. Lublin, "Health Fears on VDTs Spur Union Action," *Wall Street Journal*, October 27, 1980, p. 31. *Computerworld* quoted in "The Next Asbestos?" *VDT News*, May/June 1985, 2. On the asbestos cover-up, see Paul Brodeur, *Outrageous Misconduct: The Asbestos Industry on Trial* (New York: Pantheon, 1985).

23. Lynn Haber, "Union Contract Targets VDT Users," *Computerworld*, September 26, 1983, 2; Lois Paul, "Pregnant CRT Operators Win Work Boycott," *Computerworld*, April 20, 1981, 14; "More Protections for Pregnant Workers, VDT Users Favored in Proposed Guild Program," *Occupational Safety & Health Reporter*, June 28, 1984, 67; "Contracts in California," *VDT News*, September/October 1984, 15; Tamar Lewin, "Protecting the Baby: Work in Pregnancy Poses Legal Frontier," *New York Times*, August 2, 1988, p. A1.

24. "Special Clauses for Pregnant VDT Users, 'Hypocrisy' of Health Concerns are

Criticized," *Occupational Safety & Health Reporter,* January 25, 1989, 1519–1520.

25. LeGates quoted in Joann S. Lublin, "Fearing Radiation, Pregnant Women Win Transfers from Work on Video Terminals," *Wall Street Journal,* April 6, 1984, p. 31. James quoted in David Myers, "Pregnant Users Seek Non-VDT Reassignments," *Computerworld,* April 30, 1984, 1.

26. José M. R. Delgado, J. Leal, J. L. Monteagudo, and M. G. Gareia, "Embryological Changes by Weak, Extremely Low Frequency Electromagnetic Fields," *Journal of Anatomy* 134 (1982): 533–551; José M. R. Delgado, A. Ubeda, J. Leal, M. A. Trillo, and M. A. Majimenez, "Pulse Shape of Magnetic Fields Influence Chick Embryogenesis," *Journal of Anatomy* 137 (October 1983): 513–536.

27. Arthur Guy, *Health Assessment of Radiofrequency Electromagnetic Fields Emitted by Video Display Terminals,* report to IBM's Office of the Director of Health and Safety, October 29, 1984. Cited in DeMatteo, *Terminal Shock,* 79.

28. "IBM Report Recommends Shielding Older VDTs," *VDT News,* March/April 1985, 5.

29. "IBM Report Recommends Shielding Older VDTs," *VDT News,* March/April 1985, 5.

30. Ibid., 5–6; emphasis added.

31. The plant produced five hundred VDTs a day. See DeMatteo, *Terminal Shock,* 51.

32. Quoted in "IBM Releases Summary of Electromagnetic Radiation Assessment," *VDT News,* January/February 1985, 19.

33. See Note no. 1, and Pinsky, Zybko and Slesin, *Video Display Terminals,* 13; Brodeur, *Currents of Death,* 257–258, 260–261.

34. "Industry Group Protests Radiation Shield Ads," in Pinsky, Zybko and Slesin, *Video Display Terminals,* 23.

35. Press release, Swedish National Board of Occupational Safety and Health, Stockholm, January 30, 1986. For the Swedish study, see National Board of Occupational Safety and Health, "Effects of Pulsed Magnetic Fields on Embryonic Development in Mice," January 30, 1986.

36. "Swedish Study Renews Concern Over VDT Pregnancy Risks," *Office Health & Safety Monitor,* April 1986, 1.

37. Per Isaksson, "Computers May Pose Risk to Pregnant Women, Scientists Say," Reuters, January 30, 1986; Louis Slesin, "The (Nearly) Silent Treatment," *Columbia Journalism Review* (May/June 1986): 23–24; "U.S. Computer Industry Reacts Swiftly," *Office Health & Safety Monitor,* April 1986, 10.

38. OTA, *Automation of America's Offices* (Washington, D.C.: GPO, 1985), 20; "OTA Report on Office Automation 'Needlessly Alarming,' Group Says," *Occupational Safety & Health Reporter,* January 16, 1986, 887.

39. "News Reports of Possible VDT-Related Birth Defects Based on Incomplete Evidence," Center for Office Technology, press release, February 6, 1986, 2.

40. "Swedish Study Renews Concern," *Office Health & Safety Monitor,* 10; press release, Swedish National Board of Occupational Safety and Health, February 13,

1986, quoted in *Office Health & Safety Monitor,* April 1986, 12.

41. Breidensjo quoted in "Swedish Study Renews Concern," 10–11; Swedish scientist quoted in "Swedish Mice Study Links VDT Radiation to External Fetal Malformations," *Microwave News,* March/April 1986, 2.

42. Tony Collins, "Can VDUs Cause Cancer?" *Computer Weekly,* October 7, 1993, 16.

43. "A Government Study of Risks from VDTs Is Temporarily Derailed," *Wall Street Journal,* February 18, 1986, p. 1. For quotes, see Slesin, "(Nearly) Silent Treatment," 23–24.

44. Jukka Juutilainen and Keijo Saali, "Effects of Low Frequency Magnetic Fields on the Development of Chick Embryos," Paper given at International Symposium on Work with Display Units, Stockholm, Sweden, May 12–15, 1986. The epidemiological studies are discussed in the EPA report, *Evaluation of the Potential Carcinogenicity of Electromagnetic Fields,* review draft (Washington, D.C.: EPA, 1990).

45. Brodeur, *Currents of Death,* 279–280, 292–293.

46. "Early PMF Exposure Shows Greater Effects," *VDT News,* January/February 1989, 2.

47. Marilyn K. Goldhaber, Michael R. Polen, and Robert A. Hiatt, "The Risk of Miscarriage and Birth Defects among Women Who Use Visual Display Terminals During Pregnancy," *American Journal of Industrial Medicine* 13 (June 1988). See also Tamar Lewin, "Pregnant Women Increasingly Fearful of VDTs," *New York Times,* July 10, 1988, p. 19; and "VDT Use Linked to Increased Miscarriage Risk," *VDT News,* July/August 1988, 1.

48. "IBM Shielding Move Prompts New Conflicts," *VDT News,* January/February 1990, 4–5. "Shielding Magnetic Fields: IBM Filed for Patent in 1987," *VDT News,* November/December 1989, 1; "IBM Cuts VDT Emissions," *Computerworld,* November 27, 1989, 6.

49. "IBM Shielding Move," 4–5.

50. "Canadian Develops Radiation Shield," *VDT News,* May/June 1988, 1.

51. "IBM Shielding Move," 5.

52. "IBM Markets Low Magnetic Field VDTs Worldwide," *VDT News,* November/December 1989, 1.

53. Bill Paul, "Radiation Study Finds High Incidence of Cancer Among Phone Cable Splicers," *Wall Street Journal,* November 29, 1989, p. B4.

54. On the lack of U.S. research, see "Radiation: New Mice Study Confirms Effects," *VDT News,* November/December 1988, 9. Slesin quoted in "Editor's Notebook," *VDT News,* March/April 1990, 2.

55. Paul Brodeur, "The Magnetic Field Menace," *MacWorld,* July 1990, 136–145; "Annals of Radiation (Part III—Video Display Terminals)," *New Yorker,* June 20, 1989, 39–68. The latter was expanded and published in *Currents of Death.* Magnetic field emissions are stronger in color than in monochrome monitors.

56. "Danger from a Glowing Screen," *Time,* June 18, 1990, 76; Louis Slesin,

"Uncovering Radiation," *Columbia Journalism Review* (July/August 1990): 4, 6; David Corn, "I'm Typing As Fast As I Can," *Nation,* July 2, 1990, 8; Peter Lewis, "Worries About Radiation Continue, as Do Studies," *New York Times,* July 8, 1990, sec. 3, p. 8; and Kim Foltz, "Adversarial, Successful Macworld," *New York Times,* July 13, 1990, p. D1. CNN Business News, "Moneyline with Lou Dobbs," June 7, 12, 14, and 19, 1990. For the computer industry's reaction, see June 7, transcript no. 113, 7.

57. "Computer Industry Abuzz over Radiation Risks," *VDT News,* July/August 1990, 3; "Industry Moves to Allay EMF Fears," *VDT News,* September/October 1990, 1.

58. CNN, "Moneyline," June 12, 1990, transcript no. 116, 3–4.

59. "Editor's Notebook," *VDT News,* January/February 1991, 2.

60. "EEC Requires Safety Rules," *VDT News,* September/October 1990, 4–5.

61. "Sweden Proposes ELF EMF Guidelines for VDTs," *VDT News,* November/December 1990, 3. The Swedish MPRII guidelines suggest that the ELF (5Hz to 2 kHz) magnetic fields not exceed 2.5 milligauss measured in three rings around the monitor at a distance of 50 centimeters (19.5 inches) from its middle point, and at 25 centimeters (9.75 inches) above and below the middle of the monitor. The guideline for electric fields is 25 volts per meter measured 50 centimeters from the screen.

62. Steven Greenhouse, "Europe Stumbles in Computers," *New York Times,* April 22, 1991, p. D1.

63. "Computer Makers Push for EMF Limits," *VDT News,* May/June 1991, 8.

64. "Industry Panel Proposes First U.S. EMF Limits for VDTs," *VDT News,* March/April 1991, 1.

65. "Push for EMF Limits," *VDT News,* 1.

66. James Ledbetter, "Zap Update," *Village Voice,* July 17, 1990, 9; "EPA on Electromagnetic Fields: Radiation Threat Upgraded," *VDT News,* July/August 1990, 1. Also see Philip Shabecoff, "U.S. Sees Possible Cancer Tie to Electromagnetism," *New York Times,* May 23, 1990, p. A22; William K. Stevens, "Scientists Debate Health Hazards of Electromagnetic Fields," *New York Times,* July 11, 1989, p. C1; The EPA's ranking system is as follows: Group A—Human Carcinogens; Group B—Probable Human Carcinogens; divided into two groups (B1—Limited Epidemiological Evidence, and B2—Sufficient Animal Evidence); Group C—Possible Human Carcinogens; Group D—Not Classifiable as to Human Carcinogenicity; and Group E—Evidence of Non-Carcinogenicity for Humans.

67. "EPA on Electromagnetic Fields," *VDT News,* 1; "EPA Describes Low Frequency Radiation as a Source of Concern, but Not Cause of Cancer," *Occupational Safety & Health Reporter,* June 27, 1990, 129–130.

68. "Editors' Notebook," *VDT News,* May/June 1990, 2.

69. Bromley quoted in J. A. Savage, "Further Study of VDTs Needed, EPA Reports," *Computerworld,* December 17, 1990, 96. Barnes quoted in "E.P.A. Said to Fight

Effort to Sway Report on Electromagnetic Risks," *New York Times,* January 14, 1991, p. A15.

70. "In Washington All Eyes Are on EPA EMF–Cancer Report," *VDT News,* January/February 1991, 3; Savage, "Further Study of VDTs Needed," 96.

71. "All Eyes Are on EPA EMF-Cancer Report," *VDT News,* 3.

72. "Effort to Sway Report on Electromagnetic Risks," *New York Times,* January 14, 1991, p. A15.

73. "All Eyes Are on EPA EMF-Cancer Report," *VDT News,* 4.

74. EPA, *Evaluation of the Potential Carcinogenicity of Electromagnetic Fields;* Curt Suplee, "Electromagnetic Fields: Draft Report on Hazards Generates Controversy," *Washington Post,* December 20, 1990, p. A21; Savage, "Further Study of VDTs Needed, EPA Reports," 96; and Philip J. Hilts, "Study Says Electrical Fields Could Be Linked to Cancer," *New York Times,* December 15, 1990, p. 12.

75. "Note to Reviewers," by Erich W. Bretthauer, assistant administrator for Research and Development, EPA, December 13, 1990.

76. Natalie Angier, "Sharp Rise in Brain Cancer Rates Found Among Americans Under 45," *New York Times,* December 11, 1990, p. C3.

77. EPA, *Potential Carcinogenicity of Electromagnetic Fields,* 1–5.

78. Hilts, "Electrical Fields Could Be Linked to Cancer," 12.

79. Curt Suplee, "EPA Radiation Study Far from Release; Long Review Process Under Way; Findings Expected to Be Inconclusive," *Washington Post,* August 14, 1991, p. A19.

80. EPA, *Health Effects of Low-Frequency Electric and Magnetic Fields* (Washington, D.C.: GPO, June 1992). Cited in "White House Report: EMFs Present No Health Risk," *VDT News,* January/February 1993, 4.

81. Christopher Anderson, "EMF Report Draws Fire," *Nature,* November 26, 1992, 288; Richard Stone, "Polarized Debate: EMFs and Cancer," *Science,* December 11, 1992, 1724–1725; "Where is the FDA Hiding?" *VDT News,* 3.

82. "CRT Use Linked to Cancer: Australian Study Finds Brain Tumor Risk for Women, Not Men," *VDT News,* July/August 1992, 1.

83. Sweden, National Institute of Occupational Health, *Forskning & Praktik,* 7/1992, "Cancers Related to Strong Electromagnetic Fields," 3–5, and "Power Lines Increase Cancer Risk for Children," 8–9; Also see Christine Gorman, "Danger Overhead: Two Swedish Studies Provide the Best Evidence So Far of a Link Between Electricity and Cancer," *Time,* October 26, 1992, 70; "Swedes Recognize EMF—Cancer Link," *VDT News,* November/December 1992, 1.

84. Marja-Liisa Lindbohm, Maila Hietanen, Pentti Kyyrönen, Markku Sallmén, Patrick von Nandelstadh, and Helena Taskinen, "Magnetic Fields of Video Display Terminals and Spontaneous Abortions," *American Journal of Epidemiology* 136 (November 1, 1992): 1041–1051.

85. EPA, *Potential Carcinogenicity of Electromagnetic Fields,* 1–5.

86. "OTA Sponsors VDT EMF Review," *VDT News,* November/December 1991, 1; "Congress Tunes In," *VDT News,* March/April 1990, 4–5.

Chapter 7   THE OFFICE OF MANAGEMENT AND BUDGET:
            OMBUDSMAN TO BUSINESS

1. Public Law 96–511, 94 Stat. 2812, 6245. Only the Federal Elections Commission is exempt from this requirement. Independent regulatory agencies may override OMB rejections by a majority vote, 6242–6243.

2. The Supreme Court, however, ruled that cost/benefit analysis was prohibited by the Occupational Safety and Health Act. In *American Textile Manufacturers Institute v. Donovan* (1981), Justice William Brennan said: "Congress was fully aware that the [Occupational Safety and Health] Act would impose real and substantial costs of compliance on industry," but "it believed that such costs were part of the costs of doing business." The Reagan administration then adopted a "cost-effectiveness" analysis that turned out to be cost/benefit analysis by another name.

3. See Gary C. Bryner, *Bureaucratic Discretion: Law and Policy in Federal Regulatory Agencies* (New York: Pergamon Press, 1987).

4. Unlike independent commissions, which regulate a particular industry, social regulatory agencies, such as OSHA or EPA, cut across industry lines. As they regulate more industries than independent commissions, social regulatory agencies usually incur a broader scope of business opposition.

5. "High-Level Review Group Organized; 'Midnight Regulations' to Be Studied," *Occupational Safety & Health Reporter,* February 5, 1981, 1226–1227.

6. House Committee on Energy and Commerce, *OMB: The Role of the Office of Management and Budget in Regulation: Hearings before the Subcommittee on Oversight and Investigations,* 97th Cong., 1st sess., June 19, 1981, 97.

7. Dr. Jay Bainbridge quoted in "NIOSH Planning Reproductive Study of VDT Workers," Louis Slesin and Martha Zybko, eds., *Video Display Terminals: Health and Safety* (New York: Microwave News, 1983), 73.

8. "NIOSH Cuts Back Reproductive Hazards Study," *VDT News,* January/February 1985, 4.

9. Howard quoted in "NIOSH Appeal Planned of OMB Rejection of VDT Reproductive Hazards Research," *Occupational Safety & Health Reporter,* January 16, 1986, 885. For the Southern Bell cluster, see David Myers, "Pregnant Users Seek Non-VDT Reassignments," *Computerworld,* April 30, 1984, 6. LeGates quoted in "Pregnancy and VDT Workers," *Business Week,* April 23, 1984, 80.

10. Marjorie Sun, "Federal VDT Study Finally Wins Approval," *Science* 232 (June 27, 1986): 1595; Susan Okie, "VDT Study Endangered by OMB," *Washington Post,* June 4, 1986, p. A21.

11. Teresa M. Schnorr, "The NIOSH Study of Reproductive Outcomes Among Video Display Terminal Operators," *Reproductive Toxicology* 4 (1990): 61.

12. Landrigan quoted in Okie, "VDT Study Endangered by OMB," p. A21; "NIOSH Cuts Back," *VDT News,* 4.

13. Suzanne G. Haynes, "Presentation at the American Heart Association Science

Writers Forum," Monterey, Calif., January, 1985. This was followed by the release of the NCCOSH's report, *Office Workers: Stress Survey Results,* in March. "Angina Study Suggests Elevated Risk for VDT Users, Researchers Tell Meeting," *Occupational Safety & Health Reporter,* January 24, 1985, 624. "CWA North Carolina Study Reports Link Between VDT Use, Angina: Urges More Research," *Occupational Safety & Health Reporter,* March 28, 1985, 828.

14. "Angina Study Suggests Elevated Risk for VDT Users, Researchers Tell Meeting," *Occupational Safety & Health Reporter,* January 24, 1985, 624. North Carolina Committee for Occupational Safety and Health, *Office Workers: Stress Survey Results* (March 1985). "CWA North Carolina Study Reports Link Between VDT Use, Angina: Urges More Research," *Occupational Safety & Health Reporter,* March 28, 1985, 828. NIOSH, *Health Hazard Evaluation Report: AT&T, Southern Bell and United Telephone, North Carolina* (Cincinnati, May 1986), 2. Also, see the exchange between Teresa M. Schnorr, Michael J. Thun, William E. Halperin, "Chest Pain in Users of Video Display Terminals," and "Reply," by Andrea Z. LaCroix and Suzanne G. Haynes, *JAMA* 257 (February 6, 1987): 627–628.

15. Mark A. Pinsky, "O.M.B.'s Chokehold on Government," *Nation,* January 23, 1988, 91. In 1976, MacMahon defended DuPont against congressional charges that it obstructed the release of employee cancer rate data. "Toxic Control Law Needs Helping Hand," *Chemical Week,* December 15, 1976, 37. In 1982, he chaired a panel that criticized a proposed Veterans Administration study of Dow Chemical's Agent Orange as resting on an "insecure scientific base." Philip M. Boffey, "Panel Sees Problem in Study of Effects of Agent Orange," *New York Times,* November 10, 1982, p. A26. Despite the fact that chlordane was a known carcinogen, Dr. MacMahon testified in 1983 on behalf of the Velsicol Chemical Company's claim that its pesticide did not cause cancer. Samuel Epstein, *The Politics of Cancer* (Garden City, N.Y.: Anchor Books, 1979), 271–281. See his comments on the shortcomings of MacMahon's study, 275; "How Velsicol Pitched Its Case for Chlordane," *Chemical Week,* July 27, 1983, 34.

16. *PR Newswire,* February 10, 1986; "Proposed Standard Threatens Beryllium," *Aviation Week,* May 1, 1978, 44.

17. Okie, "VDT Study Endangered by OMB," p. A21.

18. Howard quoted in "NIOSH Appeal Planned of OMB Rejection of VDT Reproductive Hazards Research," *Occupational Safety & Health Reporter,* January 16, 1986, 885. House Committee on Education and Labor, *Oversight of OSHA with Respect to Video Display Terminals in the Workplace,* staff report, Subcommittee on Health and Safety, 99th Cong., 1st sess., August 1985.

19. Pinsky, "O.M.B.'s Chokehold," 91; Richard Corrigan, "VDT Study Is Short-Circuited," *National Journal,* May 10, 1986, 1117. LeGrande quoted in Okie, "VDT Study Endangered by OMB," p. A21.

20. House Committee on Government Operations, *Occupational Health Hazard Surveillance: 72 Years Behind and Counting,* H.R. 99–979, 99th Cong., 2d sess., October 8, 1986, 24; Schnorr quoted in "NIOSH Appeal Planned of OMB

Rejection," *Occupational Safety & Health Reporter,* 885.

21. House Committee on Government Operations, *Occupational Health Hazards: Joint Hearing before Certain Subcommittees of the Committee on Government Operations,* 99th Cong., 2d sess., April 16, 1986, 88.

22. Nussbaum quoted in "VDT Study," *9 to 5 Newsletter,* September/October 1986, 2. Weiss quoted in Corrigan, "VDT Study is Short-Circuited," 1117.

23. Wendy L. Gramm to Senator Carl Levin, n.d., (received by Levin's office on December 16, 1986), 4; Dale quoted in Okie, "VDT Study Endangered by OMB."

24. Pinsky, "O.M.B.'s Chokehold," 91.

25. "NIOSH Appeal Planned of OMB Rejection," *Occupational Safety & Health Reporter,* 885.

26. House Committee on Government Operations, *Occupational Health Hazards,* 160–161.

27. "Work on BellSouth Data Collection Starts Despite Questions on Study's Credibility," *Occupational Safety & Health Reporter,* July 31, 1986, 218.

28. Congressman Weiss to Otis R. Bowen, Secretary of Health and Human Services, October 20, 1986. Dr. Diana Zuckerman, a member of Weiss's staff, reports that BellSouth was more afraid of lawsuits based on stress than radiation at the time. Telephone conversation with author, June 15, 1991.

29. House Committee on Government Operations, *Occupational Health Hazards,* 161.

30. Millar quoted in ibid., 161. NIOSH VDT study staff members met privately with BellSouth officials on December 20, 1985. The BellSouth consultants conducted two more reviews, with OMB's approval, of the revised versions of the study protocol during the winter and spring of 1986.

31. OMB also required the documentation of all adverse reproductive cases by medical records, its approval for any follow-up studies, and the rewriting of the introductory letter to be sent to the study's participants. James B. MacRae Jr., chief, Reports Management Branch, OIRA, OMB, to Barbara S. Wamsley, HHS, June 6, 1986, in House Committee on Government Operations, *Occupational Health Hazards,* 271. Selikoff quoted on 287; Butler on 284.

32. Teresa Schnorr et al., *Response to the Third (April 2, 1986) BellSouth Review of the Protocol for the Reproductive Study of Female Video Display Terminal Operators,* Cincinnati, April 9, 1986, 3. "OMB Decision Allows VDT Study, but NIOSH Is Wary of Requirements," *Daily Labor Report,* June 11, 1986, p. A12.

33. MacRae to Wamsley, in House Committee on Government Operations, *Occupational Health Hazards,* 271.

34. Schnorr et al., *Response to the Third (April 2, 1986) BellSouth Review,* 2.

35. Selikoff to Weiss, in House Committee on Government Operations, *Occupational Health Hazards,* 287. LeGrande quoted in "OMB Decision Allows VDT Study," *Daily Labor Report,* A12.

36. OTA, *Review of Questions Deleted from a NIOSH Study of Video Display Terminal Users* (Washington, D.C.: OTA, 1986), 8.

37. "HHS Secretary Urged by Weiss to Override OMB Restrictions on NIOSH

Pregnancy Study," *Occupational Safety & Health Reporter,* Sept. 17, 1986, 406–407.

38. "Asking the Right Questions," *National Journal,* September 6, 1986, 2089; "Congressman Requests that Bowen Clarify Stand on Reproductive Study at Bell-South," *Occupational Safety & Health Reporter,* November 26, 1986; "HHS Secretary Urged by Union to Override OMB Restrictions on NIOSH Pregnancy Study," *Occupational Safety & Health Reporter,* December 24, 1986, 821–822.

39. Letter by Sally Zierler, Dr.P.H., to Congressman Ted Weiss, October 9, 1986, 5–6. Zierler said the other consultant, Brian MacMahon, agreed in spirit, but he did not come forward to change his assessment of the VDT study.

40. Ibid., 6.

41. House Committee on Government Operations, *Occupational Health Hazard Surveillance,* 18, 24.

42. "BellSouth Consultant Revises Stand on NIOSH Study Questions Deleted by OMB," *Occupational Safety & Health Reporter,* October 29, 1986, 564–565.

43. Otis R. Bowen, secretary of Health and Human Services, to Congressman Augustus F. Hawkins, November 12, 1986.

44. Hawkins to Bowen, November 17, 1986; Bowen to Hawkins, December 23, 1986.

45. Letter by Senator Carl Levin to James C. Miller, November 3, 1986, 2. Contrast Bowen's silence on the VDT issue with the *New York Times* portrayal of him a few months earlier: "Dr. Bowen . . . arrived full of his own ideas, and he has not been hesitant to speak about them." Robert Pear, "Setting Up Practice in the Health Bureaucracy: Dr. Otis R. Bowen," March 31, 1986, p. A12.

46. Letter from Gramm to Levin, 1.

47. "NIOSH Reproductive Health Study to Begin," *Occupational Safety & Health Reporter,* 1455.

48. "Industry, Worker Groups Disagree on Implications of Swedish VDT Health Study," *Occupational Safety & Health Reporter,* September 2, 1987.

49. Teresa M. Schnorr et al., "Video Display Terminals and the Risk of Spontaneous Abortion," *New England Journal of Medicine* 324 (March 14, 1991): 727.

50. "NIOSH to Study Effects of VDTs," *Occupational Safety & Health Reporter,* 565; "NIOSH Cuts Back," *VDT News,* 4–7. NIOSH decided not to include a check of EMFs in 1984 and did not measure them until the study was nearly done.

51. Dr. Michele Marcus of the Mt. Sinai School of Medicine, New York, said, "I am concerned about its limitations—particularly that it could not address ELF EMFs since the control group was exposed." In "NIOSH Finds No VDT Miscarriage Risk; EMF Conclusion Sparks Debate," *Microwave News,* March/April 1991, 1.

52. For example, see William K. Stevens, "Major U.S. Study Finds No Miscarriage Risk from Video Terminals," *New York Times,* March 14, 1991, p. A22; Michael Waldholz, "VDTs Are Said Not to Increase Miscarriage Risk," *Wall Street Journal,* March 14, 1991, p. B1. Merrill Goozner, "Study Finds No VDT Link to Miscarriages," *Chicago Tribune,* March 14, 1991, 1.

53. House Committee on Energy and Commerce, Subcommittee on Oversight and

Investigations, *OMB Review of CDC Research: Impact of the Paperwork Reduction Act,* report by Barbara Boardman, Ian A. Greaves, Charles Levenstein, and Philip J. Landrigan, 99th Cong. 2d sess., 1986.

54. Ibid.
55. Ibid.
56. Senator Gary Hart, *Congressional Record* (July 24, 1986), vol. 132, S9600.
57. Senator William Proxmire speaking on January 27, 1986, in support of S. 2025. A bill to amend Chapter IX of the Food, Drug and Cosmetic Act to require that the commissioner of food and drugs be confirmed by the Senate. *Congressional Record* (January 29, 1986), vol. 132, pt. 6, S470.
58. "Washington Wire," *Wall Street Journal,* June 6, 1983, p. 1; Michael L. Millenson, "FDA 'Politicization,' Called Hazardous to Health," *Chicago Tribune,* October 20, 1985, p. 10.
59. House Committee on Energy and Commerce, *OMB Review of CDC Research,* S11722–11724.
60. "Remarks of the Honorable John D. Dingell on Workplace Health and Safety, May 5, 1987," inserted in the record by Congressman William D. Ford, *Congressional Record* (May 5, 1987), vol. 133, pt. 71, E1737.
61. For example, see John B. Judis, "To Ginsburg, a Life Is Worth $22,094.93," *In These Times,* November 11–17, 1987, 3.
62. "Administration Moves to Give OMB Insight Into Pre-Rulemaking Planning," *Daily Report for Executives,* December 24, 1984, p. A12.
63. "Major Changes Promised in Oil/Gas Rule: Ethylene Dibromide Now Set for August," *Occupational Safety & Health Reporter,* August 15, 1985, 235–237. See EO 12498s defense by two former OIRA directors, Christopher C. DeMuth and Douglas H. Ginsburg, "White House Review of Agency Rulemaking," *Harvard Law Review* 99 (March 1986): 1075–1088.
64. "Withdrawal of Ginsburg Nomination Heads Off Brewing Controversy Over OMB Role," *Occupational Safety & Health Reporter,* November 11, 1987, 936–937. "Budget Office Will Screen New Policies: Less Regulation Goal," *Chicago Tribune,* August 9, 1985, p. 3.
65. The Reagan administration wanted even deeper cuts. House Committee on Government Operations, *Occupational Health Hazard Surveillance,* 5.
66. Congressman Ted Weiss, "Hold OMB Accountable for Review Activities," *Congressional Record* (September 20, 1989), vol. 135, no. 121, E3105.
67. Ronald Brownstein and Nina Easton, *Reagan's Ruling Class: Portraits of the President's Top One Hundred Officials* (New York: Pantheon, 1983), 414. Jonathan Lash, Katherine Gillman, and David Sheridan, *A Season of Spoils: The Story of the Reagan Administration's Attack on the Environment* (New York: Pantheon, 1984), 23.
68. "OMB is Limiting Agency Documents Released Publicly, Official Reports," *Occupational Safety & Health Reporter,* July 17, 1986, 148. Alan B. Morrison, "OMB Interference with Agency Rulemaking: The Wrong Way to Write a Regulation," *Harvard Law Review* 99 (March 1986): 1066.

69. House Committee on Government Operations, *Occupational Health Hazard Surveillance*, 24.

70. Proxmire, Congressional Record, S470.

71. "Whitten Supports Dingell's Request to Cut 1987 Funding for OMB Review Function," *Occupational Safety & Health Reporter*, July 10, 1986, 131–132; Ted Weiss's tabled bill (in 1989 and 1991) to limit OMB's regulatory review powers, see *Congressional Record* (September 20, 1989), E3105, and (January 3, 1991), E24. In the upper chamber, a bill sponsored by Senators Levin, David Durenburger (R, Minn.), and Warren Rudman (R, N.H.) called for public accountability for OMB's review activities; see "Bill Aimed at Disclosing OMB's Role in Rulemaking Introduced by Senators," *Occupational Safety & Health Reporter*, January 30, 1986, 919. David Corn, "OIRA Lives!" *Nation*, October 30, 1989. For general background, see Christopher H. Foreman Jr., "Legislators, Regulators, and the OMB," in *Divided Democracy: Cooperation and Conflict Between the President and Congress*, ed. James A. Thurber (Washington: CQ Press, 1991), 123–144.

72. Lawsuits filed by the public interest groups and unions had some success in forcing the Reagan administration to issue rules held up or weakened by OMB. The most significant victory came in the Supreme Court, which ruled seven to two in *Dole v. Steelworkers* 494 U.S. 26 (1990), that the Paperwork Reduction Act did not empower OMB to forbid OSHA from sending hazard notifications to third parties (i.e., workers). Linda Greenhouse, "High Court Decides Budget Office Exceeded Power in Blocking Rules," *New York Times*, February 22, 1990, p. A1.

73. "OMB Participation in Standards Setting Does Not Displace DOL Authority, Brief Says," *Occupational Safety & Health Reporter*, August 8, 1985, 219–220; emphasis added. See also David Burnham, "Suit Challenges U.S. in Revision of a Safety Rule," *New York Times*, April 10, 1985, p. A19.

74. MacRae to Wamsley, in House Committee on Government Operations, *Occupational Health Hazards*, 271.

75. U.S. Code, *Congress and Administrative News, 96th Congress, 2nd sess., 1980* (St. Paul: West Publishing, 1981), 6242.

76. The U.S. Constitution, Article II, Section 3. The Reagan administration made this argument in *Public Citizen Health Research Group v. Robert Rowland* (1986). The appellate court did not rule on this important constitutional question.

77. U.S. Code, *Congress and Administrative News*, 6244.

78. Ibid., 6265–6266.

79. Marianne Lavelle, "For Bush, a Subtler Approach: The Administration's Regulatory Game Plan Is Difficult to Fathom," *National Law Journal*, May 20, 1991.

80. Memorandum from President Ronald Reagan to Acting Secretary of Labor Alfred M. Zuck, January 29, 1981, in "Four Pending OSHA Actions Delayed Under Reagan Order; Review Promised," *Occupational Safety & Health Reporter*, February 5, 1981, 1225–1226. During Bush's 1988 presidential campaign, his

and Reagan's aides had OMB prepare estimates that deliberately inflated the cost of Dukakis's programs in the hopes of discrediting him in the eyes of the voters. See Richard Fly and Paul Magnusson, "How Bush Is Using OMB to Drop Bombs on Dukakis," *Business Week,* September 12, 1988, 47. President Clinton abolished the Council on Competitiveness by executive order in 1993.

81. House Committee on Government Operations, *Occupational Health Hazard Surveillance,* 28.

82. "NIOSH Reproductive Health Study to Begin," *Occupational Safety & Health Reporter,* May 27, 1987, 1455. Gramm admitted to Senator Levin that the VDT study would probably be "inconclusive, requiring another study." Gramm to Levin, 4. 1984 estimate is in "Pregnancy and VDT Workers," *Business Week,* 82.

Chapter 8   STATE AND LOCAL ARENAS: LABORATORIES OF DEMOCRACY OR LABYRINTHS OF FRUSTRATION?

1. For more on the economic blackmail, see Richard Kazis and Richard L. Grossman, *Fear at Work: Job Blackmail, Labor and the Environment* (New York: Pilgrim Press, 1982).

2. Quoted in "Reagan's 'New Federalism' is About to Have Its Day in Court," *Business Week,* October 7, 1985, 59. See also "State Regulators Rush in Where Washington No Longer Treads: Will the New Federalism Create 'a 50-Headed Hydra'?" *Business Week,* September 19, 1983, 124.

3. Mark Pinsky, Martha Zybko, and Louis Slesin, *Video Display Terminals: 1983 Health and Safety Update* (New York: Microwave News, 1984), 9. Mike Clancy, "Maine is a Testing Ground for Legislation," UPI, March 31, 1981.

4. Geri D. Palast, Director of Legislation, SEIU, Washington, D.C., letter to author, February 25, 1985.

5. "Labor Endorses, Management Opposes Proposed Connecticut VDT Health Study," *Occupational Safety & Health Reporter,* March 10, 1983, 836–837.

6. Pinsky, Zybko, and Slesin, *Video Display Terminals: 1983 Health and Safety Update,* 8–12; "Canadian VDT Ruling: No Loss of Pay for Alternative Work During Pregnancy," *Microwave News,* 2 (March 1982): 5.

7. Loren Stein and Diana Hembree, "VDT Regulation: The Publishers Counterattack," *Columbia Journalism Review* (November/December 1984): 43.

8. House Committee on Education and Labor, *OSHA Oversight: Video Display Terminals in the Workplace: Hearings before the Subcommittee on Health and Safety,* 98th Cong., 2d sess., 1984, 301.

9. OTA, *Automation of America's Offices* (Washington, D.C.: GPO, 1985); Smoot quoted in "OTA Report on Office Automation 'Needlessly Alarming,' Group Says," *Occupational Safety and Health Reporter,* January 16, 1986, 887.

10. Phil Blumenkrantz, "Activists Protest Hazards, Free Lunch," *The New Haven Register,* January 5, 1984, 48. UPI, n.h., August 25, 1982; Peggy McCarthy, "Face Race to Attract Technology," *New York Times,* April 17, 1983, Connecticut ed., sec. 11, p. 1.

11. Rick Brand, "2 GOP Leaders Get Gift from 'Grandpa,'" *Newsday,* August 12, 1988, 20.
12. "No Truce Ahead in the War over VDT Safety," *Business Week,* July 25, 1983, 86; "Campaign Against VDT Bills Organized," *VDT News,* January/February 1984, 5.
13. "Firm cites VDT bill in move to delay expansion," UPI, May 5, 1983.
14. "VDT," UPI, May 6, 1983; Oregon, *Report of the Senate Interim Labor Committee VDT Subcommittee on Video Display Terminals: Workplace Health and Safety,* 62d Legislative Assembly, September 1984.
15. Mickey Green, "VDT Safety: What's Known—and What Isn't," *Public Employee Press,* December 28, 1984.
16. Stein and Hembree, "VDT Regulation," 42.
17. Quoted in "Growing Activism on VDTs," *WOHRC News,* January/February 1985, 1. "Unions Mount Campaign," *Computerworld,* February 6, 1985, 8.
18. "Groups to Push VDT Bills," *Computerworld,* December 17, 1984, 8; "Joint Effort Is Launched by SEIU, 9 to 5 to Introduce VDT Legislation in 18 States," *Occupational Safety & Health Reporter,* December 20, 1984, 555–556.
19. New Mexico, Office of the Governor, *Executive Order No. 85-11,* Governor Toney Anaya, March 27, 1985. "New Mexico Governor Anaya Signs VDT Regulations for State Workers," *Occupational Safety & Health Reporter,* April 11, 1985, 883. 9 to 5, National Association of Working Women, *First Campaign for VDT Safety Victory; Governor of New Mexico Signs VDT Regulations for State Employees,* press release, n.d.
20. "The First State VDT Law . . . ," *Wall Street Journal,* June 18, 1985, p. 1; "Oregon Legislature Closely Passes First State VDT Worker Safety Bill," 41–42; *Occupational Safety & Health Reporter,* June 20, 1985; Maura McEnaney, "Ore: House OKs VDT bill," *Computerworld,* June 24, 1985, 14; "Oregon Governor Vetoes Legislation to set Guidelines for Buying Terminals," *Occupational Safety & Health Reporter,* July 18, 1985, 116.
21. Henry Weinstein, "Explosion in Use of VDTs Spurs Regulation Debate: Industry Denies Health Threat," *Los Angeles Times,* August 10, 1985, p. 1.
22. "A Politician's Convictions," *VDT News,* March/April 1986, 3.
23. "The Quest for High-Tech Plant Sites," *Chemical Week,* December 12, 1984, 68.
24. "Nearly every city and state is convinced that, as new industries replace old, survival will depend on attracting and nurturing high-tech industry," *Business Week* reported. "Every state and city plans to make it big." "America Rushes to High Tech for Growth," March 28, 1983, 84.
25. Ibid.; Tobi Lippin, "Hyping High Tech," *Technology Review* 89 (October 1986): 77–78.
26. "Reagan Due for Whirlwind Tour of Boston," UPI, January 25, 1983; Norman D. Sandler, "Hightech," UPI, January 29, 1983.
27. McCarthy, "Face Race to Attract Technology," sec. 11, p. 1.
28. "America Rushes to High Tech for Growth," *Business Week,* 84.

29. Vico Henriques, *The State Factor: Restricting the Use of High Technology in the Workplace* (Washington, D.C.: CBEMA, 1984), 1.
30. The board's decision was criticized by the majority of the ad hoc committee's members, who pointed out that Stranberg's recommendation mirrored the minority position of the committee's four industry representatives: two from IBM, one from Hewlett-Packard, and one from the California Newspaper Publishers Association. "Cal/OSHA Says No to Regulations," *VDT News,* July/August 1989, 8. CBEMA praised Cal/OSHA's rejection of VDT regulations as being "right on the money" (J. A. Savage, "California Board: Don't Restrict the Use of VDTs," *Computerworld,* July 3, 1989, 44).
31. Rose Marie Audette, "Help! I'm Tied to My VDT!" *Environmental Action,* November/December 1984, 25.
32. Loren Stein, "Coalition Fights VDT Legislation; Business Groups Fight Bills Intended to Safeguard Office Workers," *InfoWorld,* September 17, 1984, 47.
33. Quoted in Alan Howard, "How Corporations Took $2 Billion in State Taxes (and Nobody Noticed)," *Public Employee Press,* April 20, 1990, 5.
34. Ibid., 5. It is uncertain whether IBM paid the minimum state tax of $250; Xerox paid it at least once. The $250 minimum has since been raised, but the continued existence of loopholes permits corporations to skirt this "reform."
35. Ibid., 5. The study was conducted by the New York State Legislative Commission on the Modernization and Simplification of Tax Administration. The state tax department estimated that $383 million in ITCs would be claimed by corporations in 1992. John Riley, "Leichter Wants to Cut Investment Tax Credit," *Newsday,* May 16, 1991, 57.
36. Jeffrey H. Birnbaum and Alan S. Murray, *Showdown at Gucci Gulch: Lawmakers, Lobbyists, and the Unlikely Triumph of Tax Reform* (New York: Vintage Books, 1988), Appendix B: "The Evolution of Major Provisions Affecting Businesses."
37. Howard, "How Corporations Took $2 Billion in State Taxes," 4.
38. Quoted in Stein and Hembree, "VDT Regulation," 43; also see "Screening of VDT Stories Advised," *Guild Reporter,* November 9, 1984, 2.
39. Stein and Hembree, "VDT Regulation," 43.
40. Stein and Hembree, "VDT Regulation," 44.
41. Barbara C. Pringle, Ohio state representative, to author, January 16, 1985.
42. "Suffolk's Reckless Screen Scream," editorial, *New York Times,* May 26, 1988, p. A34.
43. "RSIs at the *New York Times,*" *VDT News,* November/December 1991, 3.
44. Interview with John Foley by author, Hauppauge, N.Y., April 12, 1988; Eric Schmitt, "Suffolk's Unusual Legislature: Incubator or Just a Hothouse?" *New York Times,* May 19, 1988, p. A1.
45. "Suffolk Legislators Vote a VDT Safety Measure," *New York Times,* June 24, 1987, p. B3; "Bill to Regulate Office VDT Use Passed by County Legislature; Signature Pending," *Occupational Safety & Health Reporter,* July 1, 1987, 179–180.

46. Advocates of VDT regulations saw two problems with the County worker law. First, it contained no enforcement provision, and second, it excluded employees in the private sector. They viewed the blue ribbon VDT panel as window dressing; Foley refused his appointment on these grounds. Realizing that the Foley bill had considerable support and that they had come so close to overriding the veto, proponents of regulation decided they had nothing to lose in going for the whole loaf. The blue ribbon panel made its recommendations (which paralleled the 1988 law) to County Executive Halpin in early 1989 and then disbanded. "VDT Task Force Report," *VDT News,* May/June 1989, 9.
47. No. 7158—A, "An Act to amend the labor law, in relation to video display terminal operators"; New York State Assembly, March 28, 1983.
48. Comparison of Resolution 1469-87 (the 1987 bill) and Resolution 1173-88 (the 1988 bill).
49. "VDT Bill Passed on Long Island," *New York Newsday,* May 11, 1988, 30; Eric Schmitt, "Suffolk Approves Video-Terminal Bill," *New York Times,* May 11, 1988, p. B2.
50. Rick Brand, "Halpin Vetoes Suffolk VDT Legislation," *New York Newsday,* June 11, 1988, 13.
51. The law called for the eye exam provision to go into effect in ninety days and training provisions to start in six months. The requirement that businesses purchase or lease equipment (i.e., furniture, lighting, glare screens) that met ergonomic standards was scheduled to go into effect on January 1, 1990. "Suffolk's V.D.T. Legislation Becomes Law," news release from the office of Legislator John J. Foley," June 14, 1988.
52. Eric Schmitt, "Suffolk Executive Vetoes a Bill for Workers at Video Terminals," *New York Times,* June 11, 1988, p. 1; Eric Schmitt, "Suffolk Overrides Veto of Video Terminal Measure," *New York Times,* June 15, 1988, p. A1; "VDT Bill Challenged in Court," WINS radio, June 23, 1988.
53. News release, New York Telephone, July 5, 1988.
54. "Dangerous Terminals?" *ABC Evening News,* August 8, 1988.
55. "Measure to Regulate VDTs Is Enacted in New York," *Wall Street Journal,* June 15, 1988, p. 10.
56. "Legal Challenge to be Mounted Against Suffolk VDT Law," press release from the Long Island Association, June 24, 1988, 2. Supporting the suit were the ABLI (which conceived the idea of a legal challenge), the LIA (which coordinated efforts to bring the suit), the Advancement for Commerce and Industry, LIFT, and the Hauppauge Industrial Association.
57. "Suffolk Law Stymied by Court Orders," *VDT News,* November/December 1988, 4–5; "Video-Display Terminal Law Blocked on L.I.," *New York Times,* October 8, 1988, p. 31.
58. Eric Schmitt, "Judge Thwarts Suffolk's Video-Terminal Law," *New York Times,* December 28, 1989, p. B3; "New York Judge Overturns Law for VDT Use,"

Wall Street Journal, December 29, 1989, p. B3.

59. "Court Rejects Suffolk Law, County Appeal Likely," *VDT News,* January/February, 1990, 2.

60. James O'Connor, *The Fiscal Crisis of the State* (New York: St. Martin's Press, 1973); *Testimony of Islip Town Supervisor Frank R. Jones: VDT Public Hearing of the Suffolk County Legislature, April 12, 1988,* 5.

61. Philip S. Gutis, "Video-Display Terminal Law Blocked," *New York Times,* July 14, 1989, p. B2.

62. "Businesses Sue to Void Nation's First VDT Law," *VDT News,* September/October 1988, 2–3.

63. Alan Bresnick, "City Thinks VDT Bill's a Pain in the Neck," *Crain's New York Business,* July 25, 1989, 2.

64. N.Y.C. Video Display Terminal Coalition, *Testimony of Diane Stein,* coordinator, Civil Service and Labor Committee, New York City Council, May 19, 1989, 5–6.

65. Arnold Lubasch, "Koch, in Veto, Discounts Risks in Computer Use," *New York Times,* December 27, 1989, p. B3; Bresnick, "City Thinks VDT Bill's a Pain," 2.

66. "Unions to Renew Push on VDT Protection Bill: Mix-up in Signals," *Chief-Leader,* March 9, 1990, p. 1. DC 37 bargains for all civilian city employees on the non-wage issues to be contained in the citywide contract. Matthew Tallmer, "City Agrees to Protect VDT Users: Under Accord with DC 37," *Chief-Leader,* June 15, 1990, p. 1; "VDT Health, Safety Accord: What It Provides," *Chief-Leader,* June 15, 1990, p. 4. "Union, City Agree on VDT Safety," *Public Employee Press,* June 22, 1990, 3.

67. It required employers with fifteen or more employees working at VDTs for more than four hours a day to provide them with work breaks, adjustable work stations, proper lighting and glare screens, and training. "San Francisco Extends Deadlines for Complying with Local Ordinance," *Occupational Safety & Health Reporter,* January 9, 1991, 1207–1208.

68. Bob Baker and Martha Groves, "Judge Overturns S.F.'s Landmark VDT Law," *Los Angeles Times,* February 14, 1992, p. D1.

69. Andrew Pollack, "San Francisco Judge Voids V.D.T. Safety Law," *New York Times,* February 14, 1992, p. A14; Harriet Chiang and Reynolds Holding, "Judge Tosses Out S.F. Ordinance on VDT Safety," *San Francisco Chronicle,* February 14, 1992, p. A1.

70. "Proposed California State VDT Standard Threatens New San Francisco Ordinance," *Daily Report for Executives,* June 3, 1991, A7. "It's a victory for employers, because they shouldn't have to deal with city-by-city, county-by-county regulations," said Jeffrey Tanenbaum, the lawyer for the two firms that filed the suit, Zack Electronics and Data Processing and Accounting Services. Chiang and Holding, "Judge Tosses Out S.F. Ordinance on VDT Safety," A1.

71. VDT advocates persevere in the hope of achieving a state-level breakthrough; forty-one bills were submitted in twenty states during 1991. Albert R. Karr, "Labor Letter," *Wall Street Journal,* December 31, 1991, p. A1.

72. "Maine Governor Signs Legislation Setting Strict Limits on Drug Tests," *Daily Labor Report,* July 13, 1989, p. A9; "Maine Training Law & More," *VDT News,* September/October 1989, 5. The law was amended to include employers with only five VDTs, effective January 1, 1992. "Editor's Notebook," *VDT News,* January/February 1992, 2.

73. Title 26, Chapter 5, *Maine Revised Statutes,* 1991; in 1986, Maine passed a law granting all workers, including VDT operators, rest breaks. Title 28, Chapter 20, *General Laws of Rhode Island,* 1991. The eight states are California, Colorado, Massachusetts, New Mexico, New Jersey, New York, Washington, and Wisconsin.

Chapter 9   WORKERS' SAFETY AND HEALTH IN POSTINDUSTRIAL SOCIETY

1. See AFL-CIO, *The Future of Work* (Washington, D.C.: AFL-CIO, 1983) and Kevin Phillips, *The Politics of Rich and Poor* (New York: Random House, 1990).

2. The NIOSH recommendations are contained in House Committee on Education and Labor, *OSHA Oversight: Video Display Terminals in the Workplace: Hearings before the Subcommittee on Health and Safety,* 98th Cong., 2d sess., 1984, 16–19. See also International Labour Office, *Working with Visual Display Units,* Occupational Safety and Health Series, No. 61 (Geneva: ILO, 1989), 8–9.

3. "Computer Makers Push for EMF Limits," *VDT News,* May/June 1991, 1; "'Green' Computing Comes to Sweden," *VDT News,* January/February 1993, 1; and "Clinton Directs US Agencies to buy Energy Star Computers," executive order, April 21, 1993.

4. On the failure of the self-regulating market, see Karl Polanyi, *The Great Transformation: The Political and Economic Origins of Our Time* (Boston: Beacon Press, 1957) and K. William Kapp, *The Social Costs of Private Enterprise* (New York: Schocken Books, 1971).

5. "Adapt Work Stations to Workers' Needs, Experts Encourage Industrial Hygienists," *Occupational Safety and Health Reporter,* November 5, 1986, 599–600.

6. Shoshana Zuboff, *In the Age of the Smart Machine: The Future of Work and Power* (New York: Basic Books, 1988), especially "Office Technology as Exile and Integration," 124–173.

7. "The MacNeil/Lehrer News Hour," PBS telecast, "Big Brother in the Workplace," December 28, 1983, 13.

8. "What the Health Researchers Say," *OUCH!* Spring 1993, 3.

9. See Larry Hirschhorn, *Beyond Mechanization* (Cambridge: MIT Press, 1984), 4.

10. Carole Pateman, *Participation and Democratic Theory* (Cambridge: Cambridge University Press, 1970), 62.

11. Benjamin R. Barber, *Strong Democracy: Participatory Democracy for a New Age* (Berkeley and Los Angeles: University of California Press, 984), 305.

12. See Thomas Byrne Edsall, *The New Politics of Inequality* (New York: W. W. Norton, 1984); Thomas Geoghegan, *Which Side Are You On? Trying to be for Labor When It's Flat on Its Back* (New York: Farrar, Straus, and Giroux, 1991); Patricia

Cayo Sexton, *The War on Labor and the Left: Understanding America's Unique Conservatism* (Boulder, Colo.: Westview Press, 1991).

13. Kim Moody, "Is There a Future for Unions in the Clinton Administration's Plans?" *Labor Notes,* October 1993, 16.

14. For advances in organizing and opening leadership opportunities for women, see Dorothy Sue Cobble, ed., *Women and Unions* (Ithaca, N.Y.: ILR Press, 1993).

15. Charles C. Heckscher, *The New Unionism: Employee Involvement in the Changing Corporation* (New York: Basic Books, 1988), 8–9. See also Casey Ichniowski and Jeffrey S. Zax, "Today's Associations, Tomorrow's Unions," *Industrial and Labor Relations Review* 43 (January 1990): 191–208.

16. Heckscher, *New Unionism,* 4–5.

17. Ichniowski and Zax, "Today's Associations, Tomorrow's Unions," 191–208; Deborah Bell, "Unionized Women in State and Local Government," in *Women, Work and Protest,* ed. Ruth Milkman (Boston: Routledge and Kegan Paul, 1985), 280–299.

18. Mary Hollens, "Workers Centers: Organizing in Both the Workplace and Community," *Labor Notes,* September 1994, 8–9.

19. See Frances Fox Piven and Richard C. Cloward, *Poor People's Movements: Why They Succeed, How They Fail* (New York: Vintage Books, 1977), especially chaps. 2–3.

20. See David B. Truman, *The Governmental Process* (New York: Alfred A. Knopf, 1965), 256–261; and Edwin M. Epstein, *The Corporation in American Politics* (Englewood Cliffs, N.J.: Prentice-Hall, 1969), especially chap. 8.

21. For more on the pluralist belief that policy issues arise separately, see Robert A. Dahl, *Who Governs? Democracy and Power in an American City* (New Haven, Conn.: Yale University Press, 1961), especially 85ff, 228.

22. Daniel M. Berman, *Death on the Job: Occupational Health and Safety Struggles in the United States* (New York: Monthly Review Press, 1978), 74ff.

Selected Bibliography

GOVERNMENT SOURCES

Federal Government

Congressman Ted Weiss. "Hold OMB Accountable for Review Activities." 102d Cong., 1st sess. *Congressional Record* (January 3, 1991), vol. 137, no. 1, E24–26.

———. *Health Effects of Low-Frequency Electric and Magnetic Fields.* Washington, D.C.: GPO, June 1992.

Library of Congress. Congressional Research Service. *Video Display Terminals: The Controversy about Health and Safety Issues,* by Christopher H. Dodge. Washington, D.C.: Congressional Research Service, January 6, 1984.

Library of Congress. Office of Technology Assessment. *Potential Office Hazards and Controls,* by Robert Arndt and Larry Chapman. Washington, D.C.: Office of Technology Assessment, September 1984.

———. *Automation of America's Offices.* Washington, D.C.: GPO, 1985.

———. *Preventing Illness and Injury in the Workplace.* Washington, D.C.: GPO, April 1985.

———. *Review of Questions Deleted from a NIOSH Study of Video Display Terminal Users.* Washington, D.C.: Office of Technology Assessment, August 1986.

———. *The Electronic Supervisor: New Technology, New Tensions.* Washington, D.C.: GPO, September 1987.

Science Advisory Board. *An SAB Report: Potential Carcinogenicity of Electric and Magnetic Fields: Review of the ORD's "Potential Carcinogenicity of Electromagnetics Fields" by the Radiation Advisory Committee's Nonionizing Electric and Magnetic Fields Subcommittee.* Washington, D.C.: EPA, January 1992.

U.S. Congress. House. *Committee on Education and Labor. New Technologies in the American Workplace: Hearings before the Subcommittee on Labor Standards.* 97th Cong., 2d sess., 1982.

———. *OSHA Oversight: Video Display Terminals in the Workplace: Hearings before the Subcommittee on Health and Safety.* 98th Cong., 2d sess., 1984.

———. *Oversight of OSHA with Respect to Video Display Terminals in the Workplace.* A Staff Report. Subcommittee on Health and Safety. 99th Cong., 1st sess., August 1985.

———. *National Institute for Occupational Safety and Health Oversight: OMB*

Involvement in VDT Study: Hearings before the Subcommittee on Health and Safety. 99th Cong., 2d sess., June 4, 1986.

U.S. Congress. House. Committee on Energy and Commerce. *OMB: The Role of the Office of Management and Budget in Regulation: Hearings before the Subcommittee on Oversight and Investigations.* 97th Cong., 1st sess., June 19, 1981.

————. *OMB Review of CDC Research: Impact of the Paperwork Reduction Act.* Report prepared by Barbara Boardman et al. for the Subcommittee on Oversight and Investigations. 99th Cong., 2d sess., 1986.

————. *NIH Reauthorization and Protection of Health Facilities: Hearings before the Subcommittee on Health and the Environment.* 101st Cong., 2d sess., February 8, June 18, 1990.

U.S. Congress. House. Committee on Government Operations. *Pros and Cons of Home-Based Clerical Work: Hearing before the Employment and Housing Subcommittee.* 99th Cong., 2d sess., February 26, 1986.

————. *Occupational Health Hazards: Joint Hearing before Certain Subcommittees of the Committee on Government Operations.* 99th Cong., 2d sess., April 16, 1986.

————. *Home-Based Clerical Workers: Are They Victims of Exploitation?* 39th Report by the Committee on Government Operations. H.R. 99-677. 99th Cong., 2d sess., July 16, 1986.

————. *Occupational Health Hazard Surveillance: 72 Years Behind and Counting.* H.R. 99-979, 99th Cong., 2d sess., October 8, 1986.

————. *Dramatic Rise in Repetitive Motion Injuries and OSHA's Response: Hearing before the Employment and Housing Subcommittee.* 101st Cong., 1st sess., June 6, 1989.

U.S. Congress. House. Committee on Science and Technology. *Potential Health Effects of Video Display Terminals and Radio Frequency Heaters and Sealers: Hearings before the Subcommittee on Investigations and Oversight.* 97th Cong., 1st sess., May 12–13, 1981.

————. *The Human Factor in Innovation and Productivity: Hearings before the Subcommittee on Science, Research and Technology.* 97th Cong., 1st sess., September 16, 1981.

U.S. Congress. House. Select Committee on Aging. *Women Health Care Consumers: Shortchanged on Medical Research and Treatment: Hearings before the Subcommittee on Housing and Consumer Interests.* 101st Cong., 2d sess., July 24, 1990.

U.S. Congress. Senate. Committee on Government Affairs. *Structure of Corporate Concentration: Institutional Shareholders and Interlocking Directorates among Major U.S. Corporations.* A Staff Study. 96th Cong., 2d sess. 2 vols., December 1980.

U.S. Department of Health, Education and Welfare. National Institute for Occupational Safety and Health. Division of Biomedical and Behavioral Science. *A Report on Electromagnetic Radiation Surveys of Video Display Terminals,* by C. Eugene Moss et al. Washington, D.C.: GPO, 1977.

U.S. Department of Health and Human Services. *Potential Health Hazards of Video Display Terminals.* DHHS Rept. 81-129, June 1981.

————. National Institute for Occupational Safety and Health. *Health Hazard Evaluation Report: General Telephone Company of Michigan, Alma, MI.* DHHS

Rept. HETA 84-297-1609, July 1985.

———. *Health Hazard Evaluation Report: AT&T, Southern Bell and United Telephone, North Carolina.* DHHS Rept. HETA 85-452-1698, May 1986.

———. *Response to the Third (April 2, 1986) BellSouth Review of the Protocol for the Reproductive Study of Female Video Display Terminal Operators.* Unpublished report by Teresa Schnorr, Michael Thun, and William Halperin, April 9, 1986.

———. Division of Biomedical and Behavioral Science. *An Investigation of Health Complaints and Job Stress in Video Display Operations,* by Michael J. Smith et al. Cincinnati: Public Health Service, 1981.

U.S. Department of Labor. Women's Bureau. *Women and Office Automation: Issues for the Decade Ahead.* Washington, D.C.: GPO, 1985.

———. *Women, Clerical Work, and Office Automation: Issues for Research.* Washington, D.C.: GPO, 1986.

U.S. Environmental Protection Agency. Office of Research and Development. *Evaluation of Potential Carcinogenicity of Electromagnetic Fields.* Review draft. Washington, D.C., October 1990.

U.S. Food and Drug Administration. Bureau of Radiological Health. *An Evaluation of Radiation Emission from Video Display Terminals.* Washington, D.C.: GPO, 1981.

U.S. Occupational Safety and Health Administration. *Ergonomics: The Study of Work.* OSHA 3125. Washington, D.C.: GPO, 1991.

State and Local Governments

City of New York. City Council. A Local Law to Amend the Administrative Code of the City of New York, in Relation to Standards Governing the Health and Safety of Video Display Terminal Operators. 1088-A. December 5, 1989.

New Mexico. Office of the Governor. Executive Order No. 85-11. Governor Toney Anaya, March 27, 1985.

New York. State Legislature. Legislative Commission on Science and Technology. *Proceedings: Computer Conference I: The Impacts on Management . . . Office . . . Industry, April 29, 1982.* Albany, N.Y.: New York State Legislature, 1983.

New York. County of Suffolk. *A Local Law Providing Employee Protection Against Video Display Terminals.* Local Law 21-1988.

New York. Department of Health Services. Division of Public Health. *Hearing: Interim Regulations for Suffolk County Local Law 21-1988.* Hauppauge, N.Y.: County of Suffolk, November 21, 1988.

———. *Regulations for Suffolk County Local Law 21-1988.* Hauppauge, N.Y.: County of Suffolk, January 12, 1989.

———. *Report on the Enforcement of Local Law 21-1988: Providing Employee Protection Against Video Display Terminals.* Hauppauge, N.Y.: County of Suffolk, May 1989.

Oregon. State Legislature. *Report of the Senate Interim Labor Committee VDT Subcommittee on Video Display Terminals: Workplace Health and Safety.* 62d Legislative Assembly, September 1984.

Foreign Governments

European Community. "Council Directive of 29 May 1990 on the Minimum Safety and Health Requirements for Work with Display Screen Equipment." *Official Journal of the European Communities,* June 21, 1990, 14–18.

Norway. National Labour Inspection. *Regulations for Working with Display Screen Equipment.* Oslo, 1995.

Sweden. National Board of Occupational Safety and Health. *Office Work and Office Automation: Influence over the Work Environment and Work Organization.* Solna, Sweden, September 1985.

———. "Effects of Pulsed Magnetic Fields on Embryonic Development in Mice." Press release, Stockholm [c. 1986].

———. "Regulations Regarding Work with VDTs Will Not Be Changed." Press release, Stockholm, February 13, 1986.

———. National Institute of Occupational Health. "New Evidence of Cancer from Electromagnetic Fields." *Forskning & Praktik,* 7/1992.

United Nations. International Labour Office. *Working with Visual Display Units.* Occupational Safety and Health Series, No. 61. Geneva: ILO, 1989.

BOOKS AND REPORTS

American Civil Liberties Union. *Liberty at Work: Expanding the Rights of Employees in America.* New York: ACLU, 1988.

American Federation of Labor–Congress of Industrial Organizations. *The Future of Work.* Washington, D.C.: AFL-CIO, August 1983.

———. *The Changing Situation of Workers and Their Unions.* Washington, D.C.: AFL-CIO, February 1985.

American Federation of State, County, and Municipal Employees. *Warning: Office Work May Be Hazardous to Your Health.* Washington, D.C.: AFSCME, 1982.

American Optometric Association. *Vision and the VDT Operator.* St. Louis: AOA [c. 1983].

Andolsen, Barbara Hilkert. *Good Work at the Video Display Terminal.* Knoxville: University of Tennessee Press, 1989.

Bachrach, Peter, and Morton S. Baratz. *Power and Poverty: Theory and Practice.* New York: Oxford University Press, 1970.

Bagdikian, Ben H. *The Media Monopoly.* 4th ed. Boston: Beacon Press, 1992.

Barber, Benjamin R. *Strong Democracy.* Berkeley and Los Angeles: University of California Press, 1984.

Berman, Daniel M. *Death on the Job: Occupational Health and Safety Struggles in the United States.* New York: Monthly Review Press, 1978.

Brod, Craig. *Technostress: The Human Cost of the Computer Revolution.* Reading, Mass.: Addison-Wesley, 1984.

Brodeur, Paul. *The Zapping of America: Microwaves, Their Deadly Risk, and the*

Cover-Up. New York: W. W. Norton, 1977.

———. *Currents of Death: Power Lines, Computer Terminals, and the Attempt to Cover Up Their Threat to Your Health*. New York: Simon and Schuster, 1989.

Bryner, Gary C. *Bureaucratic Discretion: Law and Policy in Federal Regulatory Agencies*. New York: Pergamon Press, 1987.

Bureau of National Affairs. *VDTs in the Workplace: A Study of the Effects on Employment*. Washington, D.C.: Bureau of National Affairs, 1984.

Cassedy, Ellen, and Karen Nussbaum. *9 to 5: The Working Woman's Guide to Office Survival*. New York: Penguin Books, 1983.

Center for Office Technology. *Working with Displays: A Practical Guide for VDT Users*. Washington, D.C. [c. 1985–86].

———. "Management Perspectives on VDT Issues." Presented by Renee S. Ross at the International Symposium: Work with Display Units, Stockholm, May 12–15, 1986. Washington, D.C., 1986.

Cobble, Dorothy Sue, ed. *Women and Labor*. Ithaca, N.Y.: ILR Press, 1994.

Computer and Business Equipment Manufacturers Association. *Factsheet 1: Health and Safety Aspects of Visual Displays*. Washington, D.C., 1984.

———. *Fact Sheet 2: Comfort Aspects of Visual Displays*. Washington, D.C., 1984.

———. *Fact Sheet 3: Employee Relations and Visual Displays*. Washington, D.C., 1984.

———. "The State Factor: Restricting the Use of High Technology in the Workplace," by Vico Henriques, president, CBEMA, 1984.

Crompton, Rosemary, and Gareth Jones. *White-Collar Proletariat: Deskilling and Gender in Clerical Work*. Philadelphia: Temple University Press, 1984.

Dahl, Robert A. *Who Governs? Democracy and Power in an American City*. New Haven, Conn.: Yale University Press, 1961.

Davies, Margery W. *Women's Place is at the Typewriter*. Philadelphia: Temple University Press, 1982.

DeLamarter, Richard Thomas. *Big Blue: IBM's Use and Abuse of Power*. New York: Dodd, Mead, 1986.

DeMatteo, Bob. *Terminal Shock: The Health Hazards of Video Display Terminal Workers*. 2d ed. Toronto: NC Press, 1986.

Dickson, David. *The New Politics of Science*. Chicago: University of Chicago Press, 1988.

Edelman, Murray. *The Symbolic Uses of Politics*. Urbana: University of Illinois Press, 1964.

Edsall, Thomas Byrne. *The New Politics of Inequality*. New York: Norton, 1984.

Epstein, Edwin M. *The Corporation in American Politics*. Englewood Cliffs, N.J.: Prentice-Hall, 1969.

Epstein, Samuel S. *The Politics of Cancer*. Rev. ed. Garden City, N.Y.: Anchor Books, 1979.

Garson, Barbara. *The Electronic Sweatshop: How Computers Are Transforming the Office of the Future into the Factory of the Past*. New York: Simon and Schuster, 1988.

Geoghegan, Thomas. *Which Side Are You On? Trying to Be for Labor When It's Flat on Its Back.* New York: Farrar, Straus, and Giroux, 1991.

Glassberg, Elyse, Naomi Baden, and Karin Gerstel. *Absent from the Agenda: A Report on the Role of Women in American Unions.* New York: Coalition of Labor Union Women, 1980.

Guy, Arthur W. *Health Assessment of Radiofrequency Electromagnetic Fields Emitted by Video Display Terminals.* Report to IBM's Office of the Director of Health and Safety, October 29, 1984.

Heckscher, Charles C. *The New Unionism: Employee Involvement in the Changing Corporation.* New York: Basic Books, 1988.

Herman, Edward S. *Corporate Control, Corporate Power: A Twentieth Century Fund Study.* New York: Cambridge University Press, 1981.

Hirschhorn, Larry. *Beyond Mechanization: Work and Technology in the Postindustrial Age.* Cambridge: MIT Press, 1984.

Howard, Robert. *Brave New Workplace.* New York: Viking Books, 1986.

Human Factors Society. *The American National Standard for Human Factors Engineering of Visual Display Terminal Workstations.* Santa Monica, Calif.: Human Factors Society, 1988.

Kapp, K. William. *The Social Costs of Private Enterprise.* New York: Schocken Books, 1971.

Kazis, Richard, and Richard L. Grossman. *Fear at Work: Job Blackmail, Labor and the Environment.* New York: Pilgrim Press, 1982.

Kelman, Steven. *Regulating America, Regulating Sweden.* Cambridge, Mass.: MIT Press, 1981.

Kessler-Harris, Alice. *Out to Work: A History of Wage-Earning Women in the United States.* New York: Oxford University Press, 1982.

Knave, Bengt, and Gunnar Per, eds. *Work with Display Units 86.* Holland: Elsevier Science Publishers, 1987.

Kuhn, Thomas S. *The Structure of Scientific Revolutions.* 2d ed. enl. Chicago: University of Chicago Press, 1970.

Leffingwell, William H. *Office Management: Principles and Practice.* New York: McGraw-Hill, 1925.

Leontief, Wassily, and Faye Duchin. *The Impacts of Automation on Employment, 1963–2000: Final Report.* New York: Institute for Economic Analysis, New York University, 1984.

McCaffrey, David P. *OSHA and the Politics of Health Regulation.* New York: Plenum Press, 1982.

McQuaid, Kim. *Big Business and Presidential Power: From FDR to Reagan.* New York: William Morrow, 1982.

Makower, Joel. *Office Hazards.* Washington, D.C.: Tilden Press, 1981.

Marschall, Daniel, and Judith Gregory. *Office Automation: Jekyll or Hyde?* Cleveland: Working Women Education Fund, 1983.

Mills, C. Wright. *White Collar: The American Middle Classes.* New York: Oxford University Press, 1951.

National Academy of Sciences. National Research Council. Committee on Vision. *Video Displays, Work, and Vision.* Washington, D.C.: National Academy Press, 1983.

———. Committee on Women's Employment and Other Related Social Issues. *Computer Chips and Paper Clips: Technology and Women's Employment.* Washington, D.C.: National Academy Press, 1986.

National Association of Public Health Policy. Council on Occupational and Environmental Health. Women's Committee. *Women's Occupational Health Agenda for the 1990's.* Working Draft. March 1988.

National Council on Compensation Insurance. *VDTs and Office Safety: An Overview, Radiation, Stress, Vision and Ergonomics.* New York: National Council on Compensation Insurance, 1986.

New York Committee for Occupational Safety and Health. *The VDT Book: A Computer User's Guide to Health and Safety.* New York: NYCOSH, 1987.

The Newspaper Guild. *A Model State Act to Provide Occupational Safeguards for Operators of Video Display Terminals.* Washington, D.C.: Newspaper Guild, 1983.

9 to 5, National Association of Working Women. *Race Against Time: Automation of the Office.* Cleveland: 9 to 5, 1980.

———. *Warning: Health Hazards for Office Workers.* Cleveland: 9 to 5, 1981.

———. *The Human Factor: 9 to 5's Consumer Guide to Word Processors.* Cleveland: 9 to 5, 1982.

———. *Nine to Five Campaign on VDT Risks: Analysis of VDT Operator Questionnaires of VDT Hotline Callers.* Cleveland: 9 to 5, 1984.

———. *Hidden Victims: Clerical Workers, Automation, and the Changing Economy.* Cleveland: 9 to 5, 1985.

———. *Computer Monitoring and Other Dirty Tricks.* Cleveland: 9 to 5, 1986.

O'Connor, James. *The Fiscal Crisis of the State.* New York: St. Martin's Press, 1973.

Offe, Claus. *Disorganized Capitalism.* Cambridge, Mass.: MIT Press, 1985.

Oppenheimer, Martin. *White Collar Politics.* New York: Monthly Review Press, 1985.

Pateman, Carole. *Participation and Democratic Theory.* Cambridge: Cambridge University Press, 1970.

Phillips, Kevin. *The Politics of Rich and Poor.* New York: Random House, 1990.

Pinsky, Mark, Martha Zybko, and Louis Slesin. *Video Display Terminals: 1983 Health and Safety Update.* New York: Microwave News, 1984.

Piven, Frances Fox, ed. *Labor Parties in Postindustrial Societies.* New York: Oxford University Press, 1992.

Piven, Frances Fox, and Richard A. Cloward. *Poor People's Movements: Why They Succeed, How They Fail.* New York: Vintage Books, 1979.

Polanyi, Karl. *The Great Transformation: The Political and Economic Origins of Our Time.* Boston: Beacon Press, 1957.

Putz-Anderson, Vern, ed. *Cumulative Trauma Disorders.* Philadelphia: Taylor and Francis, 1988.

Schattschneider, E. E. *The Semisovereign People: A Realist's View of Democracy.* Hinsdale, Ill.: Dryden Press, 1975.

Service Employees International Union. District 925. *Working Women Groups Say More Links Found Between VDTs and Pregnancy Problems, Ask Congress for Action on Health/Safety Regs.* Press release, February 28, 1984.

Sexton, Patricia Cayo. *The War on Labor and the Left: Understanding America's Unique Conservatism.* Boulder, Colo.: Westview Press, 1991.

Slesin, Louis, and Martha Zybko, eds. *Video Display Terminals: Health and Safety.* New York: Microwave News, 1983.

Smith, Robert Stewart. *The Occupational Safety and Health Act: Its Goals and Achievments.* Washington, D.C.: American Enterprise Institute, 1976.

Sobel, Robert. *IBM: Colossus in Transition.* New York: Time Books, 1981.

SRI International. Information Systems Management Department. *Office Automation: Consulting and Research.* Menlo Park, Calif. [c. 1980].

Steelcase, Inc. *Office Environment Index: Detailed Findings.* Grand Rapids, Mich.: Steelcase, Inc., 1989, 1991.

Stellman, Jeanne M., and Mary Sue Henifin. *Office Work Can Be Dangerous to Your Health.* New York: Pantheon, 1983.

Stern, Philip M. *The Best Congress Money Can Buy.* New York: Pantheon, 1988.

Sturmthal, Adolph, ed. *White-Collar Trade Unions: Contemporary Developments in Industrialized Societies.* Urbana: University of Illinois Press, 1966.

Sweeney, John J., and Karen Nussbaum. *Solutions for the New Work Force: Policies for a New Social Contract.* Cabin John, Md.: Seven Locks Press, 1989.

TCO: Central Organization of Salaried Employees in Sweden. *VDU Work: The Right Way.* Stockholm: TCO, 1984.

Tepperman, Jean. *Not Servants, Not Machines: Office Workers Speak Out.* Boston: Beacon Press, 1976.

———. *60 Words a Minute and What Do You Get? Clerical Workers Today.* Somerville, Mass.: New England Free Press, 1976.

Truman, David B. *The Governmental Process.* New York: Alfred A. Knopf, 1965.

Valli, Linda. *Becoming Clerical Workers.* Boston: Routledge and Kegan Paul, 1986.

Wertheimer, Barbara Mayer. *We Were There: The Story of Working Women in America.* New York: Pantheon, 1977.

Westin Alan, F., Heather A. Schweder, Michael A. Baker, and Sheila Lehman. *The Changing Workplace: A Guide to Managing the People, Organizational and Regulatory Aspects of Office Technology.* White Plains, N.Y.: Knowledge Industry Publications, 1985.

Wilson, Graham K. *The Politics of Safety and Health.* New York: Oxford University Press, 1985.

The Women's Work Project. *Women Organizing the Office.* A Union for Radical Political Economics Political Education Project. Washington, D.C.: Women in Distribution, 1978.

Zuboff, Shoshana. *In the Age of the Smart Machine: The Future of Work and Power.* New York: Basic Books, 1988.

ESSAYS AND ARTICLES

Political and Social Analysis

Anderson, Christopher. "EMF Report Draws Fire." *Nature,* November 26, 1992, 288.

Bachrach, Peter, and Morton S. Baratz. "Two Faces of Power." *American Political Science Review* 56 (December 1962): 947–952.

———. "Decisions and Nondecisions: An Analytical Framework." *American Political Science Review* 57 (1963): 641–651.

Baran, Barbara, and Suzanne Teegarden. "Women's Labor in the Office of the Future." Paper presented at the conference on "Women and Structural Transformation: The Crisis of Work and Family Life," Rutgers University, New Brunswick, N.J., November 18–19, 1983.

Bell, Deborah. "Unionized Women in State and Local Government." In *Women, Work and Protest,* edited by Ruth Milkman, 280–299. Boston: Routledge and Kegan Paul, 1985.

Benston, Margaret Lowe. "For Women, the Chips Are Down." In *The Technological Woman,* edited by Jan Zimmerman, 44–54. New York: Praeger, 1983.

Branscum, Deborah. "Washington Rethinks ELF Emissions: The FDA Presses Computer Manufacturers for Action." *MacWorld,* December 1990, 85–88.

Brodeur, Paul. "The Magnetic-Field Menace: Computer Monitors May Pose a Very Real Threat to Users." *MacWorld,* July 1990, 136–145.

Davies, Margery. "Women's Place is at the Typewriter: The Feminization of the Clerical Labor Force." *Radical America,* July/August 1974, 1–28.

DeMuth, Christopher C., and Douglas H. Ginsberg. "White House Review of Agency Rulemaking." *Harvard Law Review* 99 (March 1986): 1075–1088.

Dickson, David, and David Noble. "By Force of Reason: The Politics of Science and Technology Policy." In *The Hidden Election,* edited by Thomas Ferguson and Joel Rogers. New York: Pantheon, 1981.

Feldberg, Roselyn L., and Evelyn N. Glenn. "Clerical Work: The Female Occupation." In *Women: A Feminist Perspective,* edited by Jo Freeman, 316–336. 3d ed. Palo Alto, Calif.: Mayfield Publishing, 1984.

———. "Proletarianizing Clerical Work: Technology and Organizational Control in the Office." In *Case Studies on the Labor Process,* edited by Andrew Zimbalist, 51–72. New York: Monthly Review Press, 1979.

"Few VDT Rules Around the World: Despite Massive Use Sweden Alone Has Broad Law." *Women's Occupational Health Resource Center Newsletter,* April/July 1986, 1.

Foreman, Christopher H., Jr. "Legislators, Regulators, and the OMB." In *Divided Democracy: Cooperation and Conflict Between the President and Congress,* edited by James A. Thurber, 123–144. Washington, D.C.: CQ Press, 1991.

Giuliano, Vincent E. "The Mechanization of Office Work." *Scientific American* 247 (September 1982): 148–164.

Henifin, Mary Sue. "The Particular Problems of Video Display Terminals." In *Double Exposure: Women's Health Hazards on the Job and at Home,* edited by Wendy Chavkin, 69–80. New York: Monthly Review Press, 1984.

Hilaski, Harvey J. "Understanding Statistics on Occupational Illnesses." *Monthly Labor Review,* March 1981, 25–29.

Ichniowski, Casey, and Jeffrey S. Zax. "Today's Associations, Tomorrow's Unions." *Industrial and Labor Relations Review* 43 (January 1990): 191–208.

Kessler-Harris, Alice. " 'Where Are the Organized Workers?' " In *A Heritage of Her Own: Toward a New Social History of American Women,* edited by Nancy F. Cott and Elizabeth H. Pleck, 343–366. New York: Simon and Schuster, 1979.

McCloud, Sheryl Gordon. "VDTs in the Workplace." *Southern California Law Review* 58 (1985): 1493–1499.

Matlack, Carol. "Tapping into Trouble?" *National Journal,* December 3, 1988, 3070–3073.

Matteis, Richard. "The New Back Office Focuses on Customer Service." *Harvard Business Review* (March–April 1979): 146–159.

Melcher, Dale, Jennifer L. Eichstedt, Shelley Eriksen, and Dan Clawson. "Women's Participation in Local Union Leadership: The Massachusetts Experience." *Industrial and Labor Relations Review* 45 (January 1992): 267–280.

Morrison, Alan B. "OMB Interference with Agency Rulemaking: The Wrong Way to Write a Regulation." *Harvard Law Review* 99 (March 1986): 1059–1074.

Murphree, Mary C. "Brave New Office: The Changing World of the Legal Secretary." In *My Troubles Are Going to Have Trouble with Me: Everyday Trials and Triumphs of Women Workers,* edited by Karen Brodkin Sacks and Dorothy Remy, 140–159. New Brunswick, N.J.: Rutgers University Press, 1984.

Northrup, Herbert R. "The AFL-CIO Blue Cross–Blue Shield Campaign: A Study of Organizational Failure." *Industrial and Labor Relations Review* 43 (July 1990): 525–541.

Otos, Sally, and Ellen Levy. "Word Processing: 'This is Not a Final Draft.' " In *The Technological Woman,* edited by Jan Zimmerman, 149–157. New York: Praeger, 1983.

Rapport, Sara. "Health Rights of Video Display Terminal Operators." *Harvard Women's Law Journal* 8 (1985): 247–264.

Smith, Michael J., Pascale Sainfort, Katherine Rogers, and David LeGrande. *Electronic Performance Monitoring and Job Stress in Telecommunications Jobs.* Madison: University of Wisconsin, Department of Industrial Engineering and the Communications Workers of America, 1990.

Sorensen, Jeff, and Jon Swan. "VDT's: The Overlooked Story Right in the Newsroom." *Columbia Journalism Review,* January/February 1981, 32–38.

Stellman, Jeanne Mager, and Joan Bertin. "Science's Anti-Female Bias." *New York Times,* June 4, 1990, p. A23.

Stein, Loren, and Diana Hembree. "VDT Regulation: The Publishers Counterattack." *Columbia Journalism Review,* November/December 1984, 42

Stone, Richard. "Polarized Debate: EMFs and Cancer." *Science,* December 11, 1992, 1724–1725.

Strom, Sharon Hartman. " 'We're No Kitty Foyles': Organizing Office Workers for the Congress of Industrial Organizations, 1937–1950." In *Women, Work and Protest: A Century of Women's Labor History,* edited by Ruth Milkman, 206–234. New York: Routledge and Kegan Paul, 1985.

Wallach, Charles. "Employer Liability in Video Display Operators' Health Complaints." *Glendale Law Review* 6 (1985): 1–14.

West, Jackie. "New Technology and Women's Office Work." In *Work, Women and the Labour Market,* by Jackie West. London: Routledge and Kegan Paul, 1982, 61–79.

Zisman, Michael D. "Office Automation: Revolution or Evolution?" *Sloan Management Review* (Spring 1978): 1–17.

Medical and Scientific

American Medical Association. Council on Scientific Affairs. "Council Report: Health Effects of Video Display Terminals." *JAMA* 257 (March 20, 1987): 1508–1512.

———. "Health Effects of Video Display Terminals: An Update." Paper presented by George H. Bohigian, M.D., April 1989.

Dainoff, Marvin J. "The Illness of the Decade." *Computerworld,* April 13, 1992, 27.

Delgado, José M. R., A. Ubeda, J. Leal, M. A. Trillo, and M. A. Majimenez. "Pulse Shape of Magnetic Fields Influence Chick Embryogenesis." *Journal of Anatomy* 137 (October 1983): 513–536.

Delgado, José M. R., J. Leal, J. L. Monteagudo, and M. G. Gareia. "Embryological Changes by Weak, Extremely Low Frequency Electromagnetic Fields." *Journal of Anatomy* 134 (1982): 533–551.

Goldhaber, Marilyn K., Michael R. Polen, and Robert A. Hiatt, "The Risk of Miscarriage and Birth Defects Among Women Who Use Visual Display Terminals During Pregnancy." *American Journal of Industrial Medicine* 13 (June 1988).

Juutilainen, Jukka, and Keijo Saali. "Effects of Low Frequency Magnetic Fields on the Development of Chick Embryos." Paper given at the International Symposium on Work with Display Units, Stockholm, Sweden, May 12–15, 1986.

Lindbohm, Marja-Liisa, Maila Hietanen, Pentti Kyyrönen, Markku Sallmén, Patrick von Nandelstadh, and Helena Taskinen. "Magnetic Fields of Video Display Terminals and Spontaneous Abortions." *American Journal of Epidemiology* 136 (November 1, 1992): 1041–1051.

Marha, Karel, and David Charron. *The Very Low Frequency (VLF) Testing of CCOHS Terminals.* Hamilton, Ontario: Canadian Centre for Occupational Health and Safety, 1983.

Marha, Karel, Barry Spinner, and Jim Purdham. *The Case for Concern about Very Low Frequency Fields from Visual Display Terminals.* Hamilton, Ontario: Canadian Centre for Occupational Health and Safety, 1983.

Ostberg, Olov. "CRT's Pose Health Problems for Operators." *International Journal of Occupational Health and Safety,* November/December 1975.

————. "The Health Debate." *Reprographics Quarterly* 12 (1979): 80–82.

Piche, André, and Jacques Piche. "Health Problems of Data Entry Clerks and Related Job Stressors." *Journal of Occupational Medicine* 29 (December 1987): 942–948.

Schnorr, Teresa M. "The NIOSH Study of Reproductive Outcomes Among Video Display Terminal Operators." *Reproductive Toxicology* 4 (1990): 61.

Sheedy, James E. "Vision Problems at Video Display Terminals: A Survey of Optometrists." November 1991. VDT Eye Clinic, University of California–Berkeley.

Swanbeck, Gunnar, and Thor Bleeker. "Skin Problems from Visual Display Units." *Acta Derm Venereol* 69 (1989): 46–51.

Wolbarsht, Myron L., F. A. O'Foghludha, D. H. Sliney, A. W. Guy, A. A. Smith Jr., and G. A. Johnson. "Electromagnetic Emission from Visual Display Units: A Non-Hazard." In *Ocular Effects of Non-ionizing Radiation: Proceedings of the Society of Photo-Optical Instrumentation Engineers,* edited by M. L. Wolbarsht and D. H. Sliney, 187–195. Bellingham, Wash.: Society of Photo-Optical Instrumentation Engineers, 1980.

Index

ABC Evening News, 139
Abernathy, Charles, 101
Adderley, T. E., 29
Adia Personnel Services, 17, 55
Advancement for Commerce and Industry, 193n56
Aetna Life and Casualty Insurance Company, 57
AFL-CIO: on the Commission on the Future of Worker-Management Relations, 148; and Congressional VDT hearings, 68; Equitable boycott, 46; on NAS vision report, 68; and organizing white-collar workers, 40, 48, 66, 148; on two-tier economy, 155n12
Agnos, Art, 141
Air Transport Association of America, 52, 57, 70
Akers, John, 63
Alford, Rebecca, 46
Amalgamated Meat Cutters Union, 42
Ambulatory Sentinel Practices Network, 14
American Airlines, 33
American Bankers Association, 52
American Civil Liberties Union, 25, 161n30
American Council on Life Insurance, 52, 57
American Council on Science and Health (ACSH), 72–73, 174–175
American Electronics Association, 52–53, 57, 70, 101
American Express, 57

American Federation of State, County and Municipal Employees (AFSCME), 42, 44, 48, 66, 69
American Health, 59
American Insurance Association, 57
American Journal of Epidemiology, 105
American Journal of Public Health, 74, 175n31
American National Standards Institute (ANSI), 5, 79, 80, 89, 150
American Newspaper Publishers Association (ANPA): conservatism of, 170n26; efforts to control VDT news coverage, 61; on employee vision benefits, 43; links to computer industry, 52, 57, 64; opposition to alternative work, 93; opposition to VDT regulations, 52, 56–58, 70, 131
American Optometric Association, 13
American Society of Travel Agents, 70
American Textile Manufacturers Institute v. Donovan, 184
Ameritrust Corporation, 73
AMR Caribbean Data Services, 33
Anaya, Toney, 131
Apple Computers, Inc., 52, 100, 169
asbestos, 92, 106, 120
Associated Press, 43
associational unionism, 148–149
Association for a Better Long Island (ABLI), 137, 193n56
Association of American Colleges, 123
Association of Schools of Public Health, 123
Association Trends (ANPA), 43

Accounting—
By Principle or Design?

Accounting—
By Principle or Design?

AHMED RIAHI-BELKAOUI

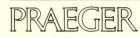

Westport, Connecticut
London

Library of Congress Cataloging-in-Publication Data

Riahi-Belkaoui, Ahmed, 1943–
    Accounting—by principle or design? / Ahmed Riahi-Belkaoui.
      p. cm.
    Includes bibliographical references and index.
    ISBN 1–56720–553–4 (alk. paper)
    1. Accounting. 2. Income accounting. 3. Corporations—Accounting. 4. Smoothing
(Statistics) 5. Fraud. I. Title.
    HF5635.R455   2003
    657—dc21   2002030332

British Library Cataloguing in Publication Data is available.

Library of Congress Catalog Card Number: 2002030332
ISBN: 1–56720–553–4

First published in 2003

Praeger Publishers, 88 Post Road West, Westport, CT 06881
An imprint of Greenwood Publishing Group, Inc.
www.praeger.com

Printed in the United States of America

The paper used in this book complies with the
Permanent Paper Standard issued by the National
Information Standards Organization (Z39.48–1984).

10 9 8 7 6 5 4 3 2 1

To Dimitra

Contents

Preface

Basically, an interested and inquisitive observer from outside the accounting establishment who examines the accounting discipline and the accounting process and output may be easily tempted to see more of various deliberate attempts to choose accounting techniques and solutions that fit a preestablished goal and picture to be conveyed as representative constructions of realities, a phenomenon that I label as "designed accounting," rather than a choice of principle-based techniques and solutions, a phenomenon that I label as "principled accounting." Aspects of this designed accounting include:

1. Income smoothing as choices of accounting techniques aimed at affecting the variance of earnings (Chapter 1).
2. Earnings management as choices of accounting techniques aimed at affecting the level of earnings (Chapter 2).
3. "Big bath" and creative accounting as choices of techniques to reduce the current level of earnings in favor of increasing the future level of earnings and to engage in various forms of "window dressing" (Chapter 3).
4. Fraud in accounting as deliberate attempts to present a false picture of reality (Chapter 4).
5. Slack in accounting as the tendency to refrain from using all of the resources available to the firm in the form of organizational slack or budgetary slack (Chapter 5).

This book should be of interest to preparers and users of accounting information and should be used in graduate courses covering the current crisis in accounting.

Many people helped in the development of this book. I received considerable assistance from the University of Illinois at Chicago, especially Ewa Thomaszewski and Maninder Bhuller. I also thank the staff at Praeger for their continuous and intelligent support.

Chapter 1

Income Smoothing

INTRODUCTION

Income smoothing is a clear form of designed accounting. It is a deliberate attempt by management to show stable earnings by reaching the variations in earnings fluctuations and securing an acceptable earnings growth. The complexity of the phenomenon warrants examination of its nature, history, the motivations behind its construction, smoothing dimensions, and variables used, as well as the objects of smoothing. Because it may take different forms depending on different contextual confirmations, income smoothing may have different impacts that also warrant examination. All of these issues are discussed in this chapter.

ACCOUNTING POLICY AND CHANGES

Firms need to make choices among the different accounting methods in recording transactions and preparing their financial statements. These choices, as dictated by generally accepted accounting principles, represent the accounting policies of the firm. They are best defined by the Accounting Principles Board (APB) in its Opinion 22, *Disclosure of Acceding Polices* (April 1972), paragraph 6:

The *accounting policies* of a reporting entity are the specific accounting principles and the methods of applying those principles that are judged by the management of the entity to be the most appropriate in the circumstances to present fairly financial position, changes in financial position, and results of operations in accordance with generally

accepted accounting principles and that accordingly have been adopted for preparing the financial statements.

Firms also make accounting changes as part of their accounting policies. The general belief is that firms make accounting changes to mask performance problems. The accounting literature explains the changes in accounting principles and estimates in terms of management's desire to reach definite objectives such as income smoothing[1] or the reduction of agency costs associated with a violation of debt covenants. A summary of existing research results suggests that as the tightness of debt covenant increases, firms are more likely to loosen the tightness of covenant restrictions through appropriate accounting changes.[2] In fact, two studies that examined the accounting changes of (1) successful and unsuccessful firms[3] and (2) firms facing or experiencing bond rating changes[4] provide some evidence consistent with the assertion that managers can modify income through judicious accounting changes.

Accounting regulators have tried to limit management's ability to use accounting changes to increase or decrease net income. Since 1970, APB No. 20 has stipulated that accounting changes should be accounted for as a cumulative effect change, requiring the reporting in the comparative income statements of the cumulative effect of change in the net income of the period of the change as well as the disclosure in the notes of the effect of adopting the new accounting principle on income before extraordinary income and net income (and on related per share amounts) of the period change. Similarly, the Securities and Exchange Commission's (SEC) accounting Release No. 177 required that accounting changes be made to more preferable accounting methods, using reasonable business judgment in the choice. While both pronouncements act as a control mechanism, they do not eliminate management's ability to increase and/or decrease income through accounting changes. SEC Chairman Arthur Levitt contended that public companies have used six accounting practices to manage corporate earnings:

1. overstatement of restructuring changes to clean up the balance sheet;

2. classification of a significant portion of the price of an acquired entity as in-process research and development so that the amount can be written off as a onetime charge;

3. creation of large liabilities for future expenses (recorded as part of the accounting for an acquisition) to protect future earnings;

4. use of unrealistic assumptions to estimate liabilities for items such as sales returns, loan losses, and warranty costs so that the overaccrual can be reversed to improve earnings during a subsequent period;

5. intentional inclusion of errors in the company's books and justifying the failure to correct the errors by arguing materiality; and

6. recognition of revenue before the earnings process is complete.[5]

INCOME SMOOTHING HYPOTHESIS

Nature of Income Smoothing

Income smoothing may be viewed as the deliberate normalization of income in order to reach a desired trend or level. As far back as 1953, Heyworth observed "more of the accounting techniques which may be applied to affect the assignment of net income successive accounting periods . . . for smoothing or leveling the amplitude of periodic net income fluctuations."[6] What followed were arguments made by Monsen and Downs[7] and Gordon[8] that corporate managers may be motivated to smooth their own income security, with the assumption that stability in income and rate of growth will be preferred over higher average income streams with greater variability. More specifically, Gordon theorized on income smoothing as follows:

Proposition 1: The criterion that a corporate management uses in selecting among accounting principles is the maximization of its utility or welfare.

Proposition 2: The utility of management increases with (1) its job security, (2) the level and rate of growth in the management's income, and (3) the level and rate of growth in the corporation's size.

Proposition 3: The achievement of the management goals stated in Proposition 2 is dependent in part on the satisfaction of stockholders with the corporation's performance; that is, other things being equal, the happier the stockholders, the greater the job security, income, and so on of the management.

Proposition 4: Stockholders' satisfaction with a corporation increases with the average rate of growth in the corporation's income (or the average rate of return on its capital) and the stability of its income. This proposition is as readily verified as Proposition 2. Theorem: Given that the above four propositions are accepted or found to be true, it follows that management would, within the limits of its power, that is, the latitude allowed by accounting rules, (1) smooth reported income and (2) smooth the rate of growth in income. By "smooth the rate of growth in income" we mean the following: if the rate of growth is high, accounting practices that reduce it should be adopted, and vice versa.[9]

The best definition of income smoothing was provided by Beidleman as follows:

Smoothing of reported earnings may be deemed as the intentional dampening or fluctuations about some level of earnings that is currently considered to be normal for a firm. In this sense smoothing represents an attempt on the part of the firm's management to reduce abnormal variations in earnings to the extent allowed under sound accounting and management principles.[10]

Given the above definition, what needs to be explicated are the motivation of smoothing, the dimensions of smoothing, and the instruments of smoothing.

History of Income Smoothing

Most of the literature on income smoothing attributes the origin of the concept to one of the three works by Gordon et al.,[11] Hepworth,[12] and White.[13] However, an article by Buckmaster[14] on income smoothing in accounting and business literature prior to 1954 identifies up to thirty-four works from 1893 to 1953 that contain some kind of reference to the smoothing properties of an accounting method or to an accounting practice used in such a way as to dampen the fluctuations of reported income. The article reports on pages that focus on the balance sheet and secret reserves that result in the reduction of the volatility of income time-series and those that examined the last in, first out (LIFO) base-stock inventory debate as it related to income smoothing.

Secret reserves were created by management in order to "avoid the distribution of firm assets as dividends, by creating a contra asset account or a liability or by failing to record assets and/or writing them off as expenses or directly to surplus (retained earnings)."[15] The secret reserves can also be created by the recording of unusually large amounts of depreciation in good years,[16] the write-down of assets,[17] the classification of extraordinary losses as extraordinary depreciation,[18] the use of flexibility in the capitalize/expense decisions for plant and equipment related costs,[19] the charging of large amounts of capital expenditures to expenses in periods of high profits,[20] the practice of overly excessive repairs in good years and inadequate repairs in bad years,[21] and the making of excessive provisions for bad debt and valuing inventories at below cost.[22]

Base-stock inventory was also used for smoothing purposes and dampening of business cycles. As Warshaw explains:

The leveling of inventory gains and losses, with the comparative stability of yearly profits which this method brings about . . . exerts a subconscious effect upon business policy which is very desirable. Prices of manufacturing articles are kept in more proper relation to prices of raw material. The management is not elated by apparent profits or depressed by apparent losses. Such elation and depression are responsible for most business follies. The normal stock inventory automatically creates a reserve that strengthens the basis for credit, gives stability, and makes expansion safe. Moreover, it has the great advantage of being a concrete suggestion for mitigating the security of business cycles.[23]

Warshaw's arguments were later supported by Davis[24] and Cotter.[25] Cotter mentioned the smoothing properties of LIFO and the advantages of (a) dampening the business cycles, (b) avoiding overexpansion of credit, (c) avoiding demands for excessive dividends, and (d) better information for pricing decisions.[26]

Motivations of Smoothing

As early as 1953 Heyworth claimed that motivations behind smoothing include the improvements of relations with creditors, investors, and workers, as

well as dampening of business cycles through psychological processes.[27] Gordon proposed that:

1. The criterion that a corporate management uses in selecting among accounting principles is to maximize its utility or welfare.
2. The same utility is a function of job security, the level and rate of growth of salary, and the level and growth rate in the firm's size.
3. Satisfaction of shareholders with the corporation's performance enhances the status and rewards of managers.
4. The same satisfaction depends on the rate of growth and stability of the firm's income.[28]

These propositions culminate in the need to smooth as explained in the following theorem:

Given that the above four propositions are accepted or found to be true, it follows that a management should, within the limits of its power, i.e., the latitude allowed by accounting rules, (1) smooth reported income and (2) smooth the rate of growth in income. By smoothing the rate of growth in income we mean the following: If the rate of growth is high, accounting practices which reduce it should be adopted and vice-versa.[29]

Beidelman considers two reasons for management to smooth reported earnings.[30] The first argument rests on the assumption that a stable earnings stream is capable of supporting a higher level of dividends than a more variable earnings stream, having a favorable effect on the value of the firm's shares as overall riskiness of the firm is reduced. He states:

To the extent that the observed variability about a trend of reported earnings influences investors' subjective expectations for possible outcomes of future earnings and dividends, management might be able favorably to influence the value of the firm's shares by smoothing earnings.[31]

The second argument attributes to smoothing the ability to counter the cyclical nature of reported earnings and likely reduce the correlation of a firm's expected returns with returns on the market portfolio. He states:

To the degree that auto-normalization of earnings is successful, and that the reduced covariance of returns with the market is recognized by investors and incorporated into their evaluation process, smoothing will have added beneficial effects in share values.[32]

It results from the need felt by management to neutralize environmental uncertainty and dampen the wide fluctuations in the operating performance of the firm subject to an intermittent cycle of good and bad times. To do so, management may resort to organizational slack behavior,[33] budgetary slack behavior,[34]

or risk-avoiding behavior.[35] Each of these behaviors necessitates decisions affecting the incurrence and /or allocation of discretionary expenses (costs) that result in income smoothing.

In addition to these behaviors intended to neutralize environmental uncertainty, it is possible to identify organizational characterizations that differentiate firms in their extent of smoothing. For example, Kamin and Ronen[36] examined the effects of the separation of ownership and control on income smoothing, under the hypothesis that management-controlled firms are more likely to be engaged in smoothing as a manifestation of managerial discretion and budgetary slack. Their results confirmed that income smoothing is higher among management-controlled firms with high barriers to entry.

Management was also assigned to circumvent news of the constraints of generally accepted accounting principles by attempting to smooth income numbers so as to convey their expectations of future cash flows, enhancing in the process the apparent reliability of predictions based on the observed smoothed series of numbers.[37] Three constraints are presumed to lead managers to smooth:

1. the competitive market mechanisms, which reduce the options available to management;
2. the management compensation scheme, which is linked directly to the firm's performance; and
3. the threat of management displacement.

This smoothing is not limited to high-level management and external accounting; it is also presumed to be used by lower-level management and internal accounting in the form of organizational slack and slack budgeting.[38]

Types of Smoothing

An early definition of income smoothing states that it "moderates year-to-year fluctuations in income by shifting earnings from peak years to less successful periods."[39] A more recent definition of income smoothing sees the phenomenon as "the process of manipulating the time profile of earnings or earnings reports to make the reported income less variable, while not increasing reported earnings over the long run."[40] Both definitions seem to imply that there is only one form of income smoothing used to dampen fluctuations of earnings toward an expected level of earnings. Of the studies that distinguished between potentially different types of smoothing, the article by Eckel[41] provides the more exhaustive classification of the different types of smooth income statements. The first distinction is made between an intentional or designed smoothing and a natural smoothing. The second distinction is to classify the intentional or designed smoothing with either an artificial smoothing or a real smoothing. These various types of smoothing are explicated next.

Intentional or designed smoothing refers specifically to the deliberate designing choices made to dampen earnings fluctuations around a desired level. Therefore, intentional or designed smoothing is essentially an accounting smoothing that uses the existing flexibility in generally accepted accounting principles and the choices and combinations available to smooth income. It is therefore essentially a form of the designed accounting that is the objective of this book.

Natural smoothing, unlike designed smoothing, is a natural product of the income-generating process, rather than the result of actions taken by management. Eckel gives the following example: "For example, one would expect the income generating process of public utilities to be such that income streams would be naturally smooth."[42]

Designed smoothing may be accomplished by either artificial or real smoothing. Artificial smoothing is the result of resorting to accounting manipulations to smooth income. As stated by Eckel:

These manipulations do not represent underlying economic events or affect cash flows, but shift costs and/or revenues from one period to another. For example, a firm would increase or decrease reported income smoothing by changing its actuarial assumptions concerning pension costs.[43]

Finally, real smoothing involves the deliberate choice and timing of transactions that can affect cash flows and control underlying choices of purchasing, hiring production, investment, sales, capital budgeting, research and development, advertising, and other decisions. It is basically a choice of business conduct to deliberately alter the cash flows of a corporation toward dampening earnings fluctuations. It can be either an attempt to control economic events or an attempt to construct economic events with the intention of affecting cash flows and smooth earnings. The actions taken by management in real smoothing are intended to alter the firm's production and/or investment decisions at year-end based on the knowledge of how the firm has performed up to that time of the year.[44]

The Smoothing Object

Basically, the smoothing object should be based on the most visible and used financial indication, which is the profit. Because income smoothing is not a visible phenomenon, the literature speculates on various expressions of profit as the most likely object of smoothing. These expressions include (1) net income-based indicators generally before extraordinary items and before or after tax, (2) earnings per share-based indicators generally before extraordinary gains and losses and adjusted for stock splits and dividends. The researchers choose net income- or earnings per share-based indicators as the object of smoothing because of the belief that management's long-term concern is with the net income,

and users have a kind of functional fixation on the bottom figure, whether it is income or earnings per share. This is simplistic reasoning, as management may find it necessary and practical to smooth sales, and fixed sales commitments have only the flexibility of smoothing expenses. Similarly, a firm with good control on its expenses may find it more practical to smooth its sales revenues.

The Dimensions of Smoothing

The dimensions of smoothing are basically the means used to accomplish the smoothing of income numbers. Dascher and Malcolm distinguished between real smoothing and artificial smoothing as follows:

Real smoothing refers to the actual transaction that is undertaken or not undertaken on the basis of its smoothing effect on income, whereas artificial smoothing refers to accounting procedures which are implemented to shift costs and/or revenues from one period to another.[45]

These types of smoothing may be indistinguishable. For example, the amount of reported expenses may be lower or higher than in previous periods because of either deliberate actions on the level of the expenses (real smoothing) or the reporting methods (artificial smoothing). For both types, an operational test proposed is to fit a curve to a stream of income calculated two ways, excluding a possible manipulative variable and including it.[46]

Artificial smoothing was also considered by Copeland and defined as follows:

Income smoothing involves the repetitive selection of accounting measurement or reporting rules in a particular pattern, the effect of which is to report the stream of income with a smaller variation from trend than would otherwise have appeared.[47]

Besides real and artificial smoothing, other dimensions of smoothing were considered in the literature. A popular classification adds a third smoothing dimension, namely, classificatory smoothing. Barnes et al. distinguished between three smoothing dimensions as follows:

1. *Smoothing through events' occurrence and/or recognition.* Management can time actual transactions so that their effects on reported income would tend to dampen its variations over time. Mostly, the planned timing of events' occurrences (e.g., research and development) would be a function of the accounting rules governing the accounting recognition of the events.

2. *Smoothing through allocation over time.* Given the occurrence and the recognition of an event, management has more discretionary control over the determination over the periods to be affected by the events' quantification.

3. *Smoothing through classification (hence, classifactory smoothing).* When income statement statistics other than net income (net of all revenues and expenses) are the

object of smoothing, management can classify intraincome statement items to reduce variations over time in that statistic.[48]

Basically, real smoothing corresponded to the smoothing through events' occurrence and/or recognition, while artificial smoothing corresponded to the smoothing through the allocation over time.

The Smoothing Variables

The smoothing devices or instruments are the variables used to smooth the chosen performance indicator. Copeland suggested the following five conditions as necessary for a smoothing instrument:

A. Once used, it must not commit the firm to any particular future action.
B. It must be based upon the exercise of professional judgment and be considered within the domain of "generally accepted accounting principles."
C. It must lead to material shifts relative to year-to-year differences in income.
D. It must not require a "real" transaction with second parties, but only a reclassification of internal account balances.
E. It must be used, singularly or in conjunction with other practices, over consecutive periods of time.[49]

Beidelman suggested two different and less restrictive criteria:

1. It must permit management to reduce the variability in reported earnings as it strives to achieve its long-run earnings (growth) objective.
2. Once used, it should not commit the firm to any particular action.[50]

Examples of smoothing instruments used include:

1. Switch from accelerated to straight-line depreciation[51]
2. Choice of cost or equity method[52]
3. Pension costs[53]
4. Dividend income[54]
5. Gains and losses on sale of securities[55]
6. Investment tax credit[56]

RESEARCH FINDINGS ON INCOME SMOOTHING

Sector and Country Analysis

It is possible to identify organizational characterizations, sector classifications, and country classifications that differentiate among different firms in their extent of smoothing.

1. With respect to the organizational characterizations, Kamin and Ronen[57] examined the effects of the separation of ownership and control on income smoothing under the hypothesis that management-controlled firms are more likely to be engaged in smoothing as a manifestation of managerial discretion and budgetary slack. Their results confirmed that a majority of the firms examined behave as if they were smoothers, and a particularly strong majority is included among management-controlled firms with high barriers to entry.

2. With respect to sectorial classifications, Belkaoui and Picur[58] tested the effects of a dual economy on income-smoothing behavior. The main hypothesis was that a higher degree of smoothing of income numbers will be exhibited by firms in the periphery sector than firms in the core sector as a reaction to differences in the opportunity structures, experiences, and environmental uncertainty. Their results indicated that a majority of U.S. firms may be resorting to income smoothing, with a higher number included among firms in the periphery sector. However, using an income variability method of analysis, those results could not be replicated using a U.S. sample[59] or a Canadian sample.[60] In a Finnish context, Kinnunen et al.[61] found that one-sector firms may have more opportunities and more predisposition to income-smoothing behavior than firms operating in the more peripheral sector of the Finnish economy. The following explanation is provided for the Finnish results:

As an explanation for these findings, it can be argued that compared with the periphery sector, Finnish accounting rules provide the sector firms more opportunities to exploit certain earnings management instruments (such as accounting for depreciation of fixed assets, untaxed reserves, pension liabilities, exchange losses and R&D [research and development] costs). Furthermore, because these firms sell their products in highly competitive international markets, and are very much dependent on those markets, they presumably face a higher degree of environmental uncertainty than firms in the periphery sector. Therefore, the core sector firms are more apt to use income smoothing in the conventional sense.[62]

3. With regard to country classifications excluding the United States, the evidence shows a certain degree of income smoothing in Japan,[63] the United Kingdom,[64] Canada,[65] France,[66] and Singapore.[67]

Job Security and Anticipatory Smoothing

The general idea behind income smoothing is that the manager may take actions that increase reported income when income is low and take actions that decrease reported income when income is high. This is possible through either the flexibility allowed within generally accepted accounting principles or deliberate changes in operations. We may ask about the motivations of managers engaged in income smoothing. Fudenberg and Tirole[68] analytically show that

income smoothing to increase job security arises in equilibrium if the following assumptions hold:

1. Managers enjoy nonmonetary private benefits (incumbency rents) from running the firm.
2. The firm is not committed to long-term incentive contract, which results in managers' dismissal in case of poor performance.
3. This is information decay in the sense that current earnings are more important than previous earnings in management's performance evaluation.

Because of these assumptions, managers in good times save for bad times. In other words:

First, when current earnings are relatively low, but expected future earnings are relatively high, managers will make accounting choices that increase current period discretionary accruals. In effect, managers in this setting are "borrowing" earnings from the future. Second, when current earnings are relatively high, but expected future earnings are relatively low, managers will make accounting choices that decrease current year discretionary accruals. Managers are effectively "saving" current earnings for possible use in the future.[69]

DeFond and Park[70] investigated the intuition derived from the Fudenberg-Tirole model by examining the effects of current relative premanaged earnings and expected future relative earnings on the behavior of discretionary accruals. Their evidence suggests that when current earnings are "poor," and expected future earnings are "good," managers "borrow" earnings from the future for use in the current period. Conversely, when current earnings are "good" and expected future earnings are "poor," managers "save" current earnings for possible use in the future. These findings that managers of firms experiencing poor (good) performance in the current period and expecting good (poor) performance in the next period choose income-increasing (income-decreasing) discretionary accruals in order to reduce the threat of being dismissed did not directly examine the link between job security and income smoothing. Accordingly, Ahmed et al.[71] hypothesized that the extent of income smoothing varies directly with managers' job security concern as proxied by the degree of competition in a firm's product markets, product durability, and capital-intensity. Basically, the argument is that managers of firms in more competitive industries, durable goods industries, and capital-intensive businesses are likely to have greater job security concerns than managers of other firms and therefore are more likely to engage in a greater extent of income smoothing. The results were consistent with the predictions. Using a different methodology, Elgers et al.[72] were able to provide results indicating that patterns in measured discretionary accruals and relative earnings performance are consistent with the theory that managers smooth earnings based

on both current-year results and expected next-year results, a phenomenon better labeled as "anticipatory income smoothing."

Stockholders' Wealth and Income Smoothing

The only literature in income smoothing maintained and/or established a positive relationship between income smoothing and shareholders' wealth. The statements and/or findings are as follows:

1. Stockholder satisfaction is bound to increase with the rate of growth in a firm's income and the stability of its income.[73]

2. The possibility that analysts may become more enthusiastic about self-smoothers increases the interest in the firm's market shares and may have a favorable effect on share value and cost of capital.[74]

3. Income variability may be shown to be significantly correlated with both overall and systematic risk measures.[75]

4. Smoothing may imply a direct, cause-effect relationship between earnings fluctuations and market risk.[76]

5. By allowing management to select alternative accounting techniques, owners can capitalize upon managers' expertise.[77]

6. Smooth income reduces the probability of financial ratio covenants' leading to a reduction in the cost of default and renegotiation.[78]

7. Smooth income reduces the probability of financial ratio covenants' leading to a reduction in the cost of default and renegotiation.[79]

8. Firms that do not smooth have higher unexpected returns from earnings surprises than firms that smooth income.[80]

9. Institutional investors avoid firms that exhibit large variations in earnings. A smoother income stream is preferred.[81]

Other analyses of the impact of income smoothing on stockholders' wealth were more market-based. Nichelson et al.[82] found lower returns, lower risk, and larger firm sizes for smoothing firms. Wang and Williams[83] found that firms with a smooth income series were less risky and had a market response four times as large as that for the other firms. This favorable impact of smoothing is evaluated as follows:

Contrary to the widespread view that managers engage in income smoothing to increase their own welfare at the expense of stockholders, this study documents consistent evidence indicating that accounting income smoothing can be beneficial to the firm's stockholders and prospective investors. Specifically, the analysis demonstrated that income smoothing may enhance the informational value of earnings and reduce the riskiness of the firm.[84]

Chaney et al.[85] presents evidence that managers smooth income around their arrangements of the firm's permanent earnings. Income smoothing becomes a long-term strategy to communicate a firm's permanent earnings using discretionary accruals to remove (or offset) a portion of the transitory component of reported earnings. The evidence shows that (1) if the current year's income before discretionary accruals is lower than last year's reported earnings, discretionary accruals will be positive and (2) if the current year's income before discretionary accruals is already higher than last year's reported earnings, discretionary accruals will be negative. They conclude as follows:

We suggest that smoothing income around the managers' assessment of the firm's permanent earnings enhances the market's perception of the firm whose earnings are being managed. When firms consistently manage earnings to present a smooth pattern of profits to market participants, they avoid the dips in earnings (and related reputation effects) that may follow periods of over-reported earnings. We hypothesize and present evidence that earnings response coefficients, which reflect the relation between unexpected earnings and market returns, as well as the perceived reliability of reported earnings, are higher for firms that engage consistently in income smoothing.[86]

Finally, Chaney and Lewis[87] investigated income smoothing and underperformance in initial public offerings. They found a positive association between a proxy for income smoothing and firm performance, in the sense that (1) firms that perform well tend to report earnings with less variability relative to cash from operations compared to other firms and (2) the earnings response coefficient is greater for firms that are able to smooth earnings relative to cash flows. The result is interpreted as being totally consistent with the hypothesis that the market is better able to assess the information content of earnings for firms with smoother earnings.

NOTES

1. A. Belkaoui, *Accounting and Public Policy* (Westport, CT: Quorum Books, 1995).

2. A. Christie, "Aggregation of Test Statistics: On Evaluation of the Evidence as Contracting and Size Hypotheses," *Journal of Accounting and Economics* 12 (1990).

3. S. Lilien, M. Mellman, and V. Pastena, "Accounting Changes: Successful or Unsuccessful Firms," *The Accounting Review* (October 1988), pp. 642–651.

4. A. Belkaoui, "The Effect of Bond Ratings on Accounting Changes," Working Paper, University of Illinois at Chicago, 2002.

5. "SEC Chairman Discusses Earnings Management," *Deloitte & Touche Review* (October 12, 1998), p. 1.

6. S.R. Heyworth, "Smoothing Periodic Income," *The Accounting Review* (January 1953), p. 32.

7. R.J. Monsen and A. Downs, "A Theory of Large Managerial Firms," *The Journal of Political Economy* (June 1965).

8. M.J. Gordon, "Postulates, Principles, and Research in Accounting," *The Accounting Review* (April 1964), pp. 251–263.

9. Ibid., pp. 261–262.

10. C.R. Beidleman, "Income Smoothing: The Role of Management," *The Accounting Review* (October 1973), p. 653.

11. M.J. Gordon, B.M. Horwitz, and P.T. Meyers, "Accounting Measurement and Normal Growth of the Firm," in R. Jaedicke, Y. Ijiri, and O. Nielsen (eds.), *Research in Accounting Measurement* (Evanston, IL: American Accounting Association, 1966), pp. 221–231.

12. Hepworth, "Smoothing Periodic Income," pp. 32–39.

13. G. White, "Discretionary Accounting Disclosures and Income Normalization," *Journal of Accounting Research* (Autumn 1970), pp. 260–273.

14. D. Buckmaster, "Income Smoothing in Accounting and Business Literature Prior to 1954," *The Accounting Historian's Journal* (December 1992), pp. 147–173.

15. Ibid., p. 155.

16. E. Matheson, *The Depreciation of Factories, Mines and Industrial Undertaking and Their Valuation* (London: E. and F.N. Spon, 1910; reprint, New York: Arno Press, 1976), p. 44.

17. J.P. Joplin, "Secret Reserves," *Journal of Accountancy* (December 1910), pp. 407–417.

18. A.B. Grunder and D.R. Becker, "The Straight-Line Depreciation Accounting Practice of Telephone Companies in the United States," in *International Congress on Accounting* (New York: International Congress, 1930), pp. 351–403.

19. L.R. Dicksee, *Depreciation, Reserves, and Reserve Funds* (London: Gee & Co., 1903).

20. J.F. Johnson and E.S. Meade, "Editorial: Maintenance Expenses and Concealment of Earnings," *Journal of Accountancy* (March 1906), pp. 410–412.

21. Ibid.

22. Joplin, "Secret Reserves."

23. H.T. Warshaw, "Inventory Valuation and the Business Cycle," *Harvard Business Review* (October 1924), pp. 27–34.

24. A.R. Davis, "Inventory Valuation and Business Profits: The Case for a Cost or Market Basis," *N.A.C.A. Bulletin* (December 1937), pp. 400–409.

25. A. Cotter, *Fool's Profits* (New York: Barwin's Publishing, 1940).

26. Ibid.

27. Heyworth, "Smoothing Periodic Income," p. 34.

28. Gordon, "Postulates, Principles, and Research in Accounting," pp. 251–263.

29. Ibid.

30. Beidleman, "Income Smoothing," pp. 658–667.

31. Ibid., p. 654.

32. Ibid.

33. R.M. Cyert and J.G. March, *A Behavioral Theory of the Firm* (Englewood Cliffs, NJ: Prentice-Hall, 1963).

34. M. Schiff and A.Y. Levin, "Where Traditional Budgeting Fails," *Financial Executive* (May 1968), pp. 57–62.

35. J.D. Thompson, *Organizations in Action* (New York: McGraw-Hill, 1967).

36. J.Y. Kamin and J. Ronen, "The Smoothing of Income Numbers: Some Empirical

Evidence in Systematic Differences among Management-Controlled and Owner-Controlled Firms," *Accounting, Organizations and Society* 3, 2 (1978), pp. 141–153.

37. A. Barnea, J. Ronen, and S. Sadan, "Classificatory Smoothing of Income with Extraordinary Items," *The Accounting Review* (January 1976), pp. 110–122.

38. A. Belkaoui, *Behavioral Accounting* (Westport, CT: Greenwood Press, 1989).

39. R. Copeland, "Income Smoothing," *Empirical Research in Accounting: Selected Studies*, suppl. to *Journal of Accounting Research* 6 (1968), p. 101.

40. D. Fudenberg and J. Tirole, "A Theory of Income and Dividend Smoothing Based on Incumbency Rents," *Journal of Political Economy* 1 (1995), pp. 75–93.

41. N. Eckel, "The Income Smoothing Hypothesis Revisited," *Abacus* 17 (June 1981), pp. 28–40.

42. Ibid., p. 28.

43. Ibid., p. 29.

44. R.A. Lamber, "Income Smoothing as Rational Equilibrium Behavior," *The Accounting Review* 59 (October 1984), p. 606.

45. P.E. Dascher and R.E. Malcolm, "A Note on Income Smoothing in the Chemical Industry," *Journal of Accounting Research* (Autumn 1970), pp. 253–254.

46. M.J. Gordon, "Discussions of the Effects of Alternative Accounting Rules for Nonsubsidiary Investments," *Empirical Research in Accounting: Selected Studies*, suppl. to *Journal of Accounting Research* 4 (1966), p. 223.

47. Copeland, "Income Smoothing," 6, p. 101.

48. Barnea, Ronen, and Sadan, "Classificatory Smoothing of Income with Extraordinary Items," p. 111.

49. Copeland, "Income Smoothing," p. 102.

50. Beidleman, "Income Smoothing," p. 658.

51. T.R. Archibald, "The Return to Straight-Line Depreciation: An Analysis of a Change in Accounting Method," *Empirical Research in Accounting: Selected Studies*, suppl. to *Journal of Accounting Research* 5 (1967), pp. 164–180.

52. R.M. Barefield, and E.E. Comiskey, "The Smoothing Hypothesis: An Alternative Test," *The Accounting Review* (April 1972), pp. 291–298.

53. Beidleman, "Income Smoothing," pp. 653–667.

54. Copeland, "Income Smoothing," pp. 101–116.

55. N. Dopuch and D. Drake, "The Effect of Alternative Accounting Rules for Nonsubsidiary Investments," *Empirical Research in Accounting: Selected Studies* (1966), pp. 192–219.

56. Gordon, Horwitz, and Meyers, "Accounting Measurement and Normal Growth of the Firm," pp. 220–223.

57. Kamin and Ronen, "The Smoothing of Income Numbers," pp. 141–153.

58. A. Belkaoui and R.D. Picur, "The Smoothing of Income Numbers: Some Empirical Evidence on the Systematic Differences between Core and Periphery Industrial Sectors," *Journal of Business Finance & Accounting*, 11, 4 (Winter 1984), pp. 527–545.

59. W.D. Albrecht, and F.M. Richardson, "Income Smoothing by Economic Sector," *Journal of Business Finance & Accounting* 17, 5 (Winter 1990), pp. 713–730.

60. G. Breton and Jean Pierre Chenail, "Une Etude Emperique du Lissage des Benefices dansles Enterprises Canadiennes," *Comptabilite, Controle, Audit* (March 1997), pp. 53–68.

61. J. Kinnunen, E. Kasanen, and J. Nisleanen, "Earnings Management and the Eco-

nomy Sector Hypothesis: Empirical Evidence on a Converse Relationship in the Finnish Case," *Journal of Business Finance and Accounting* (June 1995), pp. 497–520.

62. Ibid., p. 498.

63. H. Genay, "Assessing the Condition of Japanese Banks: How Informative Are Accounting Earnings?" *Economic Perspectives* 22, 4 (1998), pp. 12–34; M. Sheikkoleslami, "The Impact of Foreign Stock Exchange Listing on Income Smoothing: Evidence from Japanese Firms," *International Journal of Management* 11, 2 (1994), pp. 737–742.

64. R.E. Bragshaw and A.E.K. Elchni, "The Smoothing Hypothesis and the Role of Exchange Differences," *Journal of Business Finance and Accounting* 16, 5 (1989), pp. 621–633; V. Beattie, S. Brown, D. Ewers, B. John, S. Manson, S. Thomas, and M. Turner, "Extraordinary Items and Income Smoothing: A Positive Accounting Approach," *Journal of Business Finance and Accounting* 21, 6 (1994), pp. 791–811.

65. S.M. Saudagaran and J.F. Sepe, "Replication of Moses Income Smoothing Tests with Canadian and U.K. Data, A Note," *Journal of Business Finance and Accounting* 23, 8 (1996), pp. 1219–1222; Breton and Chenail, "Une Etude Empirique," p. 54.

66. S. Chalayer, "Le Lissage des Resultats: Elements Enqlicatifs Avances des la Literature," *Comptabilite, Controle, Audit*, 2, 1 (1995), pp. 89–104.

67. N. Ashani, H.C. Koh, S.L. Tan, and W.H. Wang, "Factors Affecting Income Smoothing among Listed Companies in Singapore," *Accounting and Business Research*, 24, 96 (1994), pp. 291–301.

68. K. Fudenberg and J. Tirole, "A Theory of Income and Dividend Smoothing Based on Incumbency Results," *Journal of Political Economy*, 103 (1995), pp. 75–93.

69. M.L. DeFond and C.W. Park, "Smoothing Income in Anticipation of Future Earnings," *Journal of Accounting and Economics* 23 (1997), p. 1116.

70. Ibid., pp. 115–139.

71. A.S. Ahmed, G.J. Lobo, and J. Zhou, "Job Security and Income Smoothing: An Empirical Test of the Fudenberg and Tirole (1995) Model," Working Paper, Syracuse University, October 2000.

72. P.T. Elgers, R.J. Pfeiffer Jr., and S.L. Porter, "Anticipatory Income Smoothing: A Re-Examination," Working Paper, University of Massachusetts, February 2000.

73. Gordon, "Postulates, Principles and Research in Accounting," p. 262.

74. Beidleman, "Income Smoothing," p. 655.

75. B. Lev and S. Kunitzky, "On the Association between Smoothing Measures and the Risk of Common Stock," *The Accounting Review* (April 1974), p. 268.

76. O.D. Moses, "Income Smoothing and Incentives: Empirical Tests Using Accounting Changes," *The Accounting Review* (April 1987), p. 366.

77. J.S. Demski, J.M. Patell, and M.A. Wolfson, "Decentralized Choice of Monitoring Systems," *The Accounting Review* 59 (1984), pp. 16–34.

78. B. Trueman and S. Titman, "An Explanation for Accounting Income Smoothing," *Journal of Accounting Research* (Supplement, 1988), pp. 127–139.

79. Beattie et al., "Extraordinary Items and Income Smoothing," pp. 791–811.

80. G.G. Booth, J. Kallanki, and T. Martikainem, "Post Announcement Drift and Income Smoothing; Finnish Evidence," *Journal of Business Finance and Accounting* 23 (1996), pp. 1197–1211.

81. S.G. Badrinath, D. Gay, and J.P. Kale, "Patterns of Institutional Investment, Prudence and the Managerial 'Safety Net' Hypothesis," *Journal of Risk and Insurance* 56 (1989), pp. 605–629.

82. S.E. Nichelson, J. Jordan-Wagner, and C.W. Wroton, "A Market Based Analysis

of Income Smoothing," *Journal of Business Finance and Accounting* 22, 8 (1995), pp. 1179–1193.

83. Z. Wang and T.H. Williams, "Accounting Income Smoothing and Stockholder Wealth," *Journal of Applied Business Research* 10, 3 (1994), pp. 96–104.

84. Ibid., p. 102.

85. P.K. Chaney, D.C. Jeter, and C.M. Lewis, "The Use of Accruals in Income Smoothing: A Permanent Earnings Hypothesis," *Advances in Quantitative Analysis of Finance and Accounting* 6 (1998), pp. 103–135.

86. Ibid., p. 131.

87. P.K. Chaney and C.M. Lewis, "Income Smoothing and Underperformance in Initial Public Offerings," *Journal of Corporate Finance* 4 (1998), pp. 1–29.

SELECTED REFERENCES

Albrecht, W.D., and F.M. Richardson. "Income Smoothing by Economic Sector." *Journal of Business Finance & Accounting* 17, 5 (Winter 1990), pp. 713–730.

American Institute of Certified Public Accountants (AICPA). *Report of the Study Group on the Objectives of Financial Statements.* New York: AICPA, October 1973.

Amihud, Y., J. Kamin, and J. Ronen. "Managerialism and Ownerism in Risk-Return Preferences." Ross Institute of Accounting Research (R.I.A.R.) Working Paper 95–4, New York University, 1975.

Archibald, T.R. "The Return to Straight-Line Depreciation: An Analysis of a Change in Accounting Method." *Empirical Research in Accounting: Selected Studies*, suppl. to *Journal of Accounting Research* 5 (1967), pp. 161–180.

Barefield, R.M., and E.E. Comiskey. "The Smoothing Hypothesis: An Alternative Test." *The Accounting Review* (April 1972), pp. 291–298.

Barnes, A., J. Ronen, and S. Sadan. "Classificatory Smoothing of Income with Extraordinary Items." *The Accounting Review* (January 1976), pp. 110–122.

———. "The Implementation of Accounting Objectives—An Application to Extraordinary Items." *The Accounting Review* (January 1975), pp. 58–68.

Baumol, W.J. *Business Behavior, Value and Growth.* New York: Macmillan, 1959.

Beidleman, C.R. "Income Smoothing: The Role of Management." *The Accounting Review* (October 1973), pp. 653–667.

Belkaoui, A., and R.D. Picur. "The Smoothing of Income Numbers: Some Empirical Evidence on the Systematic Differences between Core and Periphery Industrial Sectors." *Journal of Business Finance & Accounting* 11, 4 (Winter 1984), pp. 527–545.

Bernard, V.L., and R.S. Stober. "The Nature and Amount of Information Reflected in Cash Flows and Accruals." *The Accounting Review* (October 1989), pp. 624–652.

Copeland, R., "Income Smoothing." *Empirical Research in Accounting: Selected Studies*, suppl. to *Journal of Accounting Research* 6 (1968), pp. 101–116.

Copeland, R., and R. Licastro. "A Note on Income Smoothing." *The Accounting Review* (July 1968), pp. 540–545.

Copeland, R., and J. Wojdak. "Income Manipulation and the Purchase Pooling Choice." *Journal of Accounting Research* (Autumn 1969), pp. 188–195.

Cushing, B.E. "An Empirical Study of Changes in Accounting Policy." *Journal of Accounting Research* (Autumn 1969), pp. 196–203.

Cyert, R.M., and J.G. March. *A Behavioral Theory of the Firm*. Englewood Cliffs, NJ: Prentice-Hall, 1963.

Dascher, P.E., and R.E. Malcolm. "A Note on Income Smoothing in the Chemical Industry." *Journal of Accounting Research* (Autumn 1970), pp. 253–259.

Eckel, N. "The Income Smoothing Hypothesis Revisited." *Abacus* 17 (June 1981), pp. 28–40.

Gordon, M.J. "Postulates, Principles and Research in Accounting." *The Accounting Review* (April 1964), pp. 251–263.

Gordon, M.J., B.M. Horwitz, and P.T. Meyers. "Accounting Measurement and Normal Growth of the Firm." In R. Jaedicke, Y. Ijiri, and O. Nielsen (eds.), *Research in Accounting Measurement*. Evanston, IL: American Accounting Association, 1966, pp. 221–231.

Hepworth, S.R. "Smoothing Periodic Income." *The Accounting Review* (January 1953), pp. 32–39.

Horwitz, B.N. "Comments on Income Smoothing: A Review by J. Ronen, S. Sadan and C. Snow." *Accounting Journal* (Spring 1977), pp. 27–29.

Imhoff, E.A., Jr. "Income Smoothing—A Case for Doubt." *Accounting Journal* (Spring 1977), pp. 85–101.

———. "Income Smoothing: An Analysis of Critical Issues." *Quarterly Review of Economics and Business* (Autumn 1981), pp. 23–42.

Jeter, D.C., and P.K. Chancy. "An Empirical Investigation of Factors Affecting the Earnings Association Coefficient." *Journal of Business Finance & Accounting* 19, 6 (November 1992), pp. 839–863.

Jordan-Wagner, J., and C.W. Wootton. "An Analysis of Earnings in Oil Related Industries." *Petroleum Accounting and Financial Management Journal* (Spring 1993), pp. 110–123.

Lamber, R.A. "Income Smoothing as Rational Equilibrium Behavior." *The Accounting Review* 59 (October 1984), pp. 604–618.

Lev, B., and S. Kunitzky. "On the Association between Smoothing Measures and the Risk of Common Stock." *The Accounting Review* (April 1974), pp. 259–270.

Mason, R.D., and D.A. Lind. *Statistical Techniques in Business and Economics*, 8th ed. Homewood, IL: Irwin, 1993, pp. 136–137.

Moses, O.D. "Income Smoothing and Incentives: Empirical Tests Using Accounting Changes." *The Accounting Review* (April 1987), pp. 358–377.

O'Hanlon, J. "The Relationship in Time between Annual Accounting Returns and Annual Stock Market Returns in the UK." *Journal of Business Finance & Accounting* 18, 3 (April 1991), pp. 305–314.

Ronen, J., and S. Sadan. "Classificatory Smoothing: Alternative Income Models." *Journal of Accounting Research* (Spring 1975), pp. 133–149.

———. *Smoothing Income Numbers, Objectives, Means, and Implications*. Reading, MA: Addison Wesley, 1981.

Strong, N. "Modelling Abnormal Returns: A Review Article." *Journal of Business Finance & Accounting* 19, 4 (June 1992), pp. 531–553.

Thorne, D. "The Information Content of the Trend between Historic Cost Earnings and Current Cost Earnings (United States of America)." *Journal of Business Finance & Accounting* 18, 3 (April 1991), pp. 289–303.

Trueman, B., and S. Titman. "An Explanation for Accounting Income Smoothing." *Journal of Accounting Research* (Supplement, 1988), pp. 127–139.

Zmijewski, M.E., and R.L. Hagerman. "An Income Strategy Approach to the Positive Theory of Accounting Standard Setting/Choice." *Journal of Accounting and Economics* (August 1981), pp. 129–149.

Appendix 1A. Accrual Accounting and Cash Accounting: Relative Merits of Derived Accounting Indicator Numbers

One of the dominant characteristics in early views of the purpose of financial statements is the stewardship function. Under this view, management is entrusted with control of the financial resources provided by capital suppliers. Accordingly, the purpose of financial statements is to report to the concerned parties so as to facilitate the evaluation of management's stewardship. To accomplish this objective, the reporting system favored and deemed essentially superior to others is the accrual system. Simply, the accrual basis of accounting refers to a form of record keeping that, in addition to recording transactions resulting from the receipt and disbursement of cash, records the amounts that it owes others and that others owe it (Gross, 1972). At the core of this system is the matching of revenues and expenses (Paton and Littleton, 1940). The interest in the accrual method generated a search of the "best" accrual method in general and the "ideal income" in particular (Paton, 1922 [1962]; Canning, 1929; Alexander, 1950). For a long time, this accounting paradigm governed the evaluation of accounting alternatives and the asset valuation and income determination proposals (Edwards and Bell, 1961; Chambers, 1966; Sterling, 1970). The approach was, however, constantly challenged by cash-flow accounting. The cash-flow basis of accounting has been correctly defined as the recording not only of the cash receipts and disbursements of the period (the cash basis of accounting) but also the future cash flows owed to or by the firm as a result of selling and transferring title to certain goods (the accrual basis of accounting (Hicks, 1980)). The challenge by cash-flow accounting is more evident in some of the questioning of the importance and efficacy of accrual accounting and a shift toward cash-flow approaches in security analysis (Hawkins and Campbell, 1978).

The question about the superiority of accrual accounting over cash-flow accounting is central to the determination of the objectives and the nature of financial reporting. Consensus on criteria of superiority may be difficult to attain given the diversity of users and interests. What may be more practical to examine are the relative merits of derived accounting numbers from both accrual and cash-flow accounting. Thus, the main objective of this appendix is to examine empirically the relative merits of derived performance indicator numbers from both accrual and cash-flow accounting in terms of both the persistence and the variability of such numbers.

In the first section of this appendix, the conceptual differences and the controversy between accrual accounting and cash-flow accounting are examined. This is followed by a discussion of the sample design. The third section then

examines the impact of the choice of either cash flow or accrual on accounting indicator numbers in terms of their persistence and variability. The final section presents a brief summary and conclusion.

ISSUE: ACCRUAL VERSUS CASH ACCOUNTING

As stated earlier, accrual accounting is deemed a superior system to facilitate the evaluation of management's stewardship and is essential to the matching of revenues and expenses so that efforts and accomplishments are properly aligned. The efficacy of the accrual system has been, however, questioned. Thomas (1969, 1974) stated that all allocations are arbitrary and incorrigible and recommended the minimization of such allocations. Hawkins and Campbell (1978) reported a shift in security analysis from earnings-oriented valuation approaches to cash flow-oriented approaches. Many decision usefulness theorists advocated cash-flow accounting based on the investor's desires to predict cash flows (Staubus, 1961, 1971; American Accounting Association [AAA], 1969; American Institute of Certified Public Accountants [AICPA], 1973; Revsine, 1973). Finally, various authors recommended that financial statements be based upon a cash-flow orientation because of limitations in accrual accounting (Lawson, 1971, 1973; Lee, 1972a, 1972b; Stern, 1972; Ashton, 1976; Climo, 1976; Ijiri, 1978, 1979). Most of these authors feel that the problems of asset valuation and income determination are so formidable that another accounting system should be derived and propose the inclusion of comprehensive cash-flow statements in companies' annual reports. More recently Lee (1981) described how cash-flow accounting and net realizable value accounting can be brought together in a series of articulating statements that provide more relevant information for the report user about cash and cash management than can be given by either system on its own.[1]

Cash-flow accounting is viewed by supporters as superior to conventional accrual accounting. Lawson (1971) argues that his system of cash-flow accounting provides an analytical framework for linking past, present, and future financial performance. Lee (1972a) argues that investors could see from the projected cash flows both the ability of the company to pay its way in the future and also its planned financial policy. Ashton (1976, p. 75) maintains that a "price/discounted flow" ratio would be a more reliable investment indicator than the present "price/earnings" ratio because of the numerous arbitrary allocations used to compute the earnings per share. Ijiri (1979, p. 57) argues for the development of cash-flow accounting to correct the gap in practice between the way in which an investment decision is made (generally based on cash flows) and the ways that the results are evaluated (generally based on earnings). Finally, various authors are expressing doubt with regard to the relevance and utility of accrual accounting information for investors who are concerned mainly with decision making (Edey, 1963; Lawson, 1971; Lee, 1971, 1972b).

Objectives

Given the issue of accrual versus cash accounting, the main objective in this appendix is to evaluate the relative merits of accounting indicators derived from either an accrual accounting system or a cash-flow accounting system. The accounting indicators derived from an accrual accounting system included both a balance sheet-oriented number and an income statement-oriented number. The indicators also had two basic characteristics. First, they are computed as per share numbers, and second, they are ratios whose dominator is the market price of a share. The first characteristic is used to ensure comparability between the indicators and the companies. The second characteristic is used to ensure that the indicator reflects both accounting-based performance and market-based numbers. A second argument for dividing the accounting-based datum by the market price of a share reflects the belief that the accounting datum should be evaluated in terms of the impact on its relationships to the market price. The implied hypothesis is that of the accounting data derived from either an accrual accounting system or a cash-flow accounting system. The one most favored by the market and/or reflected in the market price will show less variability and a higher persistence than the other numbers. The rationale is that the nature of the association between the derived accounting numbers and the behavior of security prices indicates which method the market perceives to be the most related to the information used in setting equilibrium prices. The method that produces accounting numbers having the association with security prices, with the least variability and the highest persistence, is the most consistent with the information that results in an efficient determination of security prices. But as pointed out by Beaver and Dukes (1972, p. 321), the evidence on the nature of the association is also essential regardless of the efficiency of the market. It is an important factor in any accounting policy regardless of the nature of the policymakers' views about other issues, including market efficiency.

The cash flow per share/stock price of security i for time period t, is defined as:

$$CFP_{i,t} = \frac{CFO_{i,t}/CSO_{i,t}}{P_{i,t}}$$

where

$P_{i,t}$ = price of security i at the end of period t adjusted for capital changes such as stock splits and stock dividends.

$CFO_{i,t}$ = cash flows from operations calculated by adjusting net income for noncash charges (credits) and for changes in the current accounts exclusive of changes in the firm's cash position, of firm i in period t (Compustat variable No. 10).

$CSO_{i,t}$ = common shares outstanding of firm i in period t (Compustat variable No. 25).

The common equity per share/stock price of security i for time period t is defined as:

$$CEP_{i,t} = \frac{CE_{i,t}/CSO_{i,t}}{P_{i,t}}$$

where

$CE_{i,t}$ = common equity of company i at the end of period t. Common equity (Compustat variable No. 11) represents common stock plus retained earnings, capital surplus, self-insurance reserves, and capital stock premium.

The earnings per share/stock price of security i for time period t, is defined as:

$$EPSP_{i,t} = \frac{EPS_{i,t}}{P_{i,t}}$$

where

$EPS_{i,t}$ = Earnings per share (primary), excluding extraordinary items, of company i for period t.

EPS (Compustat variable No. 58) represents the primary earnings per share figure as reported by the company.

Each of these numbers, $CFP_{i,t}$, $CEP_{i,t}$, and $EPSP_{i,t}$, represents numbers that are derived from either an accrual or a cash-flow accounting system and related to the stock price and whose merits will be evaluated in terms of variability and persistence. They represent semiaccounting indices of rate of return derived from either an accrual or a cash-flow accounting system (Barley and Levy, 1979, p. 307).

The Sample Design

The study employs both accounting and market data. Market data were retrieved from the Center for Research in Security Prices (CRSP) tape developed at the University of Chicago, while accounting data were retrieved from the Compustat tape.

Two criteria were used for the selection of companies to be included in the sample. First, its accounting and market data were available on both the Compustat and the CRSP tape for a period of nineteen years beginning in 1959 and ending in 1977. This criterion was necessary to allow for the computation of each of the semiaccounting indices of rate of return. Second, the company must figure in the *Fortune* magazine's list of the 500 largest American companies.

This criterion was adopted to limit the size and profitability differences, which may affect the results of the study. Of these companies, sixty-six met the sampling requirement. A list of these companies appears in Table 1A.1.

The three semiaccounting indices of rate of return were used for a comparison of the relative merits of accrual and cash accounting.

a. A cash-flow per share/stock price ratio was used to represent the cash accounting-derived semiaccounting index of rate of return.

b. A common equity per share/stock price ratio was used to represent the accrual accounting-derived and balance sheet-oriented semiaccounting index of rate of return.

c. An earnings per share/stock price ratio was used to represent the accrual accounting-derived and income statement-oriented semiaccounting index of rate of return.

Results

Variability of the Derived Accounting Indicator Numbers

The three accounting indicators, namely, the cash flow per share/stock price (CFP), the common equity per share/stock price (CEP), and the earnings per share/stock price (EPSP), were computed for the sixty-six companies for the years 1959 to 1977. The means, standard deviation, and coefficients of variation of these numbers are presented in Table 1A.1. In addition, this table includes a ranking of the coefficients of variations of the derived accounting indicator numbers.

An examination of Table 1A.1 shows a definite difference in the variability of these numbers. The variability of the EPSP numbers exceeds the variability of the CEP and CFP numbers. More precisely, the coefficients of variation of the EPSP's numbers are higher than those of the CEP numbers in forty-two cases or those of the CFP numbers in forty-five. The coefficients of variation of the CFP numbers were higher than those of the CEP numbers in forty-four cases. Those differences are, in most cases, considerable (see Table 1A.1).

For those cases where the variability of CEP and CFP numbers exceeds those of the EPSP numbers, the differences for more than 50 percent of the cases are rather small and do not indicate any specific pattern. The variability of the EPSP numbers, as measured by their coefficients of variation, ranges from a high of 4.723 for Allegheny Airlines to a low of 0.19 for Philip Morris Inc. The variability of the CEP numbers ranges from a high of 1.84 for General Motors to a low of 0.18 for Phillips Petroleum. Finally, the variability of the CFP numbers ranges from a high of 1.31 for Lockheed to a low of 0.19 for Phillips Petroleum.

Next, the relationship between the distributions of the coefficients of variation of EPSP, CEP, and CFP was examined by computing Spearman's rank order correlation coefficient between these distributions. The computed correlation between the coefficients of variation of CEP and EPSP is equal to .5 ($t_s = 4.6$) which is significant at = .001. Finally, the computed correlation coefficient

Table 1A.1
CFP, EPSP, and CFP's Means, Standard Deviations, and Coefficients of Variation for the Sample Companies, 1959–1977

Company	CEP_i Mean	CEP_i Standard Deviation	CEP_i Coefficient of Variation	EPSP_i Mean	EPSP_i Standard Deviation	EPSP_i Coefficient of Variation	EPSP_i Ranking	CFP_i Mean	CFP_i Standard Deviation	CFP_i Coefficient of Variation	CFP_i Ranking
1. General Motors Corp.	0.000528	0.000976	1.848484849	0.088996	0.038450	0.43204189	37	0.000129	0.000052	0.403100775	38
2. Lockheed Corp.	0.001338	0.001665	1.244394619	0.097106	0.21719	2.236628015	2	0.000390	0.000514	1.317948718	25
3. EXTRA Corp.	0.000560	0.000616	1.1	0.083259	0.104938	1.260380259	5	0.000342	0.000278	0.812865497	5
4. Honeywell Inc.	0.000546	0.000533	0.976190476	0.057101	0.043605	0.763644871	9	0.000183	0.000203	1.109289618	2
5. Cities Service Co.	0.001095	0.000163	0.879452055	0.097346	0.028520	0.292975572	59	0.000229	0.000063	0.27510917	57
6. Allegheny Airlines Inc.	0.000888	0.000696	0.783783784	0.050166	0.206859	4.12349	1	0.000421	0.000375	0.890736342	4
7. NCR Corp.	0.000670	0.000453	0.676119403	0.052659	0.063827	1.212081506	6	0.000184	0.000148	0.804347826	6
8. McDonnell Douglas Corp.	0.000851	0.000575	0.675675676	0.121786	0.069912	0.574056131	16	0.000180	0.000106	0.588888889	12
9. General Tire & Rubber Co.	0.001018	0.000655	0.643418468	0.125968	0.078580	0.623809221	12	0.000808	0.000116	0.557692308	15
10. Uniroyal Inc.	0.001388	0.000866	0.623919308	0.094273	0.053926	0.57201956	17	0.000261	0.000158	0.605363985	71
11. General Dynamics Corp.	0.000965	0.000593	0.614507772	0.078956	0.164421	2.08243832	3	0.000208	0.000186	0.894230769	3
12. FMC Corp.	0.000654	0.000393	0.600917431	0.057844	0.052524	0.597923592	14	0.000162	0.000101	0.62345679	9
13. Westinghouse Electric Corp.	0.000786	0.000467	0.594147583	0.072075	0.044888	0.6227956	13	0.000130	0.000099	0.761533462	7
14. RCA Corp.	0.000439	0.000260	0.592255125	0.062512	0.031864	0.509726133	28	0.000159	0.000110	0.691823899	8
15. VSI Corp.	0.000733	0.000422	0.575716235	0.103011	0.067321	0.653532147	10	0.000170	0.000090	0.529411765	18
16. Texaco Inc.	0.000713	0.000374	0.5245418	0.096196	0.052297	0.543650464	21	0.000156	0.000081	0.519230769	19
17. Owens-Illinois Inc.	0.000762	0.000388	0.509186352	0.079463	0.038722	0.487295974	31	0.000144	0.000074	0.513888889	22
18. IBM Corp.	0.000181	0.000091	0.502762431	0.032806	0.017787	0.542187405	23	0.000066	0.000030	0.454545455	25
19. Textron Inc.	0.000603	0.000297	0.492537313	0.098990	0.044234	0.446853218	35	0.000177	0.000078	0.440677966	89
20. TRW Inc.	0.000421	0.000203	0.482185273	0.084327	0.046748	0.554363743	19	0.000170	0.000094	0.552941176	16
21. Republic Steel Corp.	0.001923	0.000924	0.48049922	0.123040	0.094391	0.767157022	8	0.000255	0.000137	0.537254902	17
22. Atlantic Richfield Co.	0.000739	0.000352	0.47631935	0.072849	0.026904	0.369311864	49	0.000185	0.000051	0.275675676	56
23. Celanese Corp.	0.000810	0.000376	0.464197531	0.091250	0.050207	0.5502136	20	0.000279	0.000159	0.569892473	14
24. Utah Power & Light	0.000724	0.000332	0.458563356	0.079384	0.033082	0.4167338	40	0.000137	0.000050	0.364963504	46
25. Coca-Cola Co.	0.000177	0.000080	0.451977401	0.037553	0.014116	0.375895401	47	0.000049	0.000017	0.346938776	48
26. Minnesota Mining & Mfg. Co.	0.000185	0.000083	0.448648649	0.034273	0.013230	0.386018148	45	0.000048	0.000019	0.4375	31
27. Warner-Lambert Co.	0.000262	0.000111	0.423664122	0.047978	0.014925	0.31108	54	0.000059	0.000019	0.322033898	50
28. Republic of Texas Corp.	0.000620	0.000262	0.422580645	0.079088	0.042522	0.5376542	26	0.000065	0.000031	0.476923077	24
29. Ford Motor Co.	0.000947	0.000393	0.418162619	0.116545	0.062840	0.53919087	24	0.000190	0.000086	0.452631579	27
30. Philip Morris Inc.	0.000440	0.000181	0.411363636	0.071162	0.014109	0.198265928	67	0.000091	0.000021	0.230769231	61

#	Company											
31.	American Shores Co.	0.001382	0.000565	0.408827786	0.109488	0.058236	0.5318939	27	0.000250	0.000126	0.504	83
32.	Owens-Corning Fiberglass Corp.	0.000423	0.000172	0.406619385	0.048238	0.023777	0.4929101	30	0.000086	0.000039	0.453488372	26
33.	Johnson & Johnson	0.000246	0.000099	0.402439024	0.031981	0.009834	0.307495075	56	0.000047	0.000016	0.340425532	49
34.	Aluminium Co. of America	0.000779	0.000311	0.399229818	0.644410	0.034966	0.542866815	22	0.000153	0.000068	0.4444	28
35.	Gulf Oil Corp.	0.000923	0.000366	0.396533044	0.109213	0.058743	0.537875528	25	0.000203	0.000105	0.517241379	20
36.	Greyhound Corp.	0.000494	0.000177	0.393858478	0.090411	0.032712	0.361814381	50	0.000152	0.000065	0.427631579	33
37.	Raytheon Corp.	0.000665	0.000256	0.384962406	0.026635	0.027031	0.352723951	51	0.000140	0.000055	0.391857143	40
38.	Champion Intl. Corp.	0.000805	0.000307	0.38136646	0.095903	0.061573	0.642034139	11	0.000197	0.000120	0.609137056	10
39.	American Home Products Corp.	0.000110	0.000041	0.372727273	0.039494	0.009948	0.251886362	64	0.000045	0.000011	0.24444444	59
40.	Getty Oil Co.	0.000966	0.000360	0.372670807	0.087845	0.026303	0.299425124	58	0.000153	0.000034	0.2222222	62
41.	General Electric Co.	0.000306	0.000114	0.37254902	0.047901	0.020719	0.432537943	36	0.000078	0.000033	0.423076923	32
42.	Emerson Electric Co.	0.000266	0.000096	0.360902256	0.046987	0.013029	0.2772894	63	0.000063	0.000017	0.26984127	51
43.	Allied Chemical Corp.	0.000735	0.000265	0.360544218	0.078056	0.030755	0.474723276	33	0.000184	0.000071	0.385869565	44
44.	National Steel Corp.	0.001202	0.000424	0.352745424	0.101600	0.050885	0.500836614	29	0.000212	0.000086	0.405660377	37
45.	Upjohn Co.	0.000270	0.000093	0.344444444	0.043755	0.014220	0.3249914	53	0.000057	0.000020	0.350877193	47
46.	Union Oil Co. of California	0.000831	0.000284	0.341756919	0.099550	0.040527	0.4071019	42	0.000286	0.000116	0.405594406	38
47.	U.S. Steel Inc.	0.001470	0.000497	0.338095238	0.101321	0.059112	0.5834131	15	0.000231	0.000090	0.38961039	43
48.	Standard Oil Co. (California)	0.000870	0.000290	0.33333333	0.104958	0.045292	0.431524991	38	0.000170	0.000090	0.405882353	36
49.	Bethlehem Steel Corp.	0.001423	0.000467	0.328179902	0.077385	0.145041	1.874277961	4	0.000218	0.000127	0.582568807	13
50.	Borden Inc.	0.000628	0.000206	0.328015478	0.073927	0.029890	0.404317773	43	0.000120	0.000049	0.408335333	36
51.	Armco Inc.	0.001201	0.000393	0.32641196	0.105100	0.050815	0.483491912	32	0.000208	0.000086	0.413461538	34
52.	Bowater Corp. Ltd. Adr.	0.00115	0.000367	0.319130435	0.088466	0.068530	0.7746478	7	0.000238	0.000123	0.516806723	1
53.	Shell Oil Co.	0.000718	0.000226	0.314763231	0.087232	0.039576	0.45368672	34	0.000188	0.000070	0.372540426	44
54.	Standard Oil Co. (Ohio)	0.000691	0.000217	0.314037627	0.064283	0.021525	0.334847471	52	0.000125	0.000055	0.44	30
55.	R.J. Reynolds Inds.	0.000477	0.000145	0.303983229	0.092009	0.028431	0.30900238	55	0.000120	0.000047	0.591666667	41
56.	Tenneco Inc.	0.000601	0.000174	0.289517471	0.091933	0.034854	0.378876654	46	0.000215	0.000065	0.502325581	55
57.	Inland Steel Co.	0.001064	0.000300	0.281954887	0.102078	0.041250	0.404102745	44	0.000202	0.000065	0.321782178	53
58.	Georgia-Pacific Corp.	0.000362	0.000100	0.276243094	0.555220	0.020491	0.371079319	48	0.000113	0.000033	0.292055398	50
59.	Standard Oil Co. (Indiana)	0.000930	0.000251	0.269892473	0.089009	0.025605	0.287667539	60	0.000199	0.000043	0.216080402	64
60.	Dow Chemical	0.000367	0.000094	0.25613079	0.056794	0.024162	0.4254322	39	0.000116	0.000039	0.336206897	50
61.	Colgate-Palmolive Co.	0.000489	0.000119	0.243353783	0.060901	0.013485	0.221424936	66	0.000092	0.000020	0.217511504	63
62.	American Brands Inc.	0.000589	0.000135	0.229202307	0.101381	0.028532	0.281433405	62	0.000131	0.000044	0.366412214	45
63.	Kraft Inc.	0.000594	0.000132	0.22222222	0.075648	0.021650	0.286193951	60	0.000115	0.000027	0.234782601	60
64.	Caterpillar Tractor Co.	0.000365	0.000073	0.2	0.062712	0.015501	0.247177574	65	0.000096	0.000020	0.208333333	65
65.	International Paper Co.	0.000665	0.000130	0.195488722	0.070480	0.028830	0.409052213	41	0.000135	0.000043	0.318518519	53
66.	Phillips Petroleum Co.	0.000667	0.000121	0.181409295	0.070019	0.021111	0.301503878	57	0.000146	0.000028	0.191780822	66

between the coefficients of variation of CEP and CFP is equal to .57 ($t_s = 5.65$), which is also significant. Thus, it may be concluded that in spite of the differences in the variability of EPSP, CEP, and CFP numbers, there is some correlation between them. The main question created by these results refers to the possible reason(s) that the variability of income statement-oriented and accrual accounting-based numbers (EPSP) exceeds for a large number of firms in the sample those of the cash accounting-based numbers (CFP) and the balance sheet-oriented and accrual accounting-based numbers (CEP).

One reason may stem from the fact that EPSP numbers are based on accounting data, which are a likelier object of discretionary accounting income smoothing, as defined by Gordon (1964) and others, and of the smoothing process inherent in the very definition of accounting income (Barley and Levy, 1979). It may be stated first that the income smoothing is easier and more dramatic with income figures than balance sheet and cash-flow accounting data, and second, that managers may have a greater incentive in smoothing income figures given the stronger links between accounting income and the firm's reward structure (Barley and Levy, 1979, p. 314). As a result, the market is efficiently reflecting a "true" income figure different from the "reported" one, which may explain the variability of income statement-oriented and accrual accounting-based numbers.

A second reason may be that the market, very much aware of the smoothing process affecting income figures, is attaching more importance to the balance sheet position first and the cash flow second. The superiority of the balance sheet over cash-flow data may be due to a selective market response due either to the higher familiarity with balance sheet data than cash-flow data or basically to a balance sheet fixation and a stronger interest in the financial position of the firms.

PERSISTENCY OF DERIVED ACCOUNTING INDICATOR NUMBERS

The persistency of the derived accounting indicator numbers was determined by examining the median rank correlation between the accounting indicator number in the year of formation and the same number in subsequent years.[2] Tables 1A.2, 1A.3, and 1A.4 show consecutively the rank correlation of all the sample companies' CEP, CFP, and EPSP with the CEP, CFP, and EPSP in subsequent years. The median correlation of each column is reported at the bottom of the tables.

The median correlation of the CEP numbers shown in Table 1A.2 decreases from .918 in the first year after formation to .250 in the fourteenth year after formation. Five years after formation the median correlation is .629, while ten years after formation the median is .385.

The median correlation of the CFP numbers shown in Table 1A.3 decreases from .835 in the first year after formation to .281 in the fourteenth year after

Table 1A.2
Rank Correlations of All the Sample Companies' CEPs with CEPs in Subsequent Years

Base Year	Years Following Base Year													
	1	2	3	4	5	6	7	8	9	10	11	12	13	14
1959	0.825	0.733	0.670	0.592	0.431	0.468	0.304	0.288	0.207	0.310	0.726	0.244	0.257	0.106
1960	0.878	0.801	0.720	0.632	0.599	.443	0.374	0.329	0.457	0.385	0.364	0.350	0.182	0.215
1961	0.920	0.808	0.722	0.687	0.495	0.433	0.383	0.467	0.386	0.368	0.335	0.122	0.196	0.250
1962	0.916	0.856	0.834	0.658	0.579	0.536	0.539	0.475	0.492	0.451	0.175	0.242	0.296	0.371
1963	0.941	0.836	0.672	0.607	0.578	0.607	0.556	0.560	0.522	0.298	0.364	0.398	0.491	0.576
1964	0.858	0.702	0.652	0.630	0.665	0.637	0.611	0.567	0.352	0.465	0.482	0.559	0.584	
1965	0.894	0.839	0.782	0.737	0.655	0.681	0.665	0.322	0.334	0.375	0.462	0.558		
1966	0.936	0.925	0.813	0.723	0.729	0.735	0.372	0.419	0.465	0.552	0.649			
1967	0.952	0.863	0.784	0.769	0.780	0.457	0.506	0.536	0.615	0.635				
1968	0.909	0.855	0.825	0.812	0.506	0.507	0.542	0.622	0.650					
1969	0.945	0.893	0.879	0.671	0.602	0.657	0.714	0.655						
1970	0.946	0.907	0.752	0.644	0.683	0.743	0.656							
1971	0.946	0.731	0.536	0.615	0.695	0.705								
1972	0.806	0.521	0.596	0.681	0.688									
1973	0.492	0.531	0.618	0.512										
1974	0.962	0.927	0.636											
1975	0.958	0.691												
1976	0.833													
1977														
Median Correlation	.918	.836	.721	.658	.629	.607	.541	.475	.461	.385	.364	.350	.276	.250

Table 1A.3
Rank Correlations of All the Sample Companies' CFPs with CFPs in Subsequent Years

Base Year	Years Following Base Year													
	1	2	3	4	5	6	7	8	9	10	11	12	13	14
1959	0.811	0.808	0.668	0.530	0.288	0.488	0.409	0.379	0.302	0.486	0.466	0.299	0.302	0.223
1960	0.675	0.627	0.655	0.367	0.465	0.429	0.377	0.214	0.496	0.494	0.146	0.187	0.196	0.271
1961	0.690	0.513	0.321	0.618	0.516	0.541	0.437	0.514	0.464	0.367	0.348	0.220	0.273	0.281
1962	0.829	0.666	0.807	0.677	0.583	0.428	0.599	0.621	0.435	0.450	0.315	0.420	0.380	0.478
1963	0.867	0.713	0.564	0.452	0.233	0.522	0.529	0.387	0.428	0.436	0.550	0.466	0.562	0.688
1964	0.642	0.508	0.328	0.190	0.403	0.453	0.350	0.399	0.388	0.561	0.564	0.557	0.477	
1965	0.912	0.815	0.674	0.786	0.734	0.580	0.610	0.397	0.486	0.467	0.530	0.383		
1966	0.861	0.780	0.793	0.716	0.550	0.628	0.373	0.426	0.375	0.448	0.350			
1967	0.767	0.742	0.651	0.594	0.631	0.352	0.369	0.338	0.408	0.307				
1968	0.763	0.643	0.674	0.206	0.415	0.383	0.370	0.432	0.130					
1969	0.868	0.567	0.600	0.300	0.366	0.345	0.424	0.383						
1970	0.520	0.509	0.203	0.371	0.342	0.368	0.347							
1971	0.924	0.794	0.746	0.779	0.783	0.368								
1972	0.841	0.765	0.780	0.800	0.438									
1973	0.895	0.808	0.888	0.600										
1974	0.909	0.905	0.665											
1975	0.929	0.482												
1976	0.673													
1977														
Median Correlation	.835	.713	.667	.600	.452	.429	.393	.397	.418	.450	.408	.383	.341	.181

28

Table 1A.4
Rank Correlations of All the Sample Companies' EPSPs with EPSPs in Subsequent Years

Base Year	Years Following Base Year													
	1	2	3	4	5	6	7	8	9	10	11	12	13	14
1959	0.574	0.545	0.394	0.327	0.257	0.377	0.296	0.148	0.200	0.428	0.208	0.292	0.181	0.179
1960	0.576	0.360	0.262	0.306	0.474	0.358	-0.018	0.161	0.425	0.263	0.282	0.235	0.136	-0.020
1961	0.536	0.366	0.537	0.583	0.439	0.409	0.375	0.473	0.005	0.456	0.307	0.165	0.133	0.260
1962	0.900	0.738	0.655	0.504	0.342	0.291	0.168	-0.243	0.442	0.376	0.331	0.205	0.273	0.324
1963	0.812	0.790	0.570	0.380	0.384	0.172	-0.278	0.492	0.500	0.481	0.349	0.391	0.444	0.182
1964	0.819	0.710	0.424	0.549	0.407	-0.349	0.450	0.588	0.546	0.473	0.369	0.391	0.012	
1965	0.880	0.567	0.664	0.612	-0.163	0.492	0.599	0.532	0.420	0.329	0.424	0.165		
1966	0.602	0.790	0.689	-0.141	0.540	0.715	0.507	0.412	0.271	0.292	-0.009			
1967	0.626	0.441	-0.059	0.498	0.446	0.215	0.296	0.424	0.250	-0.232				
1968	0.685	-0.111	0.651	0.693	0.479	0.384	0.371	0.274	-0.172					
1969	0.016	0.537	0.592	0.350	0.530	0.153	0.136	-0.141						
1970	-0.107	-0.171	-0.265	-0.363	-0.261	-0.291	0.051							
1971	0.752	0.447	0.239	0.487	0.386	-0.091								
1972	0.717	0.554	0.463	0.492	0.127									
1973	0.820	0.653	0.779	0.395										
1974	0.666	0.698	0.266											
1975	0.840	0.091												
1976	0.490													
1977														
Median Correlation	.666	.545	.500	.487	.385	.215	.296	.412	.395	.376	.319	.235	.158	.182

formation. Five years after formation the median correlation is .452, while ten years after formation the median is .281.

The median correlation of the EPSP numbers shown in Table 1A.4 decreases from .666 in the first year to .182 in the fourteenth year. Five years after formation the median correlation is .385, while ten years after formation the median is .182.

The results show a good persistency in the CEP and CFP numbers and a low persistency in the EPSP numbers. Again the main question refers to the possible reason(s) that the persistencies of the balance sheet-oriented and accrual accounting-based number (CEP) and the cash-flow accounting-based number (CFP) exceed that of the income statement-oriented and accrual accounting-based number (EPSP). The two reasons given for the variability results may apply to the persistence results, namely, the income smoothing distortion hypothesis and the selective market response hypothesis.

SUMMARY AND CONCLUSIONS

The purpose of this study was to evaluate the relative merits of accounting indicators derived from either an income statement based on accrual accounting, a balance sheet based on accrual accounting, or cash-flow accounting. The hypothesis is that the number most favored by the market and/or reflected in the market price will show less variability and a higher persistence than the other numbers. The balance sheet-oriented number and accrual accounting-based number showed a lower variability and a higher persistence than the cash-flow accounting-based number and the income statement-oriented and accrual accounting-based number. The phenomenon was attributed to both an income smoothing distortion hypothesis and a selective market response hypothesis.

One implication of these results is that the financial position of a firm is deemed more indicative of a firm's potential by the market than either cash flows or income statement numbers. A second implication for standard-setting bodies is to consider the fundamental measurement process as being the measurement of the attributes of assets and liabilities and changes in them rather than the matching process (Belkaoui, 1981, p. 83). In short, the evidence argues for an asset/liability view of earnings rather than either a revenue/expense view or the cash-flow view.

NOTES

1. Lee also showed that the Fisherian financial statement is cash flow-based, which tends to support the contention of Whittington that Fisher was the father of cash-flow accounting (Lee, 1979, p. 327; Whittington, 1977, p. 202).

2. A similar approach was used by Beaver and Morse (1978).

REFERENCES

Alexander, S. (1950). *Five Monographs on Business Income*. New York: Study Group on Business Income, AICPA.

American Accounting Association. (1969). Committee on External Reporting, *An Evaluation of External Reporting Practices*. A Report of the 1966–68 Committee on External Reporting. *The Accounting Review* (Supplement), pp. 79–123.

American Institute of Certified Public Accountants. (1973). Study Group on the *Objectives of Financial Statements*. New York: American Institute of Certified Public Accountants.

Ashton, R. (1976). "Cash Flow Accounting: A Review and Critique." *Journal of Business Finance and Accounting* (Winter), pp. 63–81.

Barley, B., and H. Levy. (1979). "On the Variability of Accounting Income Numbers." *Journal of Accounting Research* (Autumn), pp. 305–315.

Beaver, W., and D. Morse. (1978). "What Determines Price—Earnings Ratios?" *Financial Analysts Journal* (July–August), pp. 65–76.

Beaver, W.H., and R.E. Dukes. (1972). "Interperiod Tax Allocation, Earnings Expectations, and the Behavior of Security Prices." *The Accounting Review* (April), pp. 320–332.

Belkaoui, A. (1981). *Accounting Theory*. San Diego: Harcourt Brace Jovanovich.

Canning, J. (1929). *The Economics of Accountancy*. New York: The Ronald Press.

Chambers, R. (1966). *Accounting, Evaluation and Economic Behavior*. Englewood Cliffs, NJ: Prentice-Hall.

Climo, T.A. (1976). "Cash Flow Statements for Investors." *Journal of Business Finance and Accounting* (Autumn), pp. 3–16.

Edey, H.C. (1963). "Accounting Principles and Business Reality." *Accountancy* (November), pp. 998–1002; (December), pp. 1083–1088.

Edwards, E., and P. Bell. (1961). *The Theory and Measurement of Business Income*. Berkeley: University of California Press.

Financial Accounting Standards Board. (1976). "Tentative Conclusions on Objectives of Financial Statements of Business Enterprises." Stamford, CT: FASB.

———. (1978). *Statement of Financial Accounting Concepts No. 1*. Stamford, CT: FASB.

Gordon, M.J. (1964). "Postulates, Principles and Research in Accounting." *The Accounting Review* (April), pp. 221–263.

Gross, M.J., Jr. (1972). *Financial and Accounting Guide for Nonprofit Organizations*. New York: The Ronald Press.

Hawkins, D., and W. Campbell. (1978). *Equity Valuation: Models, Analysis and Implications*. New York: Financial Executives Institute.

Hicks, B.E. (1980). "The Cash Flow Basis of Accounting." Working Paper No. 13. Sudbury, Ontario: Laurentian University.

Ijiri, Y. (1978). "Cash Flow Accounting and Its Structure." *Journal of Accounting, Auditing and Finance* (Summer), pp. 331–348.

———. (1979). "A Simple System of Cash Flow Accounting," In R. Sterling and A.L. Thomas (eds.), *Accounting for a Simplified Firm Owning Depreciable Assets*. Houston, TX: Scholars Book Co., pp. 57–71.

Lawson, G.H. (1971). "Cash-Flow Accounting I & II." *Accountant* (October 28 and November 4), pp. 20–31.

————. (1973). "Some Arguments for Cash-Flow Accounting." *Certified Accountant* (April–May), pp. 15–21.

Lee, T.A. (1971). "Goodwill—An Example of Will-o-the-Wisp Accounting." *Accounting and Business Research* (Autumn), pp. 318–328.

————. (1972a). "A Case for Cash Flow Reporting." *Journal of Business Finance* 3, pp. 27–36.

————. (1972b). "The Relevance of Accounting Information Including Cash Flows." *The Accountant's Magazine* (January), pp. 122–132.

————. (1979). "The Contribution of Fisher to Cash Flow Accounting." *Journal of Business Finance and Accounting* (Autumn), pp. 321–330.

————. (1981). "Reporting Cash Flows and Net Realizable Values." *Accounting and Business Research* (Spring), pp. 163–170.

Paton, W. (1962). *Accounting Theory*. Chicago: Accounting Studies Press. Originally published in 1922.

Paton, W., and A. Littleton. (1940). *An Introduction to Corporate Accounting Standards*. Columbus, OH: American Accounting Association.

Revsine, L. (1973). *Replacement Cost Accounting*. Englewood Cliffs, NJ: Prentice-Hall.

Staubus, G. (1961). *A Theory of Accounting to Investors*. Berkeley: University of California Press.

————. (1971). "The Relevance of Cash Flows." In R.R. Sterling (ed.), *Asset Valuation*. Houston, TX: Scholars Book Co.

Sterling, R. (1970). *Theory of the Measurement of Enterprise Income*. Lawrence: University of Kansas Press.

————. (1974). "Earnings per Share Is a Poor Indicator of Performance." *Omega* 5, pp. 11–32.

Stern, J. (1972). "Let's Abandon Earnings per Share." *Barron's* (December 18), p. 2.

Thomas, A.L. (1969). *The Allocation Problem in Financial Accounting Theory*. Studies in Accounting Research No. 3. Sarasota, FL: American Accounting Association.

————. (1974). *The Allocation Problem: Part Two*. Studies in Accounting Research No. 9. Sarasota, FL: American Accounting Association.

Whittington, G. (1977). "Accounting and Economics." In *Current Issues in Accounting*. B. Carsberg and T. Hope (eds.). New York: Philip Allan.

Appendix 1.B. The Smoothing of Income Numbers: Some Empirical Evidence on the Systematic Differences between Core and Periphery Industrial Sectors

INTRODUCTION

While the subject of income smoothing was discussed and tested previously (Gordon, 1964; Gordon, Horwitz, and Meyers, 1966; Archibald, 1967; Copeland, 1968; Copeland and Licastro, 1968; Cushing, 1969; Dasher and Malcolm,

Source: A. Belkaoui and R.D. Picur, "The Smoothing of Income Numbers: Some Empirical Evidence on the Systematic Differences between Core and Periphery Sectors," *Journal of Business Finance and Accounting* (Winter 1984), pp. 527–546. Reprinted with permission.

1970; White, 1970; Barefield and Comiskey, 1972; Beidleman, 1973; Barnea, Ronen, and Sadan, 1976; Kamin and Ronen, 1978; Ronen, 1981), the effects of the dual economy on income smoothing was never tested specifically and separately.[1] Accordingly, this study attempts to discover whether managers do in fact behave as if they engage in goal-directed determination of the cues and signals conveyed to users of financial statements through income numbers and whether this behavior differs between managers in the core (cs) and managers in the periphery (ps) sectors.

INCOME SMOOTHING: RELATED RESEARCH

Income smoothing may be defined as either the intentional or deliberate dampening of fluctuations about some level of earnings that is currently considered to be normal for a firm (Beidleman, 1973; Barnea et al., 1976, p. 143).

The various empirical studies in income smoothing assumed various smoothing objects (i.e., operating income or ordinary income), various smoothing instruments (i.e., operating expenses, ordinary expenses, or extraordinary items), and various smoothing dimensions (either accounting smoothing or "real" smoothing) (Kamin and Ronen, 1978, p. 144). Accounting smoothing affects income through accounting dimensions, namely, smoothing through events' occurrence and/or recognition, smoothing through allocation over time, and smoothing through classification (Barnea et al., 1976, p. 11). Real smoothing affects income through the deliberate or intentional changing of the operating decisions and their timing.

Various motivations for smoothing are given in the literature, such as:

1. to enhance the reliability of prediction based on the observed smoothed series of accounting numbers along a trend considered best or normal by management (Barnea et al., 1976),
2. to gain tax advantages and to improve relations with creditors, employees, and investors (Hepworth, 1953),
3. to reduce the uncertainty resulting from the fluctuations of income numbers in general and reducing systematic risk in particular by reducing the covariance of the firm's returns with the market returns (Beidleman, 1973, p. 654; Lev and Kunitzky, 1974).

These reasons for motivation result from the need felt by management to neutralize environmental uncertainty and dampen the wide fluctuations in the operating performance of the firm subject to an intermittent cycle of good and bad times. To do so, management may resort to organizational slack behavior (Cyert and March, 1963), budgetary slack behavior (Schiff and Lewin, 1968), or risk-avoiding behavior (Thompson, 1967). Each of these behaviors necessitates decisions affecting the incurrence and/or allocation of discretionary expenses (costs), which result in income smoothing.

In addition to these behaviors intended to neutralize environmental uncer-

tainty, it is possible to identify *organizational characterizations* that differentiate among different firms in their extent of smoothing. Kamin and Ronen (1978) examined the effects of the separation of ownership and control on income smoothing under the hypothesis that management-controlled firms are more likely to be engaged in smoothing as a manifestation of managerial discretion and budgetary slack. Their results confirmed that a majority of the firms examined behave as if they were smoothers, and a particularly strong majority is included among management-controlled firms with high barriers to entry. Other organizational characterizations may exist that differentiate among different firms along the dimension of the attempt to smooth. One such characterization derived from theories of economic dualism divides the industrial structure into two distinct sectors—the *core* and the *periphery* sectors.

STRATIFICATION IN A DUAL ECONOMY AND INCOME SMOOTHING

Models of sectorial economic differentiation derived from theories of economic dualism include various perspectives such as theories of dual economy, labor markets, and labor force segmentation (Cain, 1976). Common to all of these perspectives is the proposal of a division of the industrial structure of the economy into two distinct sectors (at least in the two-sector model) consisting of the *core* and *periphery* sectors. These models, however, differ in their definition and conceptualization of these sectors.

In the dual labor market and labor force segmentation perspective, the sectors are defined in terms of the characteristics of labor markets and worker behavior (cf. Harrison, 1974; Spilerman, 1982). For example, Piori (1977, p. 93) defines the two sectors as follows:

The central tenet of the analysis . . . is that the role of employment and of the disposition of manpower in the perpetuation of poverty is best understood in terms of a dual labor market. One sector of that market, which I have termed elsewhere the primary market, offers jobs which possess several of the following traits; high wages, good working conditions, employment stability and job security, equity and due process in the administration of work rules, and chances for advancement. The other, or secondary sector, has jobs which, relative to those in the primary sector, are decidedly less attractive. They tend to involve low wages, poor working conditions, considerable variability in employment, harsh and often arbitrary discipline, and little opportunity to advance. The poor are confined to the secondary labor market. The elimination of poverty requires that they gain access to primary employment.

In the dual economy perspective, the sectorial classification derives from the nature of modern industrial capitalism (Beck and Horan, 1978). More precisely, the sectorial classification resulted from the creation during the late nineteenth and early twentieth centuries of a core industrial sector dominated by large

oligopolistic corporations (Baran and Sweezy, 1966). What remained, characterized by smaller firms and a less competitive environment, is considered the periphery sector (Averitt, 1968). For example, Bluestone et al. (1973, pp. 28–29) characterizes the two sectors as follows:

The core economy includes those industries that comprise the muscle of American economic and political power. . . . Entrenched in durable manufacturing, the construction trades and, to a lesser extent, the extraction industries, the firms in the core economy are noted for high productivity, high profits, intensive utilization of capital, high incidence of monopoly elements, and a high degree of unionization. What follows normally from such characteristics are high wages. The automobile, steel, rubber, aluminum, aerospace, and petroleum industries are ranking members of this part of the economy. Workers who are able to secure employment in these industries are, in most cases, assured of relatively higher wages and better than average working conditions and fringe benefits.

Beyond the fringes of the core economy lie a set of industries that lack almost all of the advantages normally found in center firms. Concentrated in agriculture, nondurable manufacturing, retail trade, and sub-professional series, the peripheral industries are noted for their small firm size, labor intensity, low profits, low productivity, intensive product market competition, lack of unionization, and low wages. Unlike core sector industries the periphery lacks the assets, size and political power to take advantage of economies of scale or to spend large sums on research and development.

Theories of dual economy suggest that these sectorial differences have important implications for the opportunity structures and environments faced by individual firms. Firms in the periphery sector face a more restricted opportunity structure and a higher degree of environmental uncertainty than firms in the core sector.

The environmental uncertainty is more evident with regard to the market for labor. The core sector is characterized by high productivity, nonpoverty wages, and employment stability, while the periphery sector is characterized by relatively low average and marginal productivity, low wages, and employment instability. The core sector uses its market power and high degree of profitability to hire and train the best workers and maintain nonpoverty wage levels without seriously eroding their profit margin. In fact, Beck and Horan examined the importance of industrial sectors as hypothesized by the dual economy literature on the process of earnings determination and found substantively and statistically significant differences in the labor force composition and economic status between core and periphery industrial sectors (Beck and Horan, 1978, p. 704). A direct result of this situation is that turnover in the core sector is likely more expensive and less attractive than in the periphery sector. As stated by Harrison:

Secondary (periphery) employers have several reasons for placing a value on turnover, in sharp contrast to their fellows in the primary market. They can, as a rule, neither afford nor do their technologies require them to invest heavily in "specific training." Instead, they tend to rely on the "general training" (e.g., literacy, basic arithmetic) provided socially. With minimal investment in their current labor force, and given the ready

availability of substitute labor outside the firm, such employers are at the very least indifferent to the rate of turnover. (Harrison, 1974, p. 280)

Given this evidence on the differences in labor composition, economic status of employees, low turnover, higher wages, and unionized labor force, the firms in the core industry face less uncertainty in their labor management than firms in the periphery industry. Firms in the periphery industry have more opportunity and more predisposition to smooth both their operating flows (e.g., through their labor management) and reported income measures than firms in the core sector. In other words, the two economic sectors rely on their differential ability to maximize profits through the structuring of their labor processes (Hodson and Kaufman, 1982, p. 729).

The test, used also by Kamin and Ronen (1978), consists of observing the behavior of these smoothing variables: (1) operating expenses (OPEX) not inducted in cost of sales, (2) ordinary expenses (OREX), and (3) operating expenses plus ordinary expenses (OPEX + OREX), vis-à-vis the behavior of two objects of smoothing, (1) operating income (OP) and (2) ordinary income (OR).

It is assumed that management knows the future streams of inflows and outflows and their time distinction and has determined what should be the normal trend of OP and OR. To determine their normal trend, two expectation models are used here, namely, a time trend model and a market trend model.

1. *The Time Trend.* Two models will be used.

(a) The series of smoothed variables OP and OR and of smoothing variables OPEX, OREX, and OPEX + OREX were detrended in a time regression over a maximum span of twenty years, 1958 to 1977 as per the equations below.

$$Y_{ijt} = \alpha_{ij} + \beta_{ijt} + \varepsilon_{ijt}, \qquad\qquad i = 1,2,3,4,5 \quad t = 1958,\ldots 1977, (1)$$

where

$i = 1$ for OP, $i = 2$ for OR, $i = 3$ for OPEX, $i = 4$ for OREX and $i = 5$ for OPEX + OREX.

Y_{ijt} = observed OP, OR, OPEX, OREX, OPEX + OREX for firm j in year t.

(b) The first differences in OPEX, OREX and OPEX + OREX were detrended in a time regression as per equation (2) below.

$$\Delta Y_{ijt} = \delta'_{ij} + Y'_{ijt}, \qquad\qquad i = 1,2,3 \quad t = 1958,\ldots 1977 (2)$$

where

$i = 1$ for OPEX, 2 for OREX and 3 for OPEX + OREX

2. *The Market Trend*

The first differences in OP, OR, OPEX, OREX, and OPEX + OREX were regressed on a macroindex of first differences measured, respectively, as the mean observed first differences of OP, OR, OPEX, OREX, and OPEX + OREX as per equation (3) below.

$$\Delta Y_{ijt} = \alpha'_{ij} + \beta'_{ij}M_{it} + \varepsilon'_{ijt} \qquad\qquad i = 1,2,3,4,5 \quad t = 1958, \ldots 1977 \,(3)$$

where

i = 1 for OP, 2 for OR, 3 for OPEX, 4 for OREX, and 5 for OPEX + OREX

M_{it} = Sample mean index of OP, OR, OPEX, OREX, and OPEX + OREX

where

$$M_{it} = \frac{1}{N}\sum_{i=1}^{N}\Delta Y_{ijt}, \text{ N being the sample size}$$

TEST CRITERION

Similarly to Kamin and Ronen (1978), the test criterion was based on the correlation coefficient between the deviations of the smoothing objects and the deviations of the smoothing variables. A positive correlation is consistent with a smoothing behavior.

Then for each subsample classified with respect to core or periphery variables as well as for the complete sample, we test if the correlation coefficients are significantly positive using a binomial test. The statistic Z_p is computed to test the null hypothesis that r is distributed symmetrically about $\bar{r} = 0$ using the alternative hypothesis $\bar{r} > 0$. Z_p is the standard normal statistic

$$Z_p = \frac{\chi \neq 0.5n - 0.5n}{0.5n} \qquad\qquad \text{(Siegel, 1956, p. 41)}$$

where

χ = small frequency

n = number of observations

A concentration of a highly positive correlation within the 0.01 level of significance would indicate that it is sensible to use the magnitude of the association in addition to its sign (Kamin and Ronen, 1978, p. 156). This was not possible in this study due to the differences in the number of observations used for each firm in the sample. This number varied between a minimum of ten years and a

maximum of twenty years. Data for the firms in the periphery sector were un-derstandably less available than for the firms in the core sector.

Instead of testing the magnitude of the association, the present authors tested the differences in smoothing behavior. A χ^2 text uses only the proportions of smoothers in each group to indicate different proportions of smoothers.

$$\chi^2 = \sum_{i=1}^{2} \frac{(\chi_i - n_i\theta)^2}{n_i\theta(1 - \theta)}$$

where

χ_i = number of firms that indicate a smoothing behavior in group i

n_i = total number of firms in group i

THE DATA SAMPLE AND THE CLASSIFICATION OF FIRMS INTO CORE AND PERIPHERY SECTORS

To detect the differences in smoothing behavior between firms in the core sector and firms in the periphery sector, it was necessary to determine the dis-tinction between core and periphery economic sectors and to classify the sample in these two main groups.

The data included 171 U.S. firms from forty-two industries (see the Appen-dix). The classification into core and periphery sectors was based on Beck and Horan's (1978) classification. Beck and Horan relied on Bluestone et al.'s (1973) analyses, as quoted above, and allocated to the core sector those industries that exhibit high levels of capital intensity, unionization, large assets, high profit margins, product diversification, and market concentration. These include min-ing, construction, durable and nondurable manufacturing, transportation, com-munications, utilities, wholesale trade, finance, professional services, and public administration. Industries were assigned to the periphery sector because of their small firm size, seasonal and other variations in product supply and demand, labor intensity, weak unionization, and low assets. These include agriculture, portions of durable and nondurable manufacturing, retail trade, business and repair, and personal and entertainment services. This classification into a core and a periphery group resulted in 114 firms in the core sector and 57 firms in the periphery sector, chosen on the basis of availability of data for the period of the analysis.[2]

RESULTS AND DISCUSSION

An overall summary of the results is shown in Table 1B.1. This shows the significant differences in the extent to which firms in the periphery sector and the core sector may be smoothing income. Under the time expectation model

Table 1B.1
Overall Summary of Results

Smoothing Object	Smoothing Variables	Income Trend	"Smoothing" Core Firms	%	Periphery Firms	%	Differences
OP	OPEX	Time (1)	57	68	33	82	S*[1]
		Market	56	71	35	83	S*
		Time (2)	57	70	35	81	NS[2]
OR	OPEX	Time (1)	54	64	28	76	S*
		Market	45	59	24	62	S**[3]
		Time (2)	46	57	26	65	NS
OR	OREX	Time (1)	55	59	28	74	S*
		Market	51	58	23	62	NS
		Time (2)	47	55	22	56	NS
OR	OREX + OPEX	Time (1)	60	61	36	78	S**
		Market	50	57	28	72	S*
		Time (2)	50	56	28	68	NS

Notes:
1. S* = Significant at 0.10 level and indicates that the results are consistent in the greater smoothing.
2. NS = Not significant.
3. S** = Significant at 0.05 level and indicates that the results are consistent with greater smoothing by periphery firms than core firms.

No. 1 and the market model, all the differences, with one exception, are significant. Under the time expectation model No. 2, based on first differences, all the differences are not significant. Two points are noteworthy. First, where the differences are not significant, the proportion of smoothers in the periphery sector is still higher than in the core sector. Second, while most of the significant differences are at $\alpha = 0.10$, the difference resulting from a smoothing of ordinary income with operating and ordinary expenses under the first time expectation model and the difference resulting from smoothing ordinary income with ordinary expenses under the market model were significant at $\alpha = 0.05$.

The extent of smoothing in each sector is shown in Tables 1B.2–1B.13 and is indicated by Z_p. With no exceptions, the extent of smoothing for the periphery sector was significant. It was significant in seven out of the twelve cases for the core sector. These points are noteworthy. First, for the periphery sector, the extent of smoothing was significant at a higher level of confidence for the smoothing of operating income with operating expense under each of the three

Table 1B.2
Smoothing of Operating Income with Operating Expenses (Time Expectation Model No. 1)

	Core Sector $r > 0$	$r > 0$	Z_p	Periphery Sector $r > 0$	$r > 0$	Z_p	Control Effect X^2
No. of firms	57	27	-2.83*	33	7	-4.26*	2.229**
%	(68)	(32)		(82)	(17)		
r	0.51			0.60			

Notes:
*Significant at 0.05; **significant at 0.10.
r > 0 indicates positive correlation coefficients (consistent with smoothing).
r is the mean of the distribution of the correlation coefficients.

Table 1B.3
Smoothing of Operating Income with Operating Expenses ("Market" Income Expectation Model)

	Core Sector $r > 0$	$r < 0$	Z_p	Periphery Sector $r > 0$	$r < 0$	Z_p	Control Effect X^2
No. of firms	56	23	-3.71*	35	7	-4.47*	1.659**
%	(71)	(29)		(83)	(17)		
r	0.38			0.48			

Notes:
*Significant at 0.05; **significant at 0.10.
r > 0 indicates positive correlation coefficients (consistent with smoothing).
r is the mean of the distribution of the correlation coefficients.

Table 1B.4
Smoothing of Operating Income with Operating Expenses (Time Expectation Model No. 2)

	Core Sector $r > 0$	$r < 0$	Z_p	Periphery Sector $r > 0$	$r < 0$	Z_p	Control Effect X^2
No. of firms	57	25	- 3.53*	33	8	- 3.96*	1.484
%	(70)	(30)		(81)	(19)		
r	0.38			0.52			

Notes:
*Significant at 0.05.
$r > 0$ indicates positive correlation coefficients (consistent with smoothing).
r is the mean of the distribution of the correlation coefficients.

Table 1B.5
Smoothing of Ordinary Income with Operating Expenses (Time Expectation Model No. 1)

	Core Sector $r > 0$	$r < 0$	Z_p	Periphery Sector $r > 0$	$r < 0$	Z_p	Control Effect X^2
No. of firms	54	30	2.618*	28	9	-2.96*	2.204**
%	(64)	(36)		(76)	(24)		
r	0.41			0.49			

Notes:
*Significant at 0.05; **significant at 0.10.
$r > 0$ indicates positive correlation coefficients (consistent with smoothing).
r is the mean of the distribution of the correlation coefficients.

Table 1B.6
Smoothing of Operating Income with Operating Expenses ("Market" Income Expectation Model)

	Core Sector $r > 0$	$r < 0$	Z_p	Periphery Sector $r > 0$	$r < 0$	Z_p	Control Effect X^2
No. of firms	45	31	- 1.605*	24	15	-1.60*	3.799*
%	(59)	(41)		(62)	(38)		
r	0.31			0.49			

Notes:
*Significant at 0.05.
r > 0 indicates positive correlation coefficients (consistent with smoothing).
r is the mean of the distribution of the correlation coefficients.

Table 1B.7
Smoothing of Operating Income with Operating Expenses (Time Expectation Model No. 2)

	Core Sector $r > 0$	$r < 0$	Z_p	Periphery Sector $r > 0$	$r < 0$	Z_p	Control Effect X^2
No. of firms	46	34	- 1.34*	26	14	-2.055*	0.351
%	(57)	(42)		(65)	(35)		
r	0.30			0.49			

Notes:
*Significant at 0.05.
r > 0 indicates positive correlation coefficients (consistent with smoothing).
r is the mean of the distribution of the correlation coefficients.

Table 1B.8
Smoothing of Ordinary Income with Operating Expenses (Time Expectation Model No. 1)

	Core Sector $r > 0$ $r < 0$ Z_p			Periphery Sector $r > 0$ $r < 0$ Z_p			Control Effect X^2
No. of firms	55	38	-1.762*	28	10	-7.08*	1.871*
%	(59)	(41)		(74)	(26)		
r	0.41			0.44			

Notes:
*Significant at 0.05.
$r > 0$ indicates positive correlation coefficients (consistent with smoothing).
r is the mean of the distribution of the correlation coefficients.

Table 1B.9
Smoothing of Ordinary Income with Operating Expenses ("Market" Income Expectation Model)

	Core Sector $r > 0$ $r < 0$ Z_p			Periphery Sector $r > 0$ $r < 0$ Z_p			Control Effect X^2
No. of firms	51	37	1.49	23	14	-1.64*	0.056**
%	(58)	(42)		(62)	(38)		
r	0.36			0.42			

Notes:
*Significant at 0.05; **significant at 0.10.
$r > 0$ indicates positive correlation coefficients (consistent with smoothing).
r is the mean of the distribution of the correlation coefficients.

Table 1B.10
Smoothing of Ordinary Income with Operating Expenses (Time Expectation Model No. 2)

	Core Sector $r > 0$ $r < 0$ Z_p			Periphery Sector $r > 0$ $r < 0$ Z_p			Control Effect X^2
No. of firms	47	39	0.863	22	17	- 0.960	0.0001
%	(55)	(45)		(56)	(44)		
r	0.38			0.43			

Notes:
*Significant at 0.05.
$r > 0$ indicates positive correlation coefficients (consistent with smoothing).
r is the mean of the distribution of the correlation coefficients.

Table 1B.11
Smoothing of Operating Income with Operating Expenses (Time Expectation Model No. 1)

	Core Sector $r > 0$ $r < 0$ Z_p			Periphery Sector $r > 0$ $r < 0$ Z_p			Control Effect X^2
No. of firms	60	39	- 2.11*	32	9	- 3.75*	3.179*
%	(61)	(39)		(78)	(22)		
r	0.41			0.49			

Notes:
*Significant at 0.05.
$r > 0$ indicates positive correlation coefficients (consistent with smoothing).
r is the mean of the distribution of the correlation coefficients.

Table 1B.12
Smoothing of Ordinary Income with Ordinary and Operating Expenses ("Market" Income Expectation Model)

	Core Sector $r > 0$ $r < 0$ Z_p			Periphery Sector $r > 0$ $r < 0$ Z_p			Control Effect X^2
No. of firms	50	38	- 1.27	28	11	- 2.88*	1.964*
%	(57)	(43)		(72)	(28)		
r	0.30			0.39			

Notes:
*Significant at 0.05.
$r > 0$ indicates positive correlation coefficients (consistent with smoothing).
r is the mean of the distribution of the correlation coefficients.

Table 1B.13
Smoothing of Operating Income with Ordinary and Operating Expenses (Time Expectation Model No. 2)

	Core Sector $r > 0$ $r < 0$ Z_p			Periphery Sector $r > 0$ $r < 0$ Z_p			Control Effect X^2
No. of firms	50	39	- 1.165	28	13	- 2.488*	1.248
%	(56)	(44)		(68)	(32)		
r	0.33			0.48			

Notes:
*Significant at 0.05.
$r > 0$ indicates positive correlation coefficients (consistent with smoothing).
r is the mean of the distribution of the correlation coefficients.

expectation models. Second, for both the core and periphery sectors the extent of smoothing was always significant under the first time expectation model. Third, the insignificant results in the core sector were mainly under the market income expectation and the second time expectation models.

What appears worth noting from the findings is that first, both core and periphery sectors lead in terms of proportion of smoothers and extent of smoothing. Second, in attempting to smooth income, managers in both sectors are more inclined to look for a "normal" time trend as a guide rather than a market trend or a first difference trend. With respect to the first identified finding, it may be advanced that the motivation to smooth is higher for managers in the periphery sector, who have to face a more restricted opportunity structure and a higher degree of environmental uncertainty than firms in the core sector. With respect to the second identified finding, it may be advanced that what management considers the normal trend of OP and OR is the easy to conceive and to compute time trend rather than the market trend or the first differences trend.

CONCLUSION

This study has tested the effects of a dual economy on income smoothing behavior. The main hypothesis was that a higher degree of smoothing of income numbers is exhibited by firms in the periphery sector than firms in the core sector as a reaction to differences in opportunity structures, experiences, and environmental uncertainty. The results indicate that a majority of the firms may be resorting to income smoothing, with a higher number included among firms in the periphery sector. These results add to other attempts to identify organizational characteristics that differentiate between firms in their extent of smoothing (Kamin and Ronen, 1978). Future research looking into the impact of other organizational characteristics of firms that have a propensity to smooth may be helpful to users of accounting numbers.

APPENDIX: SAMPLE

Agriculture, Forestry, Fisheries

American Agronomics	3735
New Hall Land and Farm	651427

Mining

Metal Mining

Amax Inc.	023127
Cyprus Mines Corp.	232813
Standard Metals	853615
Inco Ltd-Cl B Conv	453258
Cleveland-Cliffs Iron Co.	186000

Coal Mining

West Moreland Coal Co.	960878
Piston Co.	725701
McIntyre Mines Ltd.	581283
General Exploration	369784
Woods Petroleum Corp.	980140

Crude Petroleum and Natural Gas

American Petrofina	028861
Dome Petroleum Ltd.	257093
Getty Oil Co.	634280
Ranger Oil (Canada) Ltd.	752805

Nonmetal Mining and Quarrying

Arundel Corp.	043177
Florida Rock Inds.	341140
Pebble Beach Corp.	705090
Freeport Minerals Co.	356715

Construction

Morisson-Knudsen	286438
Great Lakes Dredge and Dock Co.	390604
Centex Corp.	156312
U.S. Home Corp.	912061

Durable Manufacturing

Lumber and Wood Products

Barclay Industries	067374
Boise Cascade Corp.	097383
Louisiana Pacific	546347
Pope and Talbot Inc.	732827

Furniture and Fixtures

Aberdeen Mfg. Co.	003068
Kirsh Co.	497656
Simmons Co.	828709
Weiman Co. Inc.	948662

Stone, Clay and Glass Products

Corning Glass Works	219327
Libbey-Owens Ford Co.	530000
Midland Glass Co.	597521

Glen Gery Corp.	377568
Lenox Inc.	526264
Metal Industries	
Kaiser Steel Corp.	483098
Hofmann Industries Inc.	434560
Inland Steel Co.	457470
Bethlehem Steel Co.	087509
Cyclops Corp.	232525
Machinery (except electrical)	
Binks Mfg. Co.	090527
Ingersoll-Rand Co.	456866
Torin Corp.	891067
Parker-Hannifin Corp.	701094
Electrical Machinery, Equipment, Supplies	
North American Philips Corp.	657045
Westinghouse Electric Corp.	960402
General Electric Co.	369604
Sperry Rand Corp.	848355
Transportation Equipment	
Winnebago Industries	974637
ACF Inds.	000800
Pittsburgh Forgings Co.	725106
Rohr Industries	775422
Timken Co.	887389
Professional and Photo Equipment	
Cavitron Corp.	149645
Polaroid Corp.	731095
Visual Graphics	928438
American Sterilizer Co.	030087
Ordinance	
R.E.D.M. Corp.	749482
General Recreation	370594
Remington Arms Co.	759574
Raymond Industries Inc.	754713
Miscellaneous Durable Manufacturing	
American Technical Industries	030141
Bally Manufacturing Corp.	058732

Compudyne Corp.	204795
Hillenbrand Industries	431573
Jostens Inc.	481088

Nondurable Manufacturing

Food and Kindred Products

Beatrice Foods Co.	074077
General Mills Co.	370334
Pillsbury Co.	721510
Carnation Co.	143483

Tobacco Manufacturing

American Brands Inc.	024703
Philip Morris Inc.	718167
Reynolds (R.J.) Industries	761753
U.S. Tobacco Inc.	912775
BAYUK Cigars Inc.	073239

Textile Mill Products

West Point-Pepperell	955465
Riegel Textile Corp.	766481
Graniteville Co.	387478
Belden Hemingwey	077491
Collins & Aikrnan Corp.	194828

Apparel and Other Fabricated Textiles

Puritan Fashions Corp.	746316
Levi Strauss and Co.	527364
Fairfield-Noble Corp.	304621
Wilson Brothers	972091

Paper and Allied Products

American Israeli Paper Mills	027069
Technical Tape Inc.	878504
Domtar Inc.	257561
International Paper Co.	460146

Printing, Publishing and Allied Products

Simplicity Pattern Co.	828879
Western Publishing	959265
Knight-Ridder Newspapers Inc.	499040
Affiliated Publications	008261
Times Mirror Co.	887360

Chemical and Allied Products

American Cynamic Co.	025321
Celanese Corp.	150843
Dow Chemical	260543
Diamond Shamrock Corp.	252741

Rubber and Miscellaneous Plastic Products

Rubbermaid Inc.	781088
Armstrong Rubber	042465
Mohawk Rubber	608302
Firestone Tire and Rubber Co.	318315
Aegis Corp.	007603

Leather and Leather Products

Seton Co.	817814
Jaclyn Inc.	469772
U.S. Shoe Corp.	912605
Interco Inc.	458506
Barry (RG)	068797

Transportation

Railroads and Railway Express Services

Burlington Northern Inc.	121897
IC Industries Inc.	449268
Soo Line Railroad	835716
Santa Fe Industries	802020
Saint Louis–San Francisco Railways	791808

Trucking Services

Arkansas Best Corp.	040789
Smith's Transfer	832407
Golden Cycle Corp.	380892
Tri-State Motor Transit	895691
CW Transport Inc.	126693

Water Transportation

Seatrain Lines	812557
Sea Containers	811369
Overseas Shipping Group	690368

Air Transportation

Ozark Airlines Inc.	692515
Frontiers Airlines Inc.	359064

Piedmont Airlines Inc.	720101
Southwest Airlines	844741
Capitol International Airways	140627
Petroleum and Gas Pipelines	
Bay State Gas	072612
Mountain Fuel Supply Co.	624029
Texas Oil and Gas Co.	882593
United Energy Resources	910210
Services Incidental to Transportation	
WTC Inc.	929340
Canal-Randolph Corp.	137051

Communications

Radio Broadcasting and Television	
Metromedia Inc.	591690
CBS Inc.	124845
Reeves Telecomp Corp.	759650
Sonderling Broadcasting Corp.	835427
American Broadcasting	024735
Telephone (Wire and Radio)	
General Telephone and Electronics	371028
Continental Telephone Corp.	212093
Bell Telephone of Canada	078149
American Telephone and Telegraph	030177
Mid-Continent Telephone	595390
Telegraph (Wire and Radio)	
Western Union Corp.	959805

Utility and Sanitary Services

Electric Light and Power	
Arizona Public Service Co.	040555
Wholesale Trade	
Ketchum and Co.	492620
Lloyd's Electronics	539434
Retail Trade	
Fay's Drug Co.	313035
House of Fabrics Inc.	441758
House of Vision Inc.	441726

Walgreen Co.	031422
Servomation Corp.	817715
Finance, Insurance, and Real Estate	
Wells Fargo Mtg. and Equity T.R.	949752
Mony Mortgage Investors	615339
Tri-South Mortgage Inv.	895580
Business and Repair Services	
American Consumer Industries	025231
Ryder System Inc.	783549
Allright Auto-Parks Inc.	019879
Nielsen (A.C.) Co. Cl.	654098
Personal Services	
Family Record Plan Inc.	307045
Service Corporation International	817565
Block H & R Inc.	093671
Seligman and Latz Inc.	816323
IFS Industries Inc.	449510
Entertainment and Recreation Services	
American International Pictures	026877
San Juan Racing Assoc.	798407
Metro-Goldwyn-Mayer Inc.	591605
Disney (Walt) Productions	254687
Harrah's	413615
Public Administration	
Stone and Webster Inc.	861572
Baker (Michael) Corp.	057149

NOTES

1. A new monograph on income smoothing (Ronen, 1981) and the new and active interest in the "positive" theory of accounting bear witness to the relevance and the timeliness of the income-smoothing paradigm and the urgent need for answers and solutions.

2. Since the firms in the core/periphery sectors are likely to differ significantly in size, both parametric and nonparametric tests were done to test for differences in sizes. The differences were significant at the 0.10 level for the period of analysis. The differences were not, however, restricted to size. Significant differences were found in terms of levels of capital intensity, unionization, profit margin, product differentiation, and market concentration (Beck and Horan, 1978).

REFERENCES

Archibald, T.R. "The Return to Straight-Line Depreciation: An Analysis of a Change in Accounting Method," *Empirical Research in Accounting: Selected Studies*, suppl. to *Journal of Accounting Research* 5 (1967), pp. 161–180.

Averitt, R.T. *The Dual Economy: The Dynamics of American Industry Structure*. New York: Horton, 1968.

Baran, P.A., and P.N. Sweezy. *Monopoly Capital*. New York: Monthly Review Press, 1966.

Barefield, R.M., and E.E. Comiskey. "The Smoothing Hypothesis: An Alternative Test." *The Accounting Review* (April 1972), pp. 291–298.

Barnea, A., J. Ronen, and S. Sadan. "Classificatory Smoothing of Income with Extraordinary Items." *The Accounting Review* (January 1976), pp. 110–122.

Beck, E.M., and P.M. Horan. "The Structure of American Capitalism and Status Attainment Research: A Reassessment of Contemporary Stratification Theory." Unpublished Paper, Department of Sociology, University of Georgia, Athens, 1978.

Beck, E.M., P.M. Horan, and C.M. Tolbert II. "Stratification in a Dual Economy: A Sectorial Mode of Earnings Determination." *American Sociological Review* (October 1978), pp. 704–720.

Beidleman, C.R. "Income Smoothing: The Role of Management." *The Accounting Review* (October 1973), pp. 653–667.

Bluestone, B.W., N. Murphy, and M. Stevenson. *Low Wages and the Working Poor*. Ann Arbor: Institute of Labor and Industrial Relations, University of Michigan, 1973.

Cain, G.G. "The Challenge of Segmented Labor Market Theories to Orthodox Theory." *Journal of Economic Literature* 14 (1976), pp. 1215–1257.

Copeland, R. "Income Smoothing." *Empirical Research in Accounting: Selected Studies*, suppl. to *Journal of Accounting Research* 6 (1968), pp. 101–116.

Copeland, R., and R. Licastro. "A Note on Income Smoothing." *The Accounting Review* (July 1968), pp. 540–546.

Cushing, B.E. "An Empirical Study of Changes in Accounting Policy."*Journal of Accounting Research* (Autumn 1969), pp. 196–203.

Cyert, R.N., and J.G. March. *A Behavioral Theory of the Firm*. Englewood Cliffs, NJ: Prentice Hall, 1963.

Dasher, B.E., and R.E. Malcom. "A Note on Income Smoothing in the Chemical Industry." *Journal of Accounting Research* (Autumn 1970), pp. 253–259.

Gordon, M.J. "Postulates, Principles and Research in Accounting." *The Accounting Review* (April 1964), pp. 251–263.

Gordon, M.J., B.N. Horwitz, and E.T. Meyers. "Accounting Measurements and Normal Growth of the Firm." In R. Jaedicke, Y. Ijiri, and O. Nielson (eds.), *Research and Accounting Measurement*. Evanston, IL: American Accounting Association, 1966, pp. 221–231.

Harrison, B. "The Theory of the Dual Economy." In B. Silverman and M. Yanovitch (eds.), *The Worker in "Post Industrial" Capitalism*. New York: Free Press, 1974, pp. 269–271.

Hepworth, S.R. "Smoothing Periodic Income." *The Accounting Review* (January 1953), pp. 32–39.

Hodson, R., and R.L. Kaufman. "Economic Dualism: A Critical Review." *American Sociological Review* (December 1982), pp. 727–739.

Kamin, J.Y., and J. Ronen. "The Smoothing of Income Numbers: Some Empirical Evidence on Systematic Differences among Management-Controlled and Owner-Controlled Firms." *Accounting, Organizations and Society* 3 (1978), pp. 141–153.

Lev, B., and S. Kunitzky. "On the Association between Smoothing Reasons and the Risk of Common Stock." *The Accounting Review* (April 1974), pp. 259–270.

Piori, M. "The Dual Labor Market: Theory and Implications." In D.M. Gordon (ed.), *Problems in Political Economy: An Urban Perspective*. Lexington, MA: Heath, 1977, pp. 257–270.

Ronen, J. *Smoothing Income Numbers, Objectives, Means and Implications*. Reading, MA: Addison-Wesley, 1981.

Ronen, J., and S. Sadan. *Smoothing Income Numbers: Objectives, Reasons and Implications*. Reading, MA: Addison-Wesley, 1981.

Schiff, M., and A.N. Lewin. "Where Traditional Budgeting Fails." *Financial Executive* (May 1968), pp. 57–62.

Siegel, S. *Nonparametric Statistics for the Behavioral Sciences*. New York: McGraw-Hill, 1956.

Spilerman, S. "Careers, Labor Market Structure, and Socioeconomic Achievement." *American Journal of Sociology* 93 (1982), pp. 645–665.

Thompson, J.D. *Organizations in Action*. New York: McGraw-Hill, 1967.

White, C.E. "Discretionary Accounting Decisions and Income Normalization." *Journal of Accounting Research* (Autumn 1970), pp. 260–273.

Appendix 1C: Anticipatory Smoothing and the Investment Opportunity Set: An Empirical Test of the Fudenberg and Tirole (1955) Model

1. INTRODUCTION

It is both an empirical and anecdotal fact that managers make discretionary accounting choices that "smooth" reported earnings around some predetermined target (e.g., Ronen and Sadan, 1981; Hand, 1989; Gaver et al., 1995; Chaney et al., 1998; Defond and Park, 1997; Subramanyam, 1996). Analytical results by Fudenberg and Tirole (1995) propose that concern about job security creates an incentive for managers to smooth earnings in consideration of both current and future relative performance. Defond and Park (1997) find support for this job security and anticipatory income smoothing theory. They find that managers facing poor (good) current earnings and expecting good (poor) future earnings resort to income-increasing (income-decreasing) accruals. Their results, although consistent with the Fudenberg and Tirole (1995) thesis, do not constitute a direct test of the link between job security and income smoothing. A more direct test

was provided by Ahmed et al. (2000), who hypothesized that the extent of smoothing would vary directly with managers' job security concerns as proxied by the degree of competition in firms' product markets, product durality, and capital intensity. Their results show that managers of firms in more competitive industries and durable goods engage to a greater extent in income smoothing. The results on the relations between income smoothing and capital intensity are mixed. While their attempt and results are compatible with various calls for further research to explain how business factors affect accruals, they fail to provide an integrative explanation of the link between job security and anticipatory income smoothing. The results are silent on firms' meeting different levels on each of the economic attributes. For example, what is the motivation for smoothing in firms that are highly competitive, with low capital intensity, and coming from nondurable goods industries? Given the high number of economic characteristics espoused by firms and the high number of levels of these characteristics possible, quite a number of possible links between job security and income smoothing can be found without being helpful for an understanding of the phenomenon. This study, instead, suggests a more integrative approach by looking at a variable depicting a general economic situation that is itself a composite number of economic characteristics that can be indicative of employment situation in general and job security concerns in particular and that can be linked to anticipatory income smoothing. The economic variable deemed to fit these requirements is the investment opportunity set or growth opportunities. We argue that managers of firms with lower growth opportunities as measured by the investment opportunity set are likely to have greater job security concerns than managers of other firms. A greater extent of income motivating is expected from managers of such firms.

The empirical analysis is based on a sample of 8,632 firm-year observations selected from the Compustat database. For comparative purposes, we used the same methodology for the measurement of accruals and the estimation of discretionary accruals used in previous research. Basically, the measurement of accruals was based on both the traditional balance sheet approach and the alternative cash-flow approach proposed by Collins and Hribar (1999). The estimation of the discretionary accruals relied on two different models: the modified Jones model and the Kang and Sivaramakrishnan (1995) model.

The results of the study show that managers of firms with lower investment opportunity sets engage to a greater extent in income smoothing. In other words, the evidence suggests that when current earnings are "poor" and expected future earnings are "good," managers of firms with lower growth opportunities "borrow" earnings from the future for use in the current period. Conversely, when current earnings are "good" and expected earnings are "poor," the same managers "save" current earnings for possible use in the future. The results hold after controlling for size, leverage, and prior-period discretionary accruals. The study provides a more direct and integrative examination of the link between job security concern and income smoothing. The investment opportunity set

(IOS), rather than separate and disparate economic characteristics, is shown to be related to anticipatory income smoothing.

The appendix is organized as follows: Section 2 presents the hypothesis on the association between the IOS and job security. Section 3 presents the research design. Section 4 covers the results. The summary and conclusions are presented in Section 5.

2. THE ASSOCIATION BETWEEN THE INVESTMENT OPPORTUNITY SET AND JOB SECURITY

2.1. The Investment Opportunity Set

A firm comprises assets-in-place and future investment options or growth opportunities. The lower the proportion of firm value represented by assets-in-place, the higher the growth opportunities. Myers (1977) described these potential investment opportunities as call options, whose values depend on the likelihood that management will exercise them. Like call options, these growth opportunities represent real value to the firm (Kester, 1984). Growth options include such discretionary expenditures as capacity expansion projects, new project introductions, acquisitions of other firms, investment in brand name through advertising, and even maintenance and replacement of existing assets (Mason and Merton, 1985). A significant portion of the market value of equity is accounted for by growth opportunities (Kester, 1984; Pindyck, 1988).

2.2. Hypothesis

The IOS of a firm may be viewed as a crucial characteristic of the firm with profound influence on the way that the firm is viewed by managers, owners, investors, and creditors (Kallapur and Trombley, 2001). It has been shown theoretically to be a crucial determinant of the risk characteristics of the firm (Miles, 1986), a result confirmed empirically by Riahi-Belkaoui (1999) after controlling for multinational diversification. Similarly, Kallapur and Trombley (1999) showed strong association between some investment opportunity set proxy variables and realized growth.

Smith and Watts (1992) argue that managers of firms with relatively more growth opportunities are likely to be allowed more decision-making discretion because managers have better information about the investment opportunities than the firms' stockholders. As a result, Smith and Watts (1992) predict that growth firms are more likely to use incentive compensation schemes that tie management compensation to measures of firm performance (such as accounting earnings or stock price). The evidence indicates that growth firms are more likely to use stock-option plans (Smith and Watts, 1992) but is inconclusive with respect to which firms are more likely to use bonus plans (Gaver and Gaver,

1993). In addition, Gaver and Gaver (1993)[1] find that growth firms pay significantly higher levels of cash compensation to their executives.

The fact that IOS is related to the risk characteristics of the firm (Miles, 1986; Riahi-Belkaoui, 1999), to the realized growth of the firm (Adam and Goyal, 1999; Kallapur and Trombley, 1999), and to a greater use of incentive compensation (Smith and Watts, 1992; Gaver and Gaver, 1993; Baber et al., 1996) indicates a greater job reward and job security associated with growth opportunities.[2] Therefore, in conformity with the Fudenberg and Tirole (1995) model of association between job security and income smoothing, our hypothesis relates IOS to the extent of smoothing as follows:

H_0: *The extent of income smoothing is negatively related to the level of IOS.*

3. RESEARCH DESIGN

For purposes of comparability with and replication of previous work, the research design is essentially based on previous published research. The empirical methodology, described in Section 3.1, is based on Defond and Park (1997), Ahmed et al. (2000), and Elgers et al. (2000). The methods used to estimate discretionary accruals is described in Section 3.2. Section 3.3 discusses the measurement of a proxy for IOS.

3.1. Methodology

Following the methodology of Defond and Park (1997), Ahmed et al. (2000), and Elgers et al. (2000), we classify firm-year observations into three groups: (1) firm-years in which the current relative performance is good while the expected future relative performance is poor; (2) firm-years in which the current relative performance is poor while the expected future relative performance is good; and (3) firm-years in which the current relative performance and the expected future relative performance are both either poor or good. The focus is on groups 1 and 2, where income smoothing is expected. Current relative performance is considered good when current premanaged earnings are above the sample median earnings by year and industry. It is considered bad when current premanaged earnings are below the sample median by year and industry. Expected future relative performance is considered good when expected earnings are above the sample median, by year and industry. It is bad when the expected earnings are below the sample median by year. Group 1 is expected to have negative mean and median discretionary accruals in conformity with the theory predicting that managers will have an incentive to manage earnings upward.

Using discretionary accruals as the measure of extent of smoothing and a proxy for IOS and based on our expectations that the extent of smoothing is negatively related to the level of IOS in periods of low current/high future

performance and positively related to the level of IOS in periods of high current/ low future performance, the pooled regression takes the following form:

$$DACC_{it} = \beta_o + \beta_1 IOS_{it} + \beta_2 LEV_{it} + \beta_3 SIZE_{it} + \beta_4 DACC_{it-1} + \varepsilon_{it} \qquad (1)$$

where

$DACC_{it}$ = discretionary accruals for firm i in year t

IOS_{it} = level of firm's IOS in year t

$SIZE_{it}$ = size of firm i in year t measured as log of total assets

LEV_{it} = leverage of firm i in year t

$DACC_{it-1}$ = discretionary accruals for firms in year $t - 1$

Discussion of the measurement of all these variables is presented below. Following earlier research, control variables included leverage and size as in Becker et al. (1998) and prior discretionary accruals as in Ahmed et al. (2000).

3.2. Measurement of Premanaged Earnings and Discretionary Accruals

Premanaged earnings in a given year are measured by the reported (asset-scaled) earnings before extraordinary items less discretionary accruals.

The estimation of discretionary accruals follows the approach of (1) using alternative ways of estimating discretionary accruals: the modified Jones model (1991) and the Kang and Sivaramakrishnan model (1995) and (2) using two alternative measures of accruals: the traditional balance sheet approach and the cash-flow approach proposed by Collins and Hribar (1999).

Total accruals, as based on the balance sheet approach, are as follows:

$$TAAC_{it} = (\Delta CA_{it} - \Delta CL_{it} - \Delta Cash_{it} + \Delta STDEBT_{it} - DEPTN_{it}) \qquad (2)$$

where

ΔCA_i = change in current assets during period t (Compustat No. 4)

ΔCL_{it} = change in current liabilities during period t (Compustat No. 5)

$\Delta STDEBT_{it}$ = change in the current maturities of long-term debt and other short-term debt included in current liabilities during period t (Compustat No. 34)

$DEPTN_{it}$ = depreciation and amortization expense during period t (Compustat No. 14)

Based on the findings that studies relying on the traditional balance sheet approach to the measurement of total accruals suffer from potential contamination from measurement errors in the total accruals, Collins and Hubar (1999) suggested a straightforward approach that computes total accruals as the differ-

ence between net income and operating cash flow (taken from the cash-flow statement).

Discretionary accruals are also computed using a variant of the Jones (1991) model. The model captures regularities over time in the relations among total accruals, assets, and changes in revenues of a given firm:

$$TACC_{it} = \alpha_1(1/TA_{it-1}) + \alpha_2[(\Delta REV_{it} - \Delta REC_{it})/TA_{it-1}] \quad (3)$$
$$+ \alpha_3(PPE_{it}/TA_{it-1}) + \varepsilon_{it}$$

where $TACC_{it}$ is total accruals calculated as in equation (2), TA_{it-1} is total assets, $\Delta REV_{it} - \Delta REC_{it}$ is the change in cash-basis revenue, and PPE_{it} is gross property, plant, and equipment. Discretionary accruals from the modified Jones model are the residuals from the regression in equation (3).

An alternative approach to the measurement of discretionary accruals is proposed by Kang and Sivaramakrishnan (1995). Their model estimates managed accruals using the level, rather than the change, of current assets and current liabilities. It is expressed as follows:

$$ACCB_{it} = \Phi_0 + \Phi_1 + (\delta_1 REV_{it}) + (\delta_2 EXP_{it}) + \Phi_3(\delta_3 PPE_{it}) + \varepsilon_{it} \quad (4)$$

$ACCB_{it}$ = the balance of noncash current assets (net of tax receivables) less current liabilities (net of tax payables) for firm i at the end of year y, divided by total assets for firm i at the end of year $t - 1$. The parameters δ_1, δ_2, and δ_3 are the previous year's turnover ratios, which leads to the measurement of (1) the current period's receivables as a product of the previous year's receivables-to-sale ratio (δ_1) and the current period's sales (REV_t) and (2) the current period net current assets as the product of the previous year's net current assets-to-expense ratio (δ_2) times the current period's expenses (EXP_t).

3.3. Estimation of IOS

Because the IOS is not observable, there has not been a consensus on an appropriate proxy variable (Kallapur and Trombley, 1999). Similar to Smith and Watts (1992) and Gaver and Gaver (1993), we use a corporate measure of IOS that is designed to reduce classification error in this variable. Specifically, we use a common factor analysis of three variables to construct an index of the IOS of each firm. The three variables are market-to-book assets (MASS), market-to-book equity (MVE), and the earnings price ratio (EP). These variables are designed as follows:

1. MASS = [Assets—Total equity + Shares outstanding * Share closing price]/Assets

2. MVE = [Shares outstanding * Share closing price]/Total common equity

3. EP = [Primary EPS before extraordinary items]/Share closing price

4. RESULTS

This section covers a presentation and a discussion of the results of the empirical analysis. The sample selection criterion and a discussion of the descriptive statistics are presented in section 4.1. The results of income smoothing are discussed in section 4.2. Finally, the results of the regressions relating IOS to the extent of income smoothing are discussed in section 4.3.

4.1. Data

The sample selection criteria are the same as those reported in Elgers et al. (2000), as they constitute an improvement on those reported in Defond and Park (1997). The sample is chosen from the 152,883 firm-years in the 1998 S&P Compustat PC—this database of active and research companies having a CUSIP identifier and an SIC code. The main selection criteria are as follows:

1. Firms are chosen from industries with at least twenty members in each year.
2. Firms are eliminated due to missing data from both the I/B/E/S and Compustat databases.
3. The extremes of 1 percent of firm-years based on scaled discretionary accruals, nondiscretionary accruals, operating cash flows, and IOS as well as firm-years having less than $1 million in assets were eliminated.
4. All financial institutions and unclassified firms (SIC between 5999 and 7000 and SIC = 9999) were excluded.
5. Finally, all non-December fiscal-year-end-firm-years are excluded.[3]

The final sample contains 8,632 firm-years. Table 1C.1 represents the results of the common factor analysis of the three measures of the IOS for the sample of firms. The estimated communalities of the individual measures of the investment opportunity set are shown in panel A (see Hartman, 1976).[4] The eigenvalues of the reduced correlation matrix of the three individual measures of IOS are shown in panel B. It has been suggested that the number of factors needed to approximate the original correlations among the individual measures is equal to the number of summed eigenvalues needed to exceed the sum of the communalities. In this study, the first eigenvalue exceeds the sum of the three comunalities. It appears that one common factor explains the intercorrelations among the three individual measures.

In panel C, the correlations between the common factor and the three individual measures of the IOS indicate, as expected, a positive correlation with MASS and MVE and a negative correlation with EP. It strongly suggests that the factor captures the underlying construct common to the three measures. The descriptive statistics of the common factor are presented in panel D.

Table 1C.2 reports the descriptive statistics for the sample of firm-years used

Table 1C.1
Selected Statistics Related to a Common Factor Analysis of Three Measures of the Investment Opportunity Set (IOS)

Panel A: Estimated communalities of three IOS measures[a]

MASS[b]	MVE[c]	EP[d]
0.294	0.141	0.065

Panel B: Eigenvalues of the reduced correlation matrix of three IOS measures

1	2	3
0.831	0.267	0.052

Panel C: Correlation between the common factor and three IOS measures

MASS	MVE	EP
0.789	0.622	−0.385

Panel D: Descriptive statistics of the common factor extracted from three IOS measures

Maximum	5.236	Third quartile	2.215	Median	1.123
First quartile	0.521	Minimum	0.229	Mean	0.080

Notes:
a. Communalities are equivalent to the squared multiple correlations obtained from regressing each of the IOS measures on the other two measures.
b. The ratio of the market value of the firm to the book value of assets. The market value of the firm is computed as the book value of liabilities plus the market value of common shares.
c. The ratio of the market value of common shares to the book value of common shares.
d. The ratio of primary earnings per share before extraordinary items to closing price per share.

in the study. Both total accruals and discretionary accruals are shown under both the balance sheet approach and the cash-flow approach. The total accruals have a mean (median) of − 0.031 (0.082) under the balance sheet approach (TACC1) and a mean (median) of − 0.042 (0.091) under the cash-flow approach (TACC2). Similarly, the discretionary accruals have a mean (median) of − 0.002 (0.050) under the balance sheet approach (DACC1) and a mean (median) of −0.004 (0.001) under the cash-flow approach (DACC2). The differences between DACC1 and DACC2 appear to justify the use of both of these accrual measurement methods to test the sensitivity of the results of the impact of IOS on anticipatory income smoothing.

Table 1C.2 also reports descriptive statistics on return on assets (EB), leverage (LEV) and size (SIZE). The mean (median) is 0.071 (0.052) for return on assets (EB), 0.515 (0.301) for leverage (LEV), and 3,125 (5,230) for size (SIZE).

Table 1C.2
Descriptive Statistics (n = 8,632, 1979–1996)

Variable	Mean	σ	Lower Quartile	Median	Upper Quartile
TACC1	-0.021	-0.082	-0.071	-0.032	-0.026
TACC2	-0.042	0.091	-0.085	-0.036	0.018
DACC1	-0.002	0.050	-0.032	-0.003	0.036
DACC2	-0.004	0.001	-0.041	0.000	0.041
EBI	0.071	0.052	0.037	0.051	0.096
LEV	0.515	0.301	0.381	0.539	0.632
SIZE	3,125	5,230	252	863	2,893

Note: Variables are defined as follows:
TACC1 = Total accruals using the balance sheet approach ($\Delta CA_{it} - \Delta CL_{it} - \Delta Cash_{it} + \Delta STDEBT_{it} - DEPTN_{it}/TA_{it-1}$)
TACC2 = Total accruals using the cash-flow approach
DACC1 = Discretionary accruals based on the modified Jones model and TACC1
DACC2 = Discretionary accruals based on the modified Jones model and TACC2
EB = Earnings before extraordinary items, deflated by total assets at the beginning of the year
SIZE = Total assets ($millions)

4.2. Evidence in Anticipatory Smoothing

Anticipatory smoothing evidence has been reported in Defond and Park (1997), Ahmed et al. (2000), and Elgers et al. (2000). Table 1C.3 provided results replicating prior evidence on anticipatory smoothing. As in previous studies, Table 1C.3 partitions the discretionary accruals results (based on the modified Jones model) on the basis of "poor" and "good" relative performance, on one hand, and "poor" and "good" expected future relative performance, on the other hand. Current relative performance is classified as poor (good) when current premanaged earnings (earnings before discretionary accruals) are below (above) the sample median earnings by year and by industry. Current premanaged earnings are measured by subtracting the Jones model discretionary accrual estimate from reported earnings. Expected future relative performance is classified as poor (good) when next year's premanaged earnings (earnings before discretionary accrual) are below (above) the sample median by year and industry. Expected earnings are measured by the next period's forecast earnings taken from the I/B/E/S database.

Table 1C.3

Discretionary Accruals Partitioned by Current Relative Performance and Expected Relative Performance[a]

Current Relative Performance[b]

Expected Future Relative Performance[c]		"Poor" (Current premanaged earnings below sample median earnings, by year and industry)		"Good" (Current premanaged earnings above sample median earnings, by year and industry)		Total	
"Poor" (Expected earnings below the sample median, by year and industry)	Mean	(i)	0.001 ***(d)	(ii)	-0.051 ***		-0.003 ***
	Median		0.0039 ***		-0.038 ***		-0.001 ***
	% positive		52.39 % ***		10.15% ***		46.31% ***
	N		2772		1342		4114
"Good" (Expected earnings above the sample median, by year and industry)	Mean	(iii)	0.058 ***	(iii)	-0.002 ***	0.02	0.02 ***
	Median		0.041 ***		-0.013 ***		0.00 ***
	% positive		85.21% ***		31.12% ***		51.16 ***
	N		1485		3032		4517
Total	Mean		0.036 ***		-0.029 ***		-0.001
	Median		0.017 ***		-0.016 ***		0.000
	% positive		85.21% ***		36.12 ***		50.31%
	N		4257		4374		8631

Notes:

a. Discretionary accruals are from the modified Jones model using the balance sheet approach.

b. Current relative performance is classified as poor (good) when current premanaged earnings (earnings before discretionary accruals) are below (above) the sample median earnings, by year and industry.

c. Expected future relative performance is classified as poor (good) when next period's premanaged earnings (earnings before discretionary accruals) are below (above) the sample median by year and industry.

d. ***Significantly different from 0 at less than the 0.01 level (two-tailed). Significance levels for means refer to t-tests; for medians refer to Wilcox on sign-rank tests, and for percentage positive refer to proportions.

The anticipatory smoothing hypothesis developed in Defond and Park (1997) predicts earnings management via discretionary accruals in the second and third cell of the classification matrix in Table 1C.2. The discretionary accruals are expected to be negative in the second cell as managers are expected to "save" current earnings for possible use in the future. The discretionary accruals are expected to be positive in the third cell, as managers are expected to "borrow" earnings from the future for use in the current period. The results of the replication correspond closely to those reported in Defond and Park (1997), Ahmed et al. (2000), and Elgers et al. (2000). When current performance is good and future performance is expected to be poor, the average and median discretionary accruals are −0.051 and −0.038, respectively. The prediction of anticipatory smoothing hypothesis is supported, with only 10.15 percent of 1,342 observations in cell (3) positive. Managers are assumed to be making income-decreasing discretionary accruals to reduce the threat of dismissal due to poor performance in the future.

When current performance is poor and future performance is expected to be good, the average and median discretionary accruals are 0.058 and 0.039, respectively. The predictions of the anticipatory smoothing hypothesis are again supported, with 85.21 percent of the 1,485 observations in cell (3) positive. Managers are assumed to be making income-increasing accruals to reduce the threat of dismissal due to poor performance in the current period.

4.3. Regression Results

The replication reported in Table 1C.3 corresponds closely to the anticipatory smoothing evidence reported in Defond and Park (1997), Ahmed et al. (2000), and Elgers et al. (2000). They do not, however, provide a direct test of the link between job security and income smoothing. A direct test, proposed in this study, is to evaluate the impact of the level of IOS on the extent of smoothing as the level of IOS is related to job security. The regression results reported in this section indicate that the extent of income smoothing varies with managers' job security concerns as proxied by the level of IOS. The results of the regression on equation (1) are reported in section 4.3.1 for the good current performance/poor future performance observations and in section 4.3.2 for the poor current performance/good future performance observations. To test the sensitivity of the results to the estimation procedure used, the results are presented using (1) the modified Jones model and the Kang and Sivaramakrishnan model for the estimation of discretionary accruals and (b) the traditional balance sheet and cash-flow approaches for the computation of total accruals.

4.3.1. Results for the Good Current Performance/Poor Future Performance Partition

The hypothesis is that the extent of income smoothing is negatively related to the level of IOS. The expectation is that when current earnings are "good"

and expected earnings are "poor," the managers will "save" current earnings for possible use in the future, resulting in the use of negative disclosure accruals in the current period. As the level of IOS increases, the concern for job decreases, and therefore the discretionary accruals will be less negative. As a result, we predict the coefficient on IOS, the proxy for job security concern, to be positive.

Table 1C.4 reports the regression results for discretionary accruals from the modified Jones model (panel A) and from the Kang and Sivaramakrishnan model (panel B), using both the balance sheet and cash-flow approaches for computing total accruals. The significant negative intercept in the four cases confirms the anticipatory smoothing evidence reported in Table 1C.3. In addition, the IOS variable has a positive and significant coefficient as hypothesized. It shows that the anticipatory smoothing associated with good current performance/poor future performance increases as the level of IOS decreases. As expected and as found in prior research by Defond and Park (1997) and Ahmed et al. (2000), discretionary accruals are positively related to size and negatively related to leverage and size.

The regression results for the Kang and Sivaramakrishnan model using both the balance sheet and cash-flow approaches to the computation of total accruals are similar to the results provided by the modified Jones model.

4.3.2 Results for the Poor Current Performance/Good Future Performance Partition

The managers in this group of firms are expected to use positive disclosure accruals in the current period. As the level of IOS increases, the concern for the job decreases, and therefore the discretionary accruals will be less positive. As a result, we predict the coefficient on IOS, the proxy for job security, to be negative.

Table 1C.5 reports the regression results for discretionary accruals from the modified Jones model (panel A) and from the Kang and Sivaramakrishnan model (panel B), using both the balance sheet and cash-flow approaches for computing total accruals. The significant positive intercept in the four cases confirms the anticipatory smoothing evidence reported in Table 1C.3. In addition, the IOS variable has a negative and significant coefficient as hypothesized. It shows that the anticipatory smoothing evidence associated with poor current performance/ good future performance increases as the level of IOS decreases. As expected, the results on leverage, size, and prior disclosure accruals are similar to the findings reported for the other groups in section 4.3.2. The results for the Kang and Sivaramakrishnan model are also consistent with the results from the modified Jones model.

5. SUMMARY AND CONCLUSIONS

Fudenberg and Tirole (1995) propose that concern about job security creates an incentive for managers to smooth earnings. Consistent with their model,

Table 1C.4

Regression Results for the Good Current Performance/Poor Future Performance Partition Model: $DACC_{it} = \beta_0 + \beta_1 IOS_{it} + \beta_2 LEV_{it} + \beta_3 SIZE_{it} + \beta_4 DACCLG_{it} + \varepsilon_{it}$

Panel A: Discretionary Accruals estimated with the Modified Jones Model

	Dependent Variable = DACC1 (Balance Sheet Approach)	Dependent Variable = DACC2 (Cash-Flow Approach)
Intercept (-)	-0.13 (-7.61)	(5.32)
IOS (+)	+0.19 (4.61)	-0.32 (6.01)
LEV (-)	-0.03 (6.23)	-0.05 (-10.32)
SIZE (?)	0.02 (6.32)	0.02 (7.32)
DACCLG (-)	-0.01 (-0.31)	-0.02 (-0.15)
R-sq	11.42%	16.31%

Panel B: Discretionary Accruals Estimated with the Kang and Sivaramakrishnan Model

	Dependent Variable = DACC1 (Balance Sheet Approach)	Dependent Variable = DACC2 (Cash-Flow Approach)
Intercept (-)	-0.12 (-8.67)	-0.36 (-10.96)
IOS (+)	0.20 (7.35)	-0.32 (9.50)
LEV (-)	-0.13 (-10.15)	-0.15 (15.16)
SIZE (?)	0.01 (16.32)	0.01 (13.25)
DACCLG (-)	-0.13 (8.15)	-0.08 (-3.98)
R-sq	20.16%	85.13%
N		

Table 1C.5
Regression Results for the Poor Current Performance/Good Future Performance Partition Model: $DACC_{it} = \beta_0 + \beta_1 IOS_{it} + \beta_2 LEV_{it} + \beta_3 SIZE_{it} + \beta_4 DACCLG_{it} + \varepsilon_{it}$

Panel A: Discretionary Accruals Estimated with the Modified Jones Model

	Dependent Variable = DACC1 (Balance Sheet Approach)	Dependent Variable = DACC2 (Cash-Flow Approach)
Intercept (+)	0.15 (6.23)	0.16 (6.45)
IOS (-)	-0.06 (4.82)	-0.09 (-6.15)
LEV (-)	-0.04 (8.50)	-0.05 (6.13)
SIZE (?)	-0.002 (-2.12)	-0.002 (8.13)
DACCLG (-)	0.01 (0.16)	0.08 (3.98)
R-sq	3.2%	5.6%
N		

Panel B: Discretionary Accruals Estimated with the Kang and Sivaramakrishnan Model

	Dependent Variable = DACC1 (Balance Sheet Approach)	Dependent Variable = DACC2 (Cash-Flow Approach)
Intercept (+)	0.23 (6.37)	0.26 (9.53)
IOS (-)	-0.63 (-8.15)	-0.14 (-5.25)
LEV (-)	-0.07 (-6.16)	-0.08 (-8.32)
SIZE (?)	-0.004	-0.007
DACCLG (-)	-0.04 (-2.13)	-0.02 (-0.31)
R-sq	6.5%	7.32%
N		

Defond and Park (1997) show that managers smooth earnings in consideration of both current and future relative performance. To provide a more direct evidence of anticipatory smoothing and job security, this study hypothesizes that the extent of smoothing, as measured by four different measures of discretionary accruals, varies with managers' job security concerns as proxied by the level of the investment opportunity set or growth opportunities. More explicitly, the extent of smoothing is expected to be negatively related to the level of IOS in periods of low current/high future performance and positively related to the level of IOS in periods of high current/low future performance. The empirical results confirmed our predictions.

NOTES

1. Studies that explicitly model endogeneity between IOS and compensation type find different results. Holthausen et al. (1995) find a preference for accounting-based incentive corporations, which incorporate long-term targets.

2. Results on the impact of IOS on financial and dividend policies may also be used to support the job security hypothesis. First, firms with a high level of firm value represented by IOS rather than assets in place tend to use less debt in their capital structure (Smith and Watts, 1992; Gaver and Gaver, 1993; Skinner, 1993; Gul, 1999). Second, Smith and Watts (1992), Gaver and Gaver (1993), and Gul (1999) find a strong negative relation between dividend yield and IOS.

3. This last criterion was motivated by the reasoning that when all industry members do not share the same fiscal year, management may find it difficult to identify the median firm, as it would require comparisons of industry members across many months of the year. Support for this position is provided by Murphy (1998), Byrd et al. (1998), and Elgers et al. (2000).

4. Communalities are equivalent to the squared multiple correlations obtained from regressing each of the investment opportunity set measures on the other two measures.

REFERENCES

Adam, T., and V. Goyal. 1999. The Investment Opportunity Set and Its Proxy Variables: Theory and Evidence. Working Paper, Hong Kong University of Science and Technology.

Ahmed, A.S., G.J. Lobo, and J. Zhou. 2000. Job Security and Income Smoothing: An Empirical Test of the Fudenberg and Triole (1995) Model. Working Paper, Syracause University.

Baber, W., S. Janakiaraman, and S. Kang. 1996. Investment Opportunities and the Structure of Executive Compensation. *Journal of Accounting and Economics* 3: 297–318.

Becker, C., M. Defond, J. Jiambalvo, and K.R. Subramanyam. 1998. The Effect of Audit Quality on Earnings Management. *Contemporary Accounting Research* 15 (Spring): 1–2.

Byrd, J., M. Johnson, and S. Porter. 1998. Discretion in Financial Reporting: The Vol-

untary Disclosure of Compensation Peer Groups in Proxy Statement Performance Graphs. *Contemporary Accounting Research* 15: 25–52.

Chaney, P.K., D.C. Jeter, and C.N. Lewis. 1998. The Use of Accruals in Income Smoothing: A Permanent Hypothesis. *Advances in Quantitative Analysis of Finance and Accounting* 6: 103–135.

Collins, D., and P. Hribar. 1999. Errors in Estimating Accruals: Implications for Empirical Research. Working Paper, University of Iowa.

Defond, M.L., and C.W. Park. 1997. Smoothing Income in Anticipation of Future Earnings. *Journal of Accounting and Economics* 23: 115–139.

Elgers, P.T, R.J. Pfeiffer Jr., and S.L. Porter. 2000. Anticipatory Smoothing: A Reexamination. Working Paper, University of Massachusetts.

Fudenberg, K., and J. Tirole. 1995. A Theory of Income and Dividend Smoothing Based on Incumbency Rents. *Journal of Political Economy* 103: 75–93.

Gaver, J., K. Gaver, and J. Austin. 1995. Additional Evidence on Bonus Plans and Income Management. *Journal of Accounting and Economics* 19 (February): 3–28.

Gaver, J.J., and K.M. Gaver. 1993. Additional Evidence on the Association between the Investment Opportunity Set and Corporate Financing, Dividend, and Compensation Policies. *Journal of Accounting and Economics* 16: 125–140.

Gul, F. 1999. Growth Opportunities, Capital Structure and Dividend Policies in Japan. *Journal of Corporate Finance* 5: 141–168.

Hand, J. 1989. Did Firms Undertake Debt—Equity Swaps for an Accounting Paper Profit or True Financial Gain? *The Accounting Review* 64 (October): 587–623.

Hartman, H.H. 1976. *Modern Factor Analysis*, 3rd ed. Chicago: University of Chicago Press.

Holthausen, R., D. Larcker, and R. Sloan. 1995. Business Unit Innovation and the Structure of Executive Compensation. *Journal of Accounting and Economics* 19: 279–314.

Jones, J. 1991. Earnings Management during Import Relief Investigations. *Journal of Accounting Research* 29: 193–228.

Kallapur, S., and M.A. Trombley. 1999. The Association between Investment Opportunities Set Proxies and Realized Growth. *Journal of Business Finance and Accounting* 26: 505–519.

Kallapur, S., and M.A. Trombley. 2001. The Investment Opportunity Set Determinants, Consequences and Measurement. *Managerial Finance* 27: 3–15.

Kang, S., and K. Sivaramakrishnan. 1995. Issues in Testing Earnings Management and an Instrumental Variable Approach. *Journal of Accounting Research* 33 (Autumn): 353–367.

Kester, W.C. 1984. Todays Options for Tomorrow's Growth. *Harvard Business Review* 62 (2): 153–160.

Mason, S.P., and R.C. Merton. 1985. The Role of Contingent Claims Analysis in Corporate Finance. In E.I. Altman, ed., *Recent Advances in Corporate Finance*. Homewood, IL: Irwin, 7–45.

Miles, J. 1986. Growth Options and the Real Determinants of Systematic Risk. *Journal of Business Finance and Accounting* 13: 95–105.

Murphy, K. 1998. Executive Compensation. Working Paper, Marshall School of Business, Los Angeles.

Myers, S. 1977. Determinants of Corporate Borrowing. *Journal of Financial Economics* 5: 147–177.

Pindyck, R. 1988. Irreversible Investment Capacity Choice, and the Value of the Firm. *American Economic Review* 78: 969–985.

Riahi-Belkaoui, A. 1999. The Association between Systematic Risk and Multinationality: A Growth Opportunities Perspective. *Global Business and Finance Review* (Fall): 1–10.

Ronen, J., and S. Sadan. 1981. *Smoothing Income Numbers: Objectives, Means and Implications.* Reading, MA: Addison-Wesley.

Skinner, D.J. 1993. Asset Structure, Financing Policy and Accounting Choice: Preliminary Evidence. *Journal of Accounting and Economics* 16: 407–446.

Smith, C.W., and R.L. Watts. 1992. The Investment Opportunity Set and Corporate Financing, Dividend Compensation Policies. *Journal of Financial Economics* 32: 263–292.

Subramanyam, K.R. 1996. The Pricing of Discretionary Accruals. *Journal of Accounting and Economics* 22: 249–281.

Chapter 2

Earnings Management

INTRODUCTION

Managers have the flexibility of choosing between the alternative ways to account for transactions as well as choosing between options within the same accounting treatment. This flexibility, which is intended to allow managers to adapt to economic circumstances and portray the correct economic consequences of transactions, can also be used to affect the level of earnings at any particular time with the objective of securing gains for management and the stakeholders. This is the essence of earnings management, which is the ability to "manipulate" the choices available and make the right choices that can achieve a desired level of income. It is another flagrant example of designed accounting, which is the object of this chapter.

NATURE OF EARNINGS MANAGEMENT

Conceptual Definitions of Earnings Management

Various definitions have been offered to explain earnings management as a special form of "designed" rather than "principled" accounting. Schipper sees earnings management as a purposeful intervention in the external reporting process with the intent of obtaining some private gain.[1] This is assumed to be possible through either a selection of accounting methods within Generally Accepted Accounting Principles (GAAP) or application of given methods in particular ways.[2] Schipper also views earnings management from either an economic (or true) income perspective or an informational perspective. The true income perspective assumes (1) the existence of a true economic income

that is distributed by a deliberate earnings management and/or by measurement errors embedded in accounting rules and (2) noisy unmanaged earnings acquire through earnings management new properties in terms of amount, bias, or variance. The informational perspective assumes (1) that earnings are one of the signals used for decisions and judgments and (2) that managers have private information that they can use when they choose elements within GAAP under different sets of contracts that determine their conversation and behavior.[3]

The information perspective in better explicated in the following definitions:

Earnings management occurs when managers use judgement in financial reporting and in structuring transactions to alter financial reports to either mislead some stakeholders about the underlying economic performance of the company or to influence contractual outcomes that depend on reported accounting numbers.[4]

This definition of Healy and Wahlen focuses on the exercise of judgment in financial reports to (1) either mislead the stakeholders who do not or cannot do earnings management and (2) make financial reports more informative to users. There is therefore a good and bad side to earnings management; the bad side is the cost created by the misallocation of resources, and the good side is made up of the potential improvements in management's credible communication of private information to external stakeholders, improving resource allocation decisions.[5]

Earnings Management as Accrual Management

Basically, the operational definition of earnings management is the potential use of accrual management with the intent of obtaining some private gain. The following relationships are central to an understanding of earnings management as accrual management.

1. Total accruals = Reported net income − Cash flows from operations
2. Total accruals = Nondiscretionary accruals + Discretionary accruals

The general approach for estimating discretionary accruals is to regress total accruals on variables that are proxies for normal accruals. Unexpected accruals or discretionary accruals are considered to be the unexplained (the residual) components of total accruals.

In addition to the use of unexpected accruals and discretionary accruals as a proxy for earnings management, many studies provided evidence on which specific accruals or accounting methods are used for earnings management. Examples of specific accruals proven to be used for earnings management include:

1. Depreciation estimates and bad debt provisions surrounding initial public offers[6]
2. Loan loss reserves of banks[7] and claim loss reserves of insurers[8]
3. Deferred tax valuation allowances[9]

ACCRUALS MODELS

Discretionary accruals models involve first the computation of total accruals. Therefore, total accruals models are presented first, followed by discretionary accruals models.

Total Accruals Models

Two models are generally used for the computation of accruals: the balance sheet approach and the cash-flow approach.

The balance sheet approach for the computation of total accruals (TA) is as follows:

$$TA_t = \Delta CA_t - \Delta Cash_t - \Delta CL_t + \Delta DCL_t - DEP_t$$

where ΔCA_t is the change in the current assets in year t (Compustat No. 4); $\Delta Cash_t$ is the change in cash and cash equivalent in year t (Compustat No. 1); ΔCL_t is the change in current liabilities in the year t (Compustat No. 5); ΔDCL_t is the change in debt included in current liabilities in the year t (Compustat No. 34); and DEP_t is the depreciation and amortization expense in year t (Compustat No. 14). Based on the findings that studies relying on the traditional balance sheet approach to the measurement of total accruals suffer from potential contamination from measurement of total accruals, Collins and Hribar[10] suggested a straightforward approach that computes total accruals as the difference between net income and operating cash-flow (taken from the cash-flow statement).

Discretionary Accruals Models

Six competing discretionary accruals models are considered in the literature. They are as follows:

The DeAngelo Model

The discretionary portion of accruals in the DeAngelo model[11] is the difference between total accruals in the event year t scaled by total assets (A_{t-1}) and nondiscretionary accruals (NDA_t). The measure of nondiscretionary accruals (NDA_t) rests on last period's total accruals (TA_{t-1}) scaled by lagged total assets (A_{t-2}). In other words:

$$NDA_t = TA_{t-1}/A_{t-2}$$

The Healy Model

In the Healy model[12] the nondiscretionary accruals (NDA_t) are the mean of total accruals TA_t scaled by lagged total assets (A_{t-1}) from the estimation period. In other words:

$$NDA_t = 1/n\Sigma_y(TA_y / A_{y-1})$$

where NDA_t is nondiscretionary accruals in the year t scaled by lagged total assets; n is the number of years in the estimation period; and γ is a year subscript for years $(t-n, t-n+1, \ldots, t-1)$ included in the estimation period. The discretionary portion is the difference between the total accruals in the event year scaled by A_{t-1} and NDA_t. The main difference between the DeAngelo model and the Healy model is that NDA follows a random walk process in the DeAngelo model and a mean reverting process in the Healy model.

The Jones Model[13]

The main objective of the Jones model is to control for the effect of changes in the firm's circumstances on nondiscretionary accruals. The nondiscretionary accruals in the event year are expressed as follows:

$$NDA_t = \alpha_1(1/A_{t-1}) + \alpha_2(\Delta REV_t/A_{t-1}) + \alpha_3(PPE_t/A_{t-1})$$

where NDA_t is the nondiscretionary accruals in the year t scaled by lagged total assets; ΔREV_t is the revenue in the year t less revenues in year $t-1$; PPE_t is gross property plant and equipment at the end of the year t; A_{t-1} is total assets at the end of the year $t-1$; and $\alpha_1, \alpha_2, \alpha_3$ are the firm-specific parameters.

The estimate of the firm-specific parameters is obtained by using the following model in the estimation period:

$$TA_t/A_{t-1} = \alpha_1(1/A_{t-1}) + \alpha_2(\Delta REV_t/A_{t-1}) + \alpha_3(PPE_t/A_{t-1}) + E_t$$

where α_1, α_2, and α_3 represent the OLS estimates of α_1, α_2, and α_3. The residual E_t represents the firm-specific discretionary portion of the total accruals.

The variations of the Jones model include:

1. A model that expands the Jones model by adding lagged total accruals and lagged stock returns as two additional explanatory variables.[14]
2. A model that replaces "changes in sales" in the Jones model by "change in cash sales."[15]

The Modified Jones Model

In order to eliminate the conjectured tending of the Jones model to measure discretionary accruals with error when discretion is exercised over revenue recognition, the modified model estimates nondiscretionary accruals during the event period (i.e., during periods in which earnings management is hypothesized) as follows:

$$NDA_t = \alpha_1(1/A_{t-1}) + \alpha_2[(\Delta REV_t - \Delta REC_t)/A_{t-1}] + \alpha_3(PPE_t/A_{t-1})$$

where ΔREC_t is net receivables in year t less net receivables in year $t-1$, and other variables are as in the previous equation.

The estimates of α_1, α_2, and α_3 and nondiscretionary accruals are obtained from the original Jones model, not from the modified model, during the estimation period (in which no systematic earnings management is hypothesized). The difference between the two models is explicated as follows:

Revenues are adjusted for the change in receivables in the event period. The original Jones model implicitly assumes that discretion is not exercised over revenue in either the estimation period or the event period. The modified version of the Jones model implicitly assumes that all changes in the credit sales in the event period result from earnings management. This is based on the reasoning that it is easier to manage earnings by exercising discretion over the recognition of revenue on credit sales than to manage earnings by exercising discretion over the recognition of revenue on cash sales. If this modification is successful, then the estimate of earnings management should no longer be biased toward zero in samples where earnings management has taken place through the management of revenues.[16]

The Industry Model

The industry model relaxes the assumption that nondiscretionary accruals are constant over time. Rather than attempting a modeling of the determinants of nondiscretionary accruals directly, the industry model assumes that the variations in the determinants of nondiscretionary accruals are common across firms in the same industry. The model is expressed as follows:

$$NDA_t = \beta_1 + \beta_2 median;(TA_t/A_{t-1})$$

where NDA_t is measured by the Jones model and median; TA_t/A_{t-1} is the median value of total accruals in year t scaled by lagged total assets for all non-sample firms in the same two-digit standard industrial classification (SIC) industry (industry j). The firm-specific parameters β_1 and β_2 are obtained from an ordinary least squares regression in the observation in the estimation period. The ability of the industry model to mitigate measurement error in discretionary accruals hinges critically on the following two factors:

First, the industry removes variation in nondiscretionary accruals that is common across firms in the same industry. If changes in nondiscretionary accruals largely reflect responses to changes in firm-specific circumstances, then the industry model will not extract all nondiscretionary accruals from the discretionary accrual proxy. Second, the industry removes variation in discretionary accruals that is correlated across firms in the same industry, potentially causing problem 2. The severity of this problem depends on the extent to which the earnings management stimulus is correlated across firms in the same industry.[17]

The Kang and Sivaramakrishnan Model

The Kang and Sivaramakrishnan model[18] relies on an alternative approach that (1) estimates managed accruals using the level rather than change of current assets and current liabilities, (2) includes cost of goods sold as well as other expenses, and (3) does not require the regression to be uncontaminated. The model is expressed as follows:

$$AB_{i,t} = \phi_0 + \phi_1[\delta_{1,i}REV_{i,t}] + \phi_2[\delta_{2,i}EXP_{i,t}] + \phi_3[\delta_{3,i}GPPE_{i,t}] + u_{i,t}$$

where

$AB_{i,t}$ = accrual balance
   = $AR_{i,t} + INV_{i,t} + OCA_{i,t} - CL_{i,t} - DEP_{i,t}$

$AR_{i,t}$ = receivables, excluding tax refunds

$INV_{i,t}$ = inventory

$OCA_{i,t}$ = current assets other than cash, receivables, and inventory

$CL_{i,t}$ = current liabilities excluding taxes and current maturities of long-term debt

$DEP_{i,t}$ = depreciation and amortization

$REV_{i,t}$ = net sales revenues

$EXP_{i,t}$ = operating expenses (cost of goods sold, selling, and administrative expenses before depreciation)

$GPPE_{i,t}$ = gross property plant and equipment

$NTA_{i,t}$ = net total assets

$$\delta_{1,i} = \frac{AR_{i,t} - 1}{REV_{i,t} - 1}$$

$$\delta_{2,i} = \frac{NV_{i,t-1} + OCA_{i,t-1} - CL_{i,t-1}}{EXP_{i,t-1}}$$

$$\delta_{3,i} = \frac{DEP_{i,t} - 1}{GPPE_{i,t-1}}$$

The parameters and δ_1, δ_2, and δ_3 are turnover ratios that accommodate firm-specificity and compensate for the fact that the equation is estimated from a pooled sample.

DETECTION OF EARNINGS MANAGEMENT

Financial reporting allows a distinction between best performing firms and poorly performing firms and better and more efficient resource allocation and

financial analysis by stakeholders. The U.S. accounting standards permit managers to exercise judgment in financial reporting, allowing them to provide not only timely and credible information but also relevant information under alternative standards. The situation creates opportunities, however, for "earnings management," in which managers select reporting methods and estimates that do not reflect the firm's true economic picture. This led the chairman of the Securities and Exchange Commission (SEC), Arthur Levitt, to warn about the threat to the credibility of financial reporting created by abuses of "big bath" restructuring charges, premature revenue recognition, "cookie jar" reserves, and write-offs of purchases in process R&D.[19] A good definition of earnings management follows:

Earnings Management occurs when managers use judgement in financial reporting and in structuring transactions to alter financial reports to either mislead some stakeholders about the underlying economic performance of the company or to influence contractual outcomes that depend on reporting accounting numbers.[20]

The detection of earnings management can be accomplished by:[21]

1. The use of simple analytical procedures that can reveal unusual relationships and significant changes in financial statement item relationships.
2. The use of sophisticated models to assess the risk of earnings manipulation such as the use of artificial neural network technology to assess fraud.[22]
3. The use of a profit model that can yield an earnings manipulation index as a linear combination of financial variables to be converted to a "profitability manipulation."

The third technique is of interest to international accounting and can best be illustrated by the Beneish profit model.[23] With the objective of differentiating between GAAP violators and control firms, Beneish uses a number of variables to proxy for (1) the *probability of detection* of the violation by the market through distortions in the financial statements and (2) *incentive/ability* to violate GAAP.

The six financial statement variables designed to capture distortions in financial statement data to assess the probability of detection are:[24]

1. Day's sales in receivables index—measuring whether changes in receivables are in time with changes in sales.
2. Gross margin index—assessing whether gross margins have deteriorated, a negative signal about a firm's prospects.
3. Asset quality index—measuring changes in the risk of assets realization, with an increase to be interpreted as indicating an increased propensity to capitalize and therefore defer costs.

4. Depreciation index—measuring the change in the rate of depreciation.

5. SG&A index—measuring sales general and administrative expense (SG&A) relative to sales with a disproportionate increase in SG&A relative to sales to be considered as a negative signal suggesting loss of managerial cost control or unusual sales effort.

6. Total accruals to total assets—measuring the extent to which earnings are cash-based, with high increases in noncash working capital to reflect possible manipulation.

These variables are defined in Figure 2.1.

The five variables intended to measure a firm's incentives/ability to violate GAAP are:[25]

1. Capital structure, as the incentives to violate GAAP increase with leverage.

2. Prior market performance, as the incentives to violate GAAP increase with declining stock prices.

3. Time listed, as firms may violate GAAP and manipulate earnings at the time of initially going public or shortly thereafter.

4. Sales growth, as high-growth firms may have an incentive to dispel the impression that their growth is decelerating following a stock price drop at the release of bad news.

5. Prior positive accruals decisions, as incentives to violate GAAP may increase if managers attempt to avoid accrual reversals or cannot increase earnings.

The five proxies are operationalized by six variables: leverage, abnormal return, time listed, sales growth index, declining cash sales dummy, and positive accruals dummy. They are defined in Figure 2.1.

The earnings manipulation index, proposed by Beneish probit analysis, is expressed as the following linear combination:

$$\text{Manipulation Index} = -2.224 + 0.221* \text{ (Day's Sales in Receivables Index)}$$

$+0.102*$ (Gross Margin Index) $+ 0.007*$ (Assets Quality Index)

$+0.062*$ (Depreciation Index) $+ 0.198*$ (SG&A Index)

$-2.415*$ (Total Accruals to Total Assets) $+ 0.040*$ (Sales Growth Index)

$-0.684*$ (Abnormal Return) $- 0.001*$ (Time Listed)

$+0.587*$ (Leverage Index) $+ 0.421*$ (Positive Accrual Dummy)

$-0.413*$ (Declining Cash Sales Dummy)

The probability of manipulation is then computed by looking up the manipulation index in a standard normal distribution table, where $F(x)$ is the cumulative area under the standard normal distribution. That is:

$$\text{Probability of earnings manipulation} = F \text{ (Manipulation Index)}.$$

Figure 2.1
Variables Used in the Beneish (1997) Probit Model

Variable	Definition	Hypothesized Relationship with Dependent Variable
Days Sales in Receivables Index	$$\dfrac{\dfrac{Receivables_t[2]}{Sales_t[12]}}{\dfrac{Receivables_{t-1}[2]}{Sales_{t-1}[12]}}$$	+
Gross Margin Index	$$\dfrac{\dfrac{Sales_{t-1}[12]-COGS_{t-1}[41]}{Sales_{t-1}[12]}}{\dfrac{Sales_{t-1}[12]-COGS_{t-1}[41]}{Sales_{t-1}[12]}}$$	+
Asset Quality Index	$$\dfrac{(1-\dfrac{CurrentAssets_t[4]+PPE_t[8]}{TotalAssets_t[6]})}{(1-\dfrac{CurrentAssets_{t-1}[4]+PPE_{t-1}[8]}{TotalAssets_{t-1}[6]})}$$	+
Depreciation Index	$$\dfrac{\dfrac{Depreciation_{t-1}[14-65]}{Depreciation_{t-1}[14-65+PPE_{t-1}[8]}}{\dfrac{Depreciation_t[14-65]}{Depreciation_t[14-65+PPE_t[8]}}$$	+
SG&A Index	$$\dfrac{\dfrac{SG\&AExpense_t[189]}{Sales_t[2]}}{\dfrac{SG\&AExpense_{t-1}[189]}{Sales_{t-1}[2]}}$$	+

Figure 2.1 (continued)

Variable	Definition	Hypothesized Relationship with Dependent Variable
Total Accruals to Total Assets	$$\frac{\left[\begin{array}{l}(\Delta CurrentAss_t[4] - \Delta Cash_t[1] \\ (\Delta CurrentLiab._t[5] - \Delta Short\text{-}termdebt_t[34] - \\ Deprec.\& Amort_t[14] - DefferedtaxonEarnings[50] + \\ EquityinEarnings[55]\end{array}\right]}{TotalAssets_t[6]}$$	?
Sales Growth Index	$Sales_t[12]/Sales_{t-1}[12]$	+
Abnormal Return	Size-adjusted return for a 12-month period ending on the month prior to release of the financial statements. Computed by subtracting from the firm's buy-and-hold return the buy-and-hold return on size-matched, value-weighted portfolio of the firms.	-
Time Listed	Distance in months between the fiscal year-end and the date the company was first listed on either the New York, American, or NASDAQ exchange.	-
Leverage	$$\frac{LTD_{t-1}[9] + CurrentLiabilities_{t-1}[5]}{TotalAssets_{t-1}[6]}$$	+
Positive Accruals Dummy	1 if total accruals were positive in the current and prior year; 0 otherwise.	+
Declining Sales Dummy	1 if cash sales in the current year were lower than in the previous year; 0 otherwise. $CashSales_t = Sales_t - (\Delta Receivables_t)$	?

Annual Compustat data items are provided in brackets.
Δ means the change in the account from previous year.
t refers to the year of interest.

Beneish derives cutoff values based on different relative costs of Type I versus Type II errors. A Type I error occurs when a GAAP violator is incorrectly classified as a control firm. Conversely, a Type II error occurs when a control firm is incorrectly classified as a GAAP violator.

The Beneish model relies on various cutoff values that can delineate different levels of risk of earnings manipulation. A cutoff value of 11.72 percent results in only 45 percent of GAAP violators being correctly classified as violators and only 3.6 percent of the control firms being correctly classified as violators. A cutoff value of 5.99 percent results in 67 percent of GAAP violators being correctly classified and 13.5 percent of control firms being incorrectly classified as violators. A cutoff value of 4.3 percent results in 76 percent of GAAP violators being correctly classified and 20.4 percent of control firms being incorrectly classified as violators. Finally, a cutoff value of 2.94 percent results in 83 percent of GAAP violators being correctly classified as violators and 28.6 percent of control firms being incorrectly classified as violators. Selection of the appropriate cutoff depends on different decision makers and different levels of risk.

THE MISPRICING OF DISCRETIONARY ACCRUALS

There is sufficient evidence showing that investors do correctly use available information in forecasting future earnings performance.[26] It reflects investors' naive fixation on reported earnings, rather than earnings ability to summarize value-relevant information. Most analysts would argue that since investors tend to "fixate" on reported earnings, examining the accrual and the cash-flow components of current earnings can be used to detect mispriced securities. The reasoning is that accrual and cash-flow components of earnings have different implications for the assessment of future earnings. Accordingly, Sloan[27] investigated whether stock prices reflect information about future earnings contained in the accrual and cash-flow components of current earnings. The persistence of earnings performance was found to depend on the relative magnitudes of the cash and accrual components of earnings.

However, stock prices acted as if investors failed to identify correctly the different properties of the two components of earnings. The market erroneously overestimates the persistence of the accruals component of accrual earnings while underestimating the persistence of the cash-flow component. Accruals also exhibit negative serial correlation or mean reversion tendencies. The end result is that the market responds as if surprised when seemingly predictable earnings reversal occurs in the following year. Similarly, Subramanyam[28] finds that abnormal accruals are positively related to future profitability. Xie[29] provides more evidence on the issue, estimating abnormal accruals after controlling for major unusual accruals and nonarticulation events (i.e., mergers, acquisitions, and divestitures), and found that this refined measure of abnormal accruals, which

isolates managerial discretion, is still overpriced. These results are consistent with DeFond and Park's[30] conclusion that the market overprices abnormal accruals because investors underanticipate the future reversal of these accruals.

ISSUES IN EARNINGS MANAGEMENT

1. It is very easy to suspect that earnings management is intended to meet expectations of financial analysts or management (represented by public forecasts of earnings). In fact, there is evidence of (1) managers' taking actions to manage earnings upward to avoid reporting earnings lower than an analyst's forecast,[31] (2) financial analysts' stock recommendation (e.g., buy, hold, and sell) as a good predictor of earnings management,[32] (3) firms in danger of falling short of a management earnings forecast using unexpected accruals to manage earnings upward,[33] and (4) firms with a high percentage of institutional ownership typically not cutting research and development spending to avoid a decline in reported earnings.[34]

2. There are good reasons to suspect that earnings management is intended to influence short-term price performance in various ways.

1. There is evidence of negative unexpected accruals (income-decreasing) prior to management buyout.[35]

2. There is evidence of positive (income-increasing) unexpected accruals prior to seasoned equity offering,[36] initial public offers,[37] and stock-financed acquisitions.[38] A reversal of unexpected accruals seems to follow initial public offers and stock-financed acquisitions.

3. Earnings management is due and can persist because of asymmetric information, a condition caused by management's knowing information that they are not willing to disclose. The persistence is due to blocked communication where managers cannot communicate all their private information unless the principal contractually precommits not to use the information against the managers. Incentives for managers to reveal their private information truthfully, created by blocked communication, becomes a key for earnings management.

4. Earnings management takes place in the context of a feasible reporting set and a given set of contracts that determine sharing rules among stakeholders. Both contract sets are endogenous to the earnings management question. As the environment conditions change, both the reporting and contractual sets change, also leading to different forms of earnings management over time. For example, in environmental conditions where accounting data are used in compensation contracts, there is a strong incentive for managers to manage the data used in contracts. As a result the contracting use leads to an internal or stewardship incentive for earnings management.[39]

5. Corporate strategies for earnings management follow one or more of three approaches: (1) choosing from the flexible options available within GAAP, (2)

relying on the subjective estimates and application choices available within the options, and (3) using asset acquisitions and dispositions and the timing for reporting them.[40] Note here that the choices made within GAAP constitute earnings management, while choices made outside GAAP constitute fraud. The court may be the one to decide in some cases whether some management reporting actions that are taken outside the bounds of GAAP are fraud or earnings management.[41]

6. The earnings game—or, more precisely, the quarterly earnings report game—may be a major reason for earnings management.[42] Management is tempted to issue an earnings report that satisfies Wall Street's expectations more than it reflects financial reality. DeGeorge et al.[43] found that quarterly earnings reports that meet analysts' expectations exactly or exceed them by just a penny per share happen more frequently than would be likely in a random statistical distribution, while reports that miss by just a penny occur far less frequently.

7. Earnings management is a result of attempts to exceed thresholds.[44] The three thresholds of importance to executives are:

1. "to report positive profits, that is, report earnings that are above zero;
2. to sustain recent performance, that is, make at least last year's earnings; and
3. to meet analysts' expectations, particularly the analysts' consumer earnings forecast."[45]

Empirical explorations identified earnings management to exceed each of the three thresholds, with the positive profit threshold predominating.[46]

8. Earnings management may originate as a result of meeting covenants of implicit compensation contracts. Evidence for this thesis takes the following forms:

1. Divisional managers for a large multinational firm are likely to defer income when the earnings target in their bonus plan will not be met and when they are entitled to the maximum bonuses permitted under the plan.[47]
2. Firms with caps on bonuses are more likely to report accruals that defer income when that cap is reached than firms that have comparable performance but no bonus cap.[48]
3. During a proxy contest, incumbent managers exercised accounting discretion to improve reported earnings.[49]
4. Chief executive officers (CEOs) in their final years in office reduced R&D spending, presumably to increase reported earnings.[50]

9. Earnings management arises from the threat of two forms of regulation: industry-specific regulation and antitrust regulation. The banking and insurance industries are good examples of the existence of regulatory monitoring that is tied to accounting data. As stated by Healy and Wahlen:

Banking regulations require that banks satisfy certain capital adequacy requirements that are written in terms of accounting numbers. Insurance regulations require that insurers meet conditions for minimum financial health. Utilities have historically been rate-regulated and permitted to earn only a normal return in their invested assets. It is frequently asserted that such regulations create incentives to manage the income statement and the balance sheet variables of interest to regulators.[51]

There is, in fact, a lot of evidence supporting the above hypothesis. For example:

1. Banks that are close to minimum capital requirements tend to overstate loan loss provisions, understate loan write-offs, and recognize abnormal gains on securities portfolios.[52]
2. Financially weak property casualty insurers that risk regulatory attention tend to understate claim loss reserves[53] and engage in reinsurance transactions.[54]

10. Because of the need for government subsidies or protection as well as the fear of antitrust investigations or other political consequences, managers may resort to earnings management. A lot of evidence supports this hypothesis. For example:

1. Firms under investigation for antitrust violations reported income-decreasing abnormal accruals in the investigation years.[55]
2. Firms in industries seeking import-relief tend to defer income in the year of application.[56]
3. Firms in the cable television industry tend to defer earnings during the period of congressional scrutiny.[57]
4. Firms subject to price controls will adjust their discretionary accounting accruals downward to reduce net income and to increase the likelihood of approval of the requested price increase.[58]
5. The magnitude of the discretionary component of the postretirement obligation is negatively associated with the extent of the external regulations and auditor quality.[59]
6. More unionized firms are more likely to use immediate recognition of Statement of Financial Accounting Standards No. 106 on Employer's Accounting for Postretirement Benefits Other than Pensions, which is consistent with incentives to reduce labor negotiation costs.[60]

11. Firm valuation is generally assumed to be one of the targets of earnings management. Various analytical models have tried to explicate that relationship. Gigler[61] considers the case of the firm whose trade-off, when determining which income figure to disclose, is between the cost of acquiring new capital and the cost of competition. An overstatement of disclosed income will occur if the reduced cost of capital were higher than the increased cost of competition. The credibility of the disclosed income is possible because the firm incurs a propri-

etary cost by misrepresenting income. Chaney and Lewis[62] are concerned with an explanation for why corporate offices manage the disclosure of accounting information. They show that earnings management affects firm value when value-maximizing managers and investors are asymmetrically informed. Eilifsen et al.[63] add to the previous two models by showing that if taxable income were linked to accounting income, there will exist an automatic safeguard against manipulation of earnings, a claim also made by Johansson and Ostman.[64]

CONCLUSION

Earnings management is a deliberate choice of specific accounting techniques or options intended to secure a given level of earnings and some private gains. This chapter explicated the nature of earnings management from both a conceptual and operational viewpoint, described the different accruals models used in the literature to estimate discretionary or unexpected accruals, presented a model for the detection of earnings management, and discussed various issues, theoretical and empirical, on the form of designed accounting.

NOTES

1. K. Schipper, "Earnings Management," *Accounting Horizons* (December 1989), p. 92.
2. Ibid., p. 93.
3. Ibid.
4. P.N. Healy and J.N. Wahlen, "A Review of the Earnings Management Literature and Its Implications for Standard Setting," *Accounting Horizons* 4 (1999), p. 368.
5. Ibid, p. 369.
6. S.H. Toeh, T.J. Wong, and G. Rao, "All Accruals during Initial Public Offerings Opportunistic?" *Review of Accounting Studies* 3 (1998), pp. 173–208.
7. C. Liu, S. Ryan, and J. Wahlen, "Differential Valuation Implications of Loan Across Banks and Fiscal Quarters," *The Accounting Review* (January 1997), pp. 133–146.
8. K.R. Petroni, "Optimistic Reporting in the Property Casualty Insurance Industry," *Journal of Accounting and Economics* 18 (1994), pp. 157–179.
9. G. Visvanathan, "Deferred Tax Valuation Allowances and Earnings Management," *Accrual of Financial Statement Analysis* 3 (1998), pp. 6–15.
10. D.W. Collins and S.P. Hribar, "Errors in Estimating Accruals; Implications for Empirical Research," Working paper, University of Iowa, 1999.
11. L. DeAngelo, "Accounting Numbers as Market Valuation Substitutes: A Study of Management Buyouts of Public Shareholders," *The Accounting Review* 62, 3, pp. 431–453.
12. P.M. Healey, "The Effects of Bonus Schemes in Accounting Decisions," *Journal of Accounting and Economics* 7 (1989), pp. 85–107.
13. J. Jones, "Earnings Management during Import Relief Investigations," *Journal of Accounting Research* 29 (1991), pp. 193–228.
14. R.D. Beneish, "Detecting GAAP Violations: Implications for Assessing Earnings

Management among Firms with Extreme Financial Performance," *Journal of Accounting and Public Policy* 16 (1997), pp. 271–309.

15. R.D. Beneish, "Discussion of All Accruals during the Initial Public Offerings Opportunistic?" *Review of Accounting Studies* 3 (1998), pp. 209–221.

16. P.M. Dechow, R.G. Sloan, and A.P. Sweeney, "Detecting Earnings Management," *The Accounting Review* 70 (1995), p. 199.

17. Ibid., p. 42.

18. S.-H. Kang and K. Sivaramakrishnan, "Issues in Testing Earnings Management and an Instrumental Variable Approach," *Journal of Accounting Research* 33 (1995), pp. 353–366.

19. From Chairman Levitt's remarks in speech entitled "The Numbers Game," delivered at New York University on September 28, 1998.

20. Healy and Wahlen, "A Review of Earnings Management Literature," p. 368.

21. C.I. Wiedman, "Instructional Case: Detecting Earnings Manipulation," *Issues in Accounting Education* 14, 1 (February 1999), pp. 157–158.

22. B.P. Green and J.H. Choi, "Assessing the Risk of Management Fraud through Neural Network Technology," *Auditing: A Journal of Practice and Theory* 16 (1997), pp. 14–28.

23. Beneish, "Detecting GAAP Violations," pp. 271–309.

24. Wiedman, "Instructional Case: Detecting Earnings Manipulation," p. 160.

25. Ibid., p. 161.

26. J. On and S. Penman, "Financial Statement Analysis and the Prediction of Stock Returns," *Journal of Accounting and Economics* 11 (1989), pp. 159–330; V. Bernard and J. Thomas, "Evidence That Stock Prices Do Not Fully Reflect the Implications of Current Earnings for Future Earnings," *Journal of Accounting and Economics* 13 (1990), pp. 305–340; L.A. Maines and J.R. Hand, "Individuals' Perceptions and Misperceptions of the Time Series Properties of Quarterly Earnings," *The Accounting Review* (July 1996), pp. 317–336.

27. R.G. Sloan, "The Stock Prices Fully Reflect Information in Accruals and Cash Flows about Future Earnings," *The Accounting Review* 3 (1996), pp. 289–315.

28. K.R. Subramanyam, "The Pricing of Discretionary Accruals," *Journal of Accounting and Economics* 12 (1996), pp. 149–282.

29. H. Xie, "The Mispricing of Abnormal Accruals," *The Accounting Review* 76 (2001), pp. 357–373.

30. M.L. DeFond and C.W. Park, "The Reversal of Abnormal Accruals and the Market Valuation of Earnings Surprises," *The Accounting Review* (July 2001), pp. 145–176.

31. D., Burgstahler and M. Eames, "Management of Earnings and Analyst Forecasts," Working paper, University of Washington, 1998.

32. J. Abarbanell and R. Lehavy, "Can Stock Recommendations Predict Earnings Management and Analyst's Earnings Forecast Errors?" Working paper, University of California at Berkeley, 1998.

33. R. Kaznik, "On the Association between Voluntary Disclosure and Earnings Management," *Journal of Accounting Research* 37 (1999), pp. 57–82.

34. B. Bushee, "The Influence of Institutional Investors on Myopic R&D Investment Behavior," *The Accounting Review* 3 (1998), pp. 305–333.

35. S. Perry and T. Williams, "Earnings Management Preceding Management Buyout Offers," *Journal of Accounting and Economics* 15 (1992), pp. 157–179.

36. S.H. Teoh, I. Welch, and T.J. Wong, "Earnings Management and the Long-Term

Market Performance of Initial Public Offerings," *Journal of Finance* (December 1998), pp. 1935–1974.

37. S.H. Teoh, I. Welch, and T.J. Wong, "Earnings Management and the Post Issue Performance of Seasoned Equity Offerings," *Journal of Financial Economics* (October 1998), pp. 63–99; S.H. Teoh, I. Welch, T.J. Wong, and G. Rao, "Are Accruals during Initial Public Offerings Opportunistic?" *Review of Accounting Studies* 3 (2000), pp. 175–208.

38. M. Erickson and S.W. Wang, "Earnings Management by Acquiring Firms in Stock for Stock Mergers," *Journal of Accounting and Economics* 97 (April 1999), pp. 149–176.

39. R. Dye, "Earnings Management in an Overlapping Generations Model," *Journal of Accounting Research* 26 (1998), pp. 195–235.

40. P.R. Brown, "Earnings Management: A Subtle (and Troublesome) Twist to Earnings Quality," *The Journal of Financial Statement and Analysis* (Winter 1999), p. 62.

41. Ibid.

42. H. Collingwood, "The Earnings Game," *Harvard Business Review* (June 2001), pp. 65–74.

43. F. DeGeorge, J. Patel, and R. Zeckhauser, "Earnings Management to Exceed Thresholds," *Journal of Business* 72 (1999), pp. 1–33.

44. Ibid.

45. Ibid.

46. Ibid.

47. F.A. Guidry, A. Leone, and S. Rock, "Earnings-based Bonus Plans and Earnings Management by Business Unit Managers," *Journal of Accounting and Economics* 26 (1999), pp. 113–142.

48. R. Holhausen, D. Larker, and R. Sloan, "Annual Bonus Schemes and the Manipulation of Earnings," *Journal of Accounting and Economics* 19 (1995), pp. 29–74.

49. L.E. DeAngelo, "Managerial Competition, Information Costs, and Corporate Governance: The Use of Accounting Performance Measures in Proxy Contests," *Journal of Accounting and Economics* 10 (1988), pp. 3–36.

50. P. Dechow and R.G. Sloan, "Executive Incentives and the Horizon Problem: An Empirical Investigation," *Journal of Accounting and Economics* 14 (1991), pp. 51–89.

51. P.M. Healy and J.M. Wahlen, "A Review of the Earnings Management Literature and Its Implications for Standard Setting," *Accounting Horizons* 4 (1999), pp. 365–383.

52. S. Moyer, "Capital Adequacy Ratio Regulations and Accounting Choices in Commercial Banks," *Journal of Accounting and Economics* 12 (1990), pp. 123–154; M. Scholes, G.P. Wilson, and M. Wolfson, "Tax Planning, Regulatory Capital Planning, and Financial Reporting Strategy for Commercial Banks," *Review of Financial Studies* 3 (1990), pp. 625–650; A. Beatty, S. Chamberlain, and J. Magliolo, "Managing Financial Reports of Commercial Banks: The Influence of Taxes, Regulatory Capital and Earnings," *Journal of Accounting Research* 33 (1995), pp. 231–261; J. Collins, D. Shackelford, and J. Wahlen, "Bank Differences in the Coordination of Regulatory Capital, Earnings and Taxes," *Journal of Accounting Research* 2 (1995), pp. 263–291.

53. K.R. Petroni, "Optimistic Reporting in the Property Casualty Insurance Industry," *Journal of Accounting and Economics* 15 (1992), pp. 485–508.

54. R. Adiel, "Reinsurance and the Management of Regulatory Ratios and Taxes in the Property-Casualty Insurance Industry," *Journal of Accounting and Economics* 22, 1–3 (1996), pp. 207–240.

55. S. Cahan, "The Effect of Anti-Trust Investigations on Discretionary Accruals: A Refined Test of the Political Cost Hypothesis," *The Accounting Review* 67 (1992), pp. 77–95; S. Makar and P. Alam, "Earnings Management and Antitrust Investigations: Political Costs over Business Cycles," *Journal of Business Finance and Accounting* 5 (1998), pp. 701–720.

56. J.J. Jones, "Earnings Management during Import Relief Investigations," *Journal of Accounting Research* 29 (1991), pp. 193–228.

57. K.G. Key, "Political Cost Incentives for Earnings Management in the Cable Television Industry," *Journal of Accounting and Economics* 3 (1997), pp. 309–337.

58. S. Lim and Z. Matolcsy, "Earnings Management of Firms Subject to Produce Price Controls," *Accounting and Finance* 39 (1999), pp. 131–150.

59. S. Asthana, "The Impact of Regulatory and Audit Environment on Managers' Discretionary Accounting Choices: The Case of SFAS No. 196," *Accounting for the Public Interest* 1 (2001), pp. 23–96.

60. J. D'Souza, J. Jacob, and K. Ramesh, "The Use of Accounting Flexibility to Reduce Labor Renegotiation Costs and Manage Earnings," *Journal of Accounting and Economics* 30 (2001), pp. 187–208.

61. F. Gigler, "Self-Enforcing Voluntary Disclosures," *Journal of Accounting Research* 32 (1994), pp. 224–40.

62. P.K. Chaney and C.M. Lewis, "Earnings Management and Firm Valuation under Asymmetric Information," *Journal of Corporate Finance* 1 (1995), pp. 319–345.

63. A. Eilifsen, K.H. Knivsfla, and F. Saettem, "Earnings Manipulation: Cost of Capital versus Tax," *The European Accounting Review* 8 (1999), pp. 481–491.

64. S.E. Johansson and L. Ostman, *Accounting Theory—Integrating Behavior and Measurement* (London: Pitman, 1995), p. 201.

SELECTED REFERENCES

Adiel, R. "Reinsurance and the Management of Regulatory Ratios and Taxes in the Property-Casualty Insurance Industry." *Journal of Accounting and Economics* 22, 1–3 (1996), pp. 207–240.

Ayers, B.C. "Deferred Tax Accounting under SFAS No. 109: An Empirical Investigation of Its Incremental Value-Relevance Relative to APB No. 11." *The Accounting Review* 73, 2 (1998), pp. 195–212.

Beatty, A., S. Chamberlain, and J. Magliolo. "Managing Financial Reports of Commercial Banks: The Influence of Taxes, Regulatory Capital and Earnings." *Journal of Accounting Research* 33, 2 (1995), pp. 231–261.

Beaver, W., C. Eger, S. Ryan, and M. Wolfson. "Financial Reporting, Supplemental Disclosures and Bank Share Prices." *Journal of Accounting Research* (Autumn 1989), pp. 157–178.

Beneish, M.D. "Detecting GAAP Violation: Implications for Assessing Earnings Management among Firms with Extreme Financial Performance." *Journal of Accounting and Public Policy* 16 (1997), pp. 271–309.

———. "Discussion of: Are Accruals during Initial Public Offerings Opportunistic?" *Review of Accounting Studies* 3 (1998), pp. 209–221.

Burgstahler, D., and I. Dichev. "Earnings Management to Avoid Earnings Decreases and Losses." *Journal of Accounting and Economics* 24 (1997), pp. 99–126.

————. "Incentives to Manage Earnings to Avoid Earnings Decreases and Losses: Evidence from Quarterly Earnings." Working paper, University of Washington, 1998.

Burgstahler, D., and M. Eames. "Management of Earnings and Analysts' Forecasts." Working paper, University of Washington, 1998.

Bushee, B. "The Influence of Institutional Investors on Myopic R&D Investment Behavior." *The Accounting Review* 73, 3 (1998), pp. 305–333.

Cahan, S. "The Effect of Antitrust Investigations on Discretionary Accruals: A Refined Test of the Political Cost Hypothesis." *The Accounting Review* 67 (1992), pp. 77–95.

Collins, J., D. Shackelford, and J. Wahlen. "Bank Differences in the Coordination of Regulatory Capital, Earnings and Taxes." *Journal of Accounting Research* 33, 2 (1995), pp. 263–291.

DeAngelo, L.E. "Managerial Competition, Information Costs, and Corporate Governance: The Use of Accounting Performance Measures in Proxy Contests." *Journal of Accounting and Economics* 10 (1988), pp. 3–36.

DeAngelo, L.E., H. DeAngelo, and D. Skinner. "Accounting Choices of Troubled Companies." *Journal of Accounting and Economics* 17 (January 1994), pp. 113–143.

Dechow, P. "Accounting Earnings and Cash Flows as Measure of Firm Performance: The Role of Accounting Accruals." *Journal of Accounting and Economics* 18, 1 (1994), pp. 3–40.

Dechow, P., and R.G. Sloan. "Executive Incentives and the Horizon Problem: An Empirical Investigation." *Journal of Accounting and Economics* 14 (1991), pp. 51–89.

Dechow, P., R.G. Sloan, and A.P. Sweeney. "Causes and Consequences of Earnings Manipulation: An Analysis of Firms Subject to Enforcement Actions by the SEC." *Contemporary Accounting Research* 13, 1 (1996), pp. 1–36.

Defeo, V., R. Lamber, and D. Larcker. "The Executive Compensation Effects of Equity-for-Debt Swaps." *The Accounting Review* 54 (1989), pp. 201–227.

DeFond, M.L., and J. Jiambalvo. "Debt Covenant Effects and the Manipulation of Accruals." *Journal of Accounting and Economics* 17 (January), pp. 145–176.

Degeorge, F., J. Patel, and R. Zeckhauser. "Earnings Management to Exceed Thresholds." Working paper, Boston University, 1998.

Dye, R. "Earnings Management in an Overlapping Generations Model." *Journal of Accounting Research* 6 (1988), pp. 195–235.

Erickson, M., and S-W. Wang. "Earnings Management by Acquiring Firms in Stock for Stock Mergers." *Journal of Accounting and Economics* 27 (April 1999), pp. 149–176.

Foster, G. "Briloff and the Capital Market." *Journal of Accounting Research* 17 (Spring), pp. 262–274.

Gaver, J., K. Gaver, and J. Austin. "Additional Evidence on Bonus Plans and Income Management." *Journal of Accounting and Economics* 18 (1995), pp. 3–28.

Guay, W.A., S.P. Kothari, and R.L. Watts. "A Market-Based Evaluation of Discretionary Accrual Models." *Journal of Accounting Research* 34 (Supplement, 1996), pp. 83–105.

Healy, P.M., and E. Engel. "Discretionary Behavior with Respect to Allowances for Loan Losses and the Behavior of Security Prices." *Journal of Accounting and Economics* 22 (1996), pp. 177–206.

Healy, P.M., and M. McNichols. "The Characteristics and Valuation of Loss Reserves of Property-Casualty Insurers." Working paper, Stanford University, 1998.

Healy, P.M., and J.M. Wahlen, "A Review of the Earnings Management Literature and Its Implications for Standard Setting." *Accounting Horizons* 4 (1999), pp. 365–384.

Appendix 2A. Earnings Cycles and the Pricing of Securities

INTRODUCTION

Accounting research since the late 1960s has provided ample evidence of the significant effects of accounting earnings disclosures on firms' security prices (Bernard, 1987, 1989; Lev, 1989). Earnings appear to affect equity prices, even though the effect is in most cases small. However, given the constant criticism levied at earnings because of their historical cost emphasis or because they may be subject to earnings management, research has focused on the incremental value-relevance of cash flows and on the effects of managerial discretion (i.e., discretionary accruals) on the pricing of earnings (Bowen et al., 1987; Dechow, 1994; Riahi-Belkaoui, 2000). The interesting finding from this research is the evidence of the pricing of discretionary accruals, showing that even though opportunistic and value-irrelevant, the discretionary accruals are still priced by the market (Subramanyam, 1996). Whether it is the informativeness of earnings or the informativeness of its components (i.e., cash flows, discretionary accruals, and nondiscretionary accruals), most return-earnings regression studies have restricted themselves to a mere examination of the market pricing of a complete earnings cycle, that is to say, a chain of events with an impact of earnings power that lies in the past (AICPA, 1973; Cramer and Sorter, 1973). This is in conformity with objective No. 8 of the Trueblood Report, which states:

An objective [of financial statements] is to provide a statement of periodic earnings useful for predicting, comparing and evaluating enterprise earnings power. The net result of completed earnings cycles and enterprise activities resulting in recognizable progress toward completion of incomplete cycles should be reported. (AICPA, 1973)

For an earnings cycle to be defined as complete, three conditions should be fulfilled: (1) a realized sacrifice (an actual or high disbursement of cash); (2) a related realized benefit (an actual or probable receipt of cash); and (3) no further related substantive effort (AICPA, 1973, p. 9). In addition, the seventh objective distinguishes between a complete earnings cycle, an incomplete earnings cycle (a chain of events that has commenced but is not yet complete), and a prospective cycle (a chain of events that lies wholly in the future). For example, an earnings cycle is defined as incomplete when (1) a realized sacrifice or a benefit has occurred, but the related benefit or sacrifice has not been realized, (2) both

sacrifice and benefit are not realized, or (3) the effort has not taken place (AICPA, 1973, p. 29).

It follows that the returns-earnings regression model, generally used in the accounting literature, suffers from a misspecification due to the absence of the effects of both incomplete and prospective earnings cycles.

Accordingly, this appendix empirically examined the pricing of the three components of earnings cycles: complete, incomplete, and prospective. Evidence on this issue could improve our understanding of the manner in which the capital markets process publicly available earnings and its components (cash flows, discretionary accruals, and nondiscretionary accruals) as a measure of the complete earnings cycle and other information that can act as surrogate measures of the incomplete and prospective earnings cycles. Evidence on this issue could also provide some insights into the economic incentives for discretionary accounting choice and disclosure of the results of incomplete and prospective earnings cycles.

The empirical analysis is conducted on a sample of 21,974 firm-years for 2,853 firms during 1978–1998. Discretionary accruals are obtained by decomposing total accruals into discretionary and nondiscretionary components using four models. The results of the complete earnings cycle are measured by cash flows, discretionary accruals, and nondiscretionary accruals. The results of the incomplete earnings cycle are measured by the ratio of gross margin over sales multiplied by inventory. The rationale is that, assuming the ratio of gross margin over sales to stay constant, multiplying it by inventory yields an approximate measure of the *unrealized holding gains and losses*. The results of the prospective earnings cycle are measured by the income growth for a year multiplied by income of the same year. The rationale is that a firm expects to achieve at least the same rate of income growth as in the preceding year. The results of the study show that the market attaches value to a complete earnings cycle and its components, as well as to the results of incomplete and prospective cycles.

RESEARCH DESIGN

The Model

The model relates stock returns to the results of the complete, incomplete, and prospective earnings cycle. It is estimated as follows:

$$ASR_{it} = \alpha_0 + \alpha_1 OCF_{it} + \alpha_2 NDACC_{it} + \alpha_3 DACC_{it} + URHGL_{it} + ING_{it}$$

where:

ASR_{it} = Annual stock returns for firm i and year t

OCF_{it} = Operating cash flows for firm i and year t

$NDACC_{it}$ = Nondiscretionary accruals for firm i and year t

$DACC_{it}$ = Discretionary accruals for firm i and year t

$URHGL_{it}$ = Results of the incomplete earnings cycle for firm i and year t

ING_{it} = Results of the prospective earnings cycle for firm i and year t

Annual stock returns (ASR) are measured as compounded monthly stock returns for a twelve-month period ending three months after the end of the fiscal year of the firm. Operating cash flows (OCF) are defined in Compustat No. 308.[1] All other variables are defined next.

Sample

Financial data to construct a sample of firms are obtained from the 1978 S&P Compustat, the Center for Research in Security Prices (CRSP). Both financial institutions (SIC 1999 to 7000) and observations with change in year-end are excluded. The nature of some tests required that the sample be restricted to those firms with a minimum of five consecutive years of data on all necessary variables. The available sample includes 22,532 firm-years. An elimination of observations on operating cash flows, nondiscretionary accruals, and discretionary accruals that are more than three standard deviations from their respective means resulted in a loss of 558 observations (2.47 percent of the sample). The final sample consists of 21,974 firm-years representing 2,853 firms during 1978–1998. The results with the outliers included are qualitatively unchanged.

Measurement of the Results of the Complete Earnings Cycle

The results of the complete earnings cycle are measured by net income. Following prior research in earnings management, net income (NI) can be decomposed as follows:

$$NI = OCF + DACC + NDACC \qquad (1)$$

where

OCF = Operating cash flows

DACC = Discretionary accruals

NDACC = Nondiscretionary accruals

The estimation of discretionary accruals follows the approach based on using two alternative ways of estimating them—the modified Jones model (Dechow et al., 1995) and the Kang and Sivaramakrishnan model (1995)—and using two alternative measures of accruals—the traditional balance sheet approach and the

cash-flow approach proposed by Collins and Hribar (1999). Total accruals, as based on the traditional balance sheet approach, are as follows:

$$TACC_{it} = (\Delta CA_{it} - \Delta CL_{it} - \Delta Cash + \Delta STDEBT_{it} - DEPTN_{it}) \tag{2}$$

where:

ΔCA_{it} = Change in current assets during period t (Compustat No. 4)

ΔCL_{it} = Change in current liabilities during period t (Compustat No. 5)

$\Delta Cash_{it}$ = Change in cash and cash equivalents during period t (Compustat No. 4)

$\Delta STDEBT_{it}$ = Change in the current maturities of long-term debt and other short-term debt included in current liabilities during period t (Compustat No. 34)

$DEPTN_{it}$ = Depreciation and amortization expense during period t (Compustat No. 14)

Based on the findings that studies relying on the traditional balance sheet approach to the measurement of total accruals suffer from potential contamination from measurement error in the total accruals, Collins and Hribar (1999) suggested a straightforward approach that computes total accruals as the difference between net income and operating cash flow (taken from the cash-flow statement).

Discretionary accruals are also computed using a variant of the Jones (1991) model. The model captures regularities over time for a given firm in the relations among total accruals, assets, and changes in revenues.

$$TACC_{it} = \alpha_1(1/TA_{i,t-1}) + \alpha_2 (\Delta REV_{it} - \Delta REC_{it})/TA \tag{3}$$
$$+ \alpha_3 PPE_{it}/TA_{i,t-1} + \varepsilon_{it}$$

where $TACC_{it}$ is total accruals calculated as in equation (2), A_{it-1} is total assets, $(\Delta REV_{it} - \Delta REC_{it})$ is the change in cash-basis revenue, PPE_{it} is gross property, plant, and equipment, and α_i is firm-specific parameters. Discretionary accruals from the modified Jones model are the residuals from the regression in equation (3). An alternative approach to the measurement of discretionary accruals is proposed by Kang and Sivaramakrishnan (1995). Their model estimates managed accruals using level, rather than change of current assets and current liabilities. It is expressed as follows:

$$ACCB_{it} = \Phi_0 + \Phi_1(\delta_1 REV_{it}) + \Phi_2(\delta_2 EXP_{it}) + \Phi_3(\delta_3 PPE_{it}) + \varepsilon_{it} \tag{4}$$

where:

$ACCB_{it}$ = The balance of noncash current assets (net of tax receivables) less current liabilities (net of tax payables) for firm i at the end of year t, divided by total assets for firm i at the end of year $t - 1$

EXP_{it} = The total pretax operating expense before depreciation and interest, for firm i at the end of year t, divided by total assets for firm i at the end of year $t-1$

The parameters δ_1, δ_2, and δ_3 are the previous year's turnover ratios, which lead to the measurement of (1) the current period's receivables as a product of the previous year's receivables-to-sales ratio (δ_1) and current period sales (REV_t) and (2) current period net current assets as the product of the previous year's net current asset-to-expense ratio (δ_2) times current period expenses (EXV_t).

Measurement of the Results of the Incomplete Earnings Cycle

The results of the incomplete earnings cycle stem from the decision not to liquidate ending inventory at the end of the period. If the decision were to liquidate/sell the ending inventory at the end of the period, the results of the incomplete earnings cycle would be equal to the unrealized holding gains and losses (Hanna, 1974; Chambers, 1975; Sterling, 1975). Therefore, the results of the incomplete earnings cycle represent the gains and losses that would accrue to the firm in the future when it sells its inventory (Drake and Dopuch, 1965; Barton 1974). Assuming the gross margin over sales stays constant, the results of the incomplete earnings cycle (or unrealized holding gains and losses) would be equal to gross margin over sales times the ending inventory. The variable will be denoted as $URHGL_{it}$ (to correspond to unrealized holding gains and losses).

Results of the Prospective Earnings Cycle

The prospective earnings cycle stems from the management decision to choose a rate of income growth. The most rational decision is to maintain or to increase the present rate of income growth. If the decision is to at least maintain the same rate of income growth, then the results of the prospective earnings cycle for a coming year t+1 is equal to the income of the year t times the growth of income from year t−1 to year t. This variable is referred to as ING.

Descriptive Statistics

Table 2A.1 represents descriptive statistics about the main variables used in the study. Over 80 percent of the firms included in the sample exhibit positive net income and operating cash flows, showing a slight bias toward profitable firms. Discretionary and nondiscretionary accruals are computed under four different models: (1) model 1 relies on the balance sheet approach for the computation of total accruals and the modified Jones model for the estimation of discretionary accruals; (2) model 2 relies on the balance sheet approach for the computation of total accruals and the Kang and Sivaramakrishnan model for the

Table 2A.1
Descriptive Statistics

Variable *	Mean	Std. Dev.	Median	Maximum	Minimum	% Positive
Returns (ASR)	0.175	0.518	0.097	23.11	-0.751	66
Net Income (NI)	0.064	0.091	0.051	0.753	-0.683	86
Operating Cash Flow (OCF)	0.081	0.110	0.091	0.816	-0.713	81
Discretionary Accruals 1 (DACC1)	-0.0041	0.115	-0.0011	0.864	-0.815	46
Nondiscretionary Accruals 1 (NDACC1)	-0.0220	0.0861	-0.0411	0.741	-0.682	31
Discretionary Accruals 2 (DACC2)	-0.0039	0.110	-0.0018	0.789	-0.613	45
Nondiscretionary Accruals 2 (NDACC2)	-0.0187	0.0713	-0.0391	-0.852	-0.652	33
Discretionary Accruals 3 (DACC3)	-0.0042	0.126	-0.0017	0.823	-0.728	45
Nondiscretionary Accruals 3 (NDACC3)	-0.0196	0.0812	-0.0362	0.723	-0.678	32
Discretionary Accruals 4 (DACC4)	-0.0036	0.132	-0.0018	0.759	-0.723	44
Nondiscretionary Accruals 4 (NDACC4)	-0.0175	0.0759	-0.0352	0.826	-0.625	33
Incomplete Earnings Cycle (UHGL)	0.032	0.081	0.026	0.323	-0.382	86
Prospective Earnings Cycle (ING)	0.078	0.095	0.057	0.826	-0.683	87

Notes: The original sample consists of 22,532 firm-years during the period 1978–1998 for which a minimum of five consecutive years of data is available. Observations that are more than three standard deviations from the mean for operating cash flows, nondiscretionary accruals, and discretionary accruals are excluded. This results in a loss of 558 observations, reducing the final sample to 21,924 firm-years.

*All variables are scaled by lagged total assets.

estimation of discretionary accruals; (3) model 3 relies on the cash-flow approach to the determination of total accruals and the cross-sectional modified Jones model for the estimation of discretionary accruals; and (4) model 4 relies on the cash-flow approach to the determinants of total accruals and the Kang and Sivaramakrishnan model for the estimation of discretionary accruals. Under the four models, both the nondiscretionary accruals and discretionary accruals have negative means and medians and are positive for fewer than 46 percent of the firms for discretionary accruals and for fewer than 33 percent of the firms for nondiscretionary accruals. The results of the incomplete earnings cycle and the prospective cycles show again that over 80 percent of the firms were expecting positive unrealized holding gains and losses and future income. This occurs by construction, given the positive bias toward profitability in the sample.

EARNINGS CYCLES AND STOCK RETURNS

To assess the pricing of the results of earnings cycles, returns are regressed on the level of earnings components as measures of the results of complete earnings cycles and on measures of incomplete and prospective earnings cycles. The level of earnings as the result of complete earnings is decomposed into its three component parts: operating cash flows, nondiscretionary accruals, and discretionary accruals.[2]

Table 2A.2 presents the results of the regression of returns on measures of complete, incomplete, and prospective earnings cycles. Four models are used for the computation of discretionary accruals, as explained in the preceding sections. The coefficients on OCF, NDACC, DACC, UGHL, and ING are significant at the 0.01 level. The incremental content of the incomplete and prospective earnings cycles are on the order of an incremental R^2 higher than 1.40 percent.

The results indicate that each of the components of the earnings cycle has a significant weight in each of the four models. However, the weights attached to the components of the incomplete and prospective earnings cycle are lower than the weights attached to the components of the complete earnings cycle. These results may be due to the surrogate measures used for measuring the results of incomplete and prospective earnings cycles. In summary, these results reveal (1) that discretionary accruals have information content and (2) that both results of incomplete and prospective earnings cycles have incremental information content and improve earnings' ability to explain market returns. This evidence is consistent with the market's attaching value to the results of incomplete and prospective earnings cycles, even though they are not explicitly included in accounting reports.

Table 2A.2
Regression of Returns Earnings Components and Results of Incomplete and Prospective Cycles Using Alternative Accruals Expectations Models

Description	Intercept	OCF	NDACC	DACC	UHGL	ING	Adj. R^2%	Incr. R^2%
1. Model 1	0.125	1.32	1.02	1.01	0.78	1.12	8.69	1.42%
	(20.325)	(26.15)	(15.13)	(15.23)	(7.32)	(6.32)		(6.78)
2. Model 2	0.135	1.31	1.01	0.98	0.62	1.11	8.52	1.41%
	(20.355)	(28.13)	(15.21)	(15.61)	(7.51)	(6.51)		(6.32)
3. Model 3	0.121	1.33	1.03	0.96	0.63	1.32	8.31	1.43%
	(20.526)	(26.15)	(15.72)	(15.22)	(7.52)	(6.13)		(6.51)
4. Model 4	0.12	1.31	1.07	0.97	0.61	1.15	8.21	1.44%
	(20.612)	(26.14)	(15.33)	(15.33)	(7.37)	(6.15)		(6.72)

Notes: The original sample consists of 22,532 firm-years during the period 1978–1998 for which a minimum of five consecutive years of data is available. Observations that are more than three standard deviations from the mean for operating cash flows, nondiscretionary accruals, and discretionary accruals are excluded. This results in a loss of 558 observations, reducing the final sample to n = 21,974 firm-years.

The dependent variable in all models is cumulative stock returns over a twelve-month period ending three months after the fiscal year-end. The independent variables are operating cash flows (OCF), nondiscretionary accruals (NDACC), discretionary accruals (DACC), and results of the incomplete earnings cycle (UHGL) and the prospective earnings cycle (ING). All variables are scaled by lagged total assets. The four models differ in the estimation of discretionary accruals. Model 1 relies on the balance sheet approach for the computation of total accruals and the modified Jones model for the estimation of discretionary accruals. Model 2 relies on the balance sheet approach and the Kang and Sivaramakrishnan model. Model 3 relies on the cash-flow approach to the determination of total accruals and the modified Jones model for the estimation of discretionary accruals. Model 4 relies on the cash-flow approach and the Kang and Sivaramakrishnan model.

Figures in parentheses denote t statistics (except for incremental R-square) based on the heteroskedasticity-consistent covariance matrix (White, 1980) using a two-tailed test. Incremental R-square refers to the increase in explanatory power with the inclusion of the results of both incomplete and prospective earnings cycles. A t-statistic of 2.59 implies a significance level of 0.01 using a two-tailed test.

SUMMARY AND CONCLUSION

This appendix shows that in addition to the results of complete earnings cycles, the results of both incomplete and prospective earnings cycles are priced by the stock market. This result is consistent with the pricing of relevant information by an efficient market. There is evidence of information content of incomplete and prospective earnings cycles that improves the relevance of earnings. The results show also that although discretionary accruals are priced by an inefficient market, the information content of both incomplete and prospective earnings cycles points to the efficiency of the market looking beyond the pricing of opportunistic earnings manipulation in the pricing of future earnings.

NOTES

1. For firms that had not adopted the cash flow format, operating cash flow (OCF) is determined as follows: OCF = fund (#110) $-$ Δ current assets (#4) + Δ current liabilities (#5) + Δ cash (#1) $-$ Δ current portion of long-term debt (#34) if available.

2. The use of earnings levels rather than earnings changes is supported theoretically and empirically (Easton and Harris, 1991; Kothari, 1992; Ohlson and Shroff, 1992).

REFERENCES

American Institute of Certified Public Accountants. 1973. *Objectives of Financial Statements*. New York: AICPA.

Barton, A.D. 1974. Expectations and achievements in income theory. *The Accounting Review* (October): 664–681.

Bernard, V. 1987. Cross-sectional dependence and problems in inference in market-based accounting research. *Journal of Accounting Research* (Spring): 1–48.

Bowen, R.D., D. Burgstahler, and L. Daley. 1987. The incremental information content of accrual versus cash flows. *The Accounting Review* (October): 723–747.

Chambers, R.J. 1975. NOD, COG, and PUPU: See how inflation teases. *Journal of Accounting* (February): 56–62.

Cheng, C.S., C. Liu, and T. Schaefer. 1996. Earnings permanence and the incremental information content of cash flows from operations. *Journal of Accounting Research* (Spring): 173–181.

Collins, D., and P. Hribar. 1999. Errors in estimating accruals: Implications for empirical research. Working paper, University of Iowa.

Cramer, J.J., Jr., and G.H. Sorter. 1973. *Objectives of Financial Statements: Selected Papers*, Vol. 2. New York: AICPA, 1973.

Dechow, P. 1994. Accounting earnings and cash flow as measures of firm performance: The role of accounting accruals. *Journal of Accounting and Economics* 17: 3–42.

Dechow, P., R. Sloan, and A. Sweeney. 1995. Detecting earnings management. *The Accounting Review* 70: 193–226.

Drake, D.F., and N. Dopuch. 1965. On the case of dichotomizing income. *Journal of Accounting Research* (Fall): 192–205.

Easton, P.D., and T.S. Harris. 1991. Earnings as an explanatory variable for returns. *Journal of Accounting Research* 29: 19–36.

Hanna, J.R. 1974. *Accounting Income Models: An Application and Evaluation*. Special Study No. 8. Toronto: Society of Management Accountants.

Jones, J. 1991. Earnings management during import relief investigations. *Journal of Accounting Research* (Fall): 193–228.

Kang, S., and K. Sivaramakrishnan. 1995. Issues in testing earnings management and an instrumental variable approach. *Journal of Accounting Research* 33: 353–367.

Kothari, S.P. 1992. Price earnings regressions in the presence of prices leading earnings: Implications for earnings coefficients. *Journal of Accounting and Economics* 15: 173–202.

Lev, B. 1989. On the usefulness of earnings and earnings research: Lessons and directions from two decades of empirical research. *Journal of Accounting Research* (suppl.): 153–192.

Ohlson, J., and P. Shroff. 1992. Changes versus levels in earnings as explanatory variables for returns: Some theoretical considerations. *Journal of Accounting and Research* 30: 210–226.

Riahi-Belkaoui, A. 2000. The value relevance of earnings, cash flows, multinationality, and corporate reputation as assessed by security markets. *Advances in Quantitative Analysis of Finance and Accounting* 8: 45–59.

Sterling, R.R. 1975. Relevant financial reporting in an age of price changes. *Journal of Accounting* (August): 42–51.

Subramanyam, K.R. 1996. The pricing of discretionary accruals. *Journal of Accounting Research* 22: 249–281.

White, H. 1980. A heteroskedasticity-consistent covariance matrix estimator and a direct test for heteroskedasticity. *Econometrica* 48: 817–838.

Appendix 2B. The Impact of Multinationality on the Informativeness of Earnings and Accounting Choices

INTRODUCTION

This appendix reports the results of an investigation in how the degree of multinationality affects the informativeness of accounting and the accounting choices of managers. Three theories of multinationality link multinationality to investment value, predicting either a higher or lower value (Morck and Yeung, 1991, 1992; Mishra and Gobelli, 1998). They are the internalization theory, the imperfect world capital markets theory, and the managerial objectives theory.

The internalization theory maintains that direct foreign investment occurs when a firm can increase its value by internationalizing markets for certain of its intangibles (Rugman, 1980, 1981).

The imperfect world capital markets theory maintains that because of the imperfect world markets, multinational firms offer shareholders international di-

Source: A. Riahi-Belkaoui and R.D. Picur, "The Impact of Multinationality on the Informativeness of Earnings and Accounting Choices," *Managerial Finance* 27, 2 (2001), pp. 82–94. Reprinted with the permission of the editor.

versification opportunities, which as a result enhance their share prices (Agmon and Lessard, 1977).

Finally, the managerial objectives theory predicts that the existence of divergence of objectives between managers and shareholders, with top management favoring international diversification, may reduce the value of multinationals relative to uninationals.

The three theories are silent on the role of earnings in the relationship between multinationality and investment value. Earnings are known to be informative in explaining stock returns. Therefore, the first hypothesis predicts the informativeness of earnings in explaining stock returns and varies systematically with the level of multinationality in the corporation.

The second hypothesis derives from the managerial objectives theory and postulates that managers' accounting choices are systematically related to the level of multinationality. The managerial objectives theory recognizes divergence of objectives between management and shareholders of multinational firms regarding the merits of international diversification. Accordingly, contracts must be written, often containing accounting-based constraints, to restrict managers' value-changing behavior when multinationality is high. These same accounting-based constraints may lead managers to exploit the latitude available in accepted accounting procedures to alleviate the same constraints. Therefore, for multinational firms the magnitude of discretionary accounting accrual adjustment is positively related to the level of multinationality.

The results of this study, using U.S multinational firms, shows (1) that the level of multinationality is positively associated with the informativeness of accounting earnings and (2) that the magnitude of discretionary accounting accrual adjustments is significantly higher when the level of multinationality is high. These results are robust in the presence of endogenous and exogenous determinants of accounting choices and earnings' explanatory power for returns, including firm size, systematic risk, growth opportunities, and the variability and persistence of accounting earnings.

MULTINATIONALITY, CONTRACTS, AND ACCOUNTING

The Impact of Multinationality on the Informativeness of Earnings

Both the internalization theory and the imperfect capital markets theory predict a positive association between multinationality and firm value.

The internalization theory maintains that foreign direct investment will cause the increase of the market value of the firm relative to its accounting value only if the firm can internalize markets for certain of its intangibles.[1] Examples of these firm-specific intangible assets include production skills, managerial skills, patent, marketing abilities, consumer goodwill, research and development, advertising spending, managerial incentives alignment, and corporate reputation,

to name a few (Morck and Yeung, 1991; Mishra and Gobelli, 1998). These information-based proprietary intangible assets cannot be copied or exchanged at arm's length but can only be transferred to subsidiaries, thereby internationalizing the markets for such assets. As a result the market value of a multinational firm possessing these intangibles and engaging in foreign direct investment is directly proportional to the firm's degree of multinationality.

The imperfect capital markets theory suggests that investors, with institutional constraints on international capital flows and the information asymmetries that exist in global capital markets, invest in multinational firms to gain from the international diversification opportunities provided by these multinational firms.[2] This direct valuation of multinational firms by investors as a means of diversifying their portfolios internationally is assumed to enhance the share prices of multinational firms, independently of the information-based proprietary intangible assets possessed by these firms.

Accounting research has, however, consistently showed earning's explanatory power for returns, without explicitly examining the contingent role of multinationality. What has appeared in the international business literature with regard to the association between firm value and multinationality may be an association between earnings and firm value that is more pronounced with increased multinationality (Bodnar and Weintrop, 1997). This argumentation leads to the first testable hypothesis: *The informativeness of accounting earnings as an explanatory variable for returns is systematically related to the level of multinationality.*

The Impact of Multinationality on the Behavior of Discretionary Accounting Accruals

The managerial objectives theory rests on the assumption of the differences of motives between management and shareholders. The complexity of the multinational firm and the resulting difficulty for shareholders in monitoring management's decisions allow management to act in their self-interest. They may favor international diversification because it reduces firm-specific risk. The situation is assumed to potentially reduce the market value of multinational firms (Morck and Yeung, 1991). It can be predicted that when multinationality is high, incentives arise for managers to pursue non-value-maximization behavior. The situation calls for the writing of contracts, often containing accounting-based constraints, to monitor managers' decisions. Most likely, managers will exploit the latitude offered in available accepted accounting techniques to manage these constraints in their own interest. Their accounting choices, as reflected by the behavior of the discretionary portion of total accruals, are a positive function of the level of multinationality. These arguments lead to the second hypothesis: *The magnitude of adjustments in managers' accounting choices is systematically related to the level of multinationality.*

Other Considerations Affecting Accounting Choices

Based on contracting theory and economic theories of the political process that governs managers' incentives in the selection and reporting of accounting numbers, other endogenous and exogenous determinants of accounting choices and earnings' explanatory power for returns are also examined. They include six additional factors: firm size, systematic risk, leverage, growth opportunities, earnings variability, and earnings persistence (Warfield et al., 1995).

SAMPLE SELECTION AND DATA

Multinationality was measured as foreign sales over total sales for the most international 100 American manufacturing and service firms. *Forbes* publishes every year a list of the most international 100 American manufacturing and service firms. To be included in the sample, a firm must meet the following selection criteria:

1. The firm must be included in *Forbes'* most international 100 American manufacturing and service firms from 1994 to 1998.
2. Annual earnings-per-share and dividends are available from Standard and Poor's Compustat primary, secondary, tertiary and full coverage database.
3. Data necessary to compute stock returns (including dividends) are available from Standard and Poor's Computstat price, dividends and earnings database. Both price per share and earnings per share were adjusted for stock splits and stock dividends.
4. Annual data necessary to compute discretionary accruals are available from Standard and Poor's Compustat primary, secondary, tertiary and full coverage database.

The complete sample consists of 404 firm-year observations for the first hypothesis and 368 firm-year observations for the second hypothesis.

Descriptive statistics and correlation analysis of the data used in both hypotheses are shown in Tables 2B.1 and 2B.2.

INFORMATIVENESS OF EARNINGS CONDITIONAL ON MULTINATIONALITY

Multinationality as a Determinant of Earnings' Explanatory Power

Table 2B.3 presents the correlation between earnings and returns (column 3) and the earnings coefficients (column 4) for the different ranges of multinationality measured as foreign sales over total sales. The correlation between returns and earnings is positive and significantly greater than zero for the total sample with a level of multinationality ranging from 0 to 75 percent and for each of the other multinationality ranges. These correlations range from a minimum of

0.42 for the 0–25 percent level of multinationality to a high of 0.65 for the 50–75 percent level of multinationality. In addition, the Pearson (Spearman) correlation between the level of multinationality (column 1) and the correlation between earnings and returns (column 3) for the three multinationality levels equals 0.67 (0.75), which is significantly greater than zero at the 0.05 level. The evidence from this first test points to multinationality as a determinant of the informativeness of earnings.

The second test of the informativeness of earnings conditional on multinationality levels examines the cross-sectional variation of the earnings coefficient conditional on multinationality. The following pooled cross-sectional regression model, with a multinationality interaction term, is used:

$$(R_{i,t}) = \alpha_0 + \alpha_1 \cdot E_{i,t}/P_{i,t-1} + \alpha_2 \cdot E_{i,t} \cdot MULTY_i/P_{i,t-1} + \varepsilon_{i,t}$$

where $(R_{i,t})$ is the return of firm i for annual period t, extending from nine months prior to fiscal year-end through three months after fiscal year-end, $E_{i,t}$ is earnings-per-share, $P_{i,t-1}$ is the price-per-share at the end of period $t-1$, and $MULTY_i$ is the level of multinationality as measured by foreign sales over total sales for the year. The joint relation between earnings and multinationality is measured by α_2, showing the extent to which the informativeness of earnings is affected by the level of multinationality. The regression results in Table 2B.4 indicate that the informativeness is affected by the level of multinationality as both the regression coefficient (0.575) and the earnings-multinationality coefficient (0.865) are both significantly greater than zero at the 0.0001 level.

Given that the results in Table 2B.3 imply nonlinearity with the data, the same regression was run separately for each of the three categories of multinationality levels in the table, thereby not imposing a constant residual assumption across multinationality categories. The earnings coefficients from these regressions, reported in column 4 of Table 2B.3, imply a monotonic increase in the regression coefficients. The increase of these coefficients from 0.57 for the 0–25 range of multinationality to 0.71 for the 50–75 range of multinationality verifies the results of hypothesis 1 in Table 2B.4.

Multinationality and Other Determinants of Earnings' Explanatory Power

As stated previously, additional considerations are recognized regarding both the informativeness of earnings and managerial incentives determining accounting choices. These considerations, in addition to multinationality, include firm size, systematic risk, leverage, growth opportunities, earnings variability, and earnings persistence. Accordingly, the following pooled cross-sectional regression model is formulated:

Table 2B.1
Summary for the Variables in Section 4

Panel A: Descriptive Statistics

Variable	Mean	Standard deviation	Median	First quartile	Third quartile
Stock return ($R_{i,t}$)	0.0952	0.0552	0.0897	0.0602	0.1286
Accounting earning ($E_{i,t}/P_{i,t-1}$)	0.0570	0.0854	0.0649	0.0369	0.0847
Earnings interacted with:					
a. Multinationality ($E_{i,t} . MULTY_i / P_{i,t-1}$)	0.0193	0.0514	0.0189	0.0081	0.0332
b. Size ($E_{i,t} . SIZE_i / P_{i,t-1}$)	0.5309	0.6125	0.5689	0.3171	0.7832
c. Growth opportunities ($E_{i,t} . GROWTH_i / P_{i,t-1}$)	0.0881	0.2349	0.0508	0.0331	0.0774
d. Systematic risk ($E_{i,t} . RISK_i / P_{i,t-1}$)	0.0072	0.0134	0.0028	0.0008	0.0083
e. Leverage ($E_{i,t} . DEBT_i / P_{i,t-1}$)	0.0087	0.0119	0.0072	0.0023	0.0139
f. Earnings variability ($E_{i,t} . VAR_i / P_{i,t-1}$)	0.1269	0.099	0.1028	0.0601	0.1653
g. Earnings persistence ($E_{i,t} . PERS_i / P_{i,t-1}$)	-0.0082	0.1686	-0.0010	-0.0018	0.0005

Panel B: Pearson correlation matrix (using variables from Panel A)

Variable	E	MULTY	SIZE	GROWTH	RISK	DEBT	VAR	PERS
Accounting earnings (E)	1.00	0.281	0.2633	0.2320	0.2030	0.3496	0.3328	-0.3856
Multinationality (MULTY)		1.00	0.3588	0.3727	0.1652	0.2814	0.3685	-0.4813
Size (SIZE)			1.00	0.3670	0.3489	0.2051	0.2586	-0.4788
Growth opportunities (GROWTH)				1.00	0.0690	0.0067	0.3351	0.0103
Systematic risk (RISK)					1.00	0.1172	0.3417	0.0158
Leverage (DEBT)						1.00	0.1557	-0.0596
Earnings variability (VAR)							1.00	-0.2069
Earnings persistence (PERS)								1.00

Notes: Stock returns (R) are measured for the twelve-month period from nine months prior to the fiscal year-end through three months after the fiscal year-end, earnings (E) is the accounting earnings per share, multinationality (MULTY) is measured as foreign sales/total sales, size (SIZE) is measured as the company's market value of equity (in 000s), systematic risk (RISK) is measured by the market model beta, growth opportunities (GROWTH) are measured by the market-to-book ratio for common equity, leverage (DEBT) is measured by the ratio of total debt to total assets, earnings variability (VAR) is measured by the standard deviation of earnings for the twenty quarters 1994–1998, earnings persistence (PERS) is the first-order autocorrelation in earnings for the twenty quarters 1994–1998, and price (P) is the stock price at the beginning of the period. The sample size is 404 firm-year observations.

Table 2B.2
Summary Statistics for the Variation in Section 5

Panel A: Descriptive Statistics

Variable	Mean	Standard deviation	Median	First quartile	Third quartile
Absolute Abnormal Accrual (/AAC/)	0.0190	0.0110	0.0179	0.0120	0.0092
Multinationality (MULTY)	0.3492	0.142	0.3345	0.2360	0.4520
Size (SIZE)	8.782	0.9284	8.6983	8.1616	9.4140
Systematic risk (RISK)	0.090	0.131	0.044	0.016	0.124
Leverage (DEBT)	0.1583	0.1428	0.1384	0.0541	0.2277
Growth opportunities (GROWTH)	35.893	52.129	2.460	1.5881	4.2165
Earnings variability (VAR)	0.1673	0.0789	0.1374	0.1164	0.1930
Earnings persistence (PERS)	-0.1618	0.1316	-0.015	-0.023	-0.0097

Panel B: Pearson correlation matrix

Variable	MULTY	SIZE	RISK	DEBT	GROWTH	VAR	PERS
Multinationality (MULTY)	1.00	0.0136	0.1642	-0.1576	0.0544	0.2448	0.0326
Size (SIZE)		1.00	0.1083	-0.1312	-0.0613	0.3006	0.1590
Systematic risk (RISK)			1.00	-0.1341	-0.0704	0.1606	0.0818
Leverage (DEBT)				1.00	-0.2428	-0.2193	0.1183
Growth opportunities (GROWTH)					1.00	-0.1521	-0.0651
Earnings variability (VAR)						1.00	0.0808
Earnings persistence (PERS)							1.00

Notes: Abnormal accrual (AAC) is defined as the current-period accrual less the expected normal accrual, where the difference is standardized by the beginning period stock price. Absolute abnormal accrual (/AAC/) is measured as the absolute value of AAC. All other variables are as defined in Table 2B.1.

Table 2B.3
Relation between Earnings and Returns Depending on the Level of Multinationality

Level of Multinationality	Number of Firm-Period Observations	Correlation between Earnings and Returns	Earnings Coefficient
0–75	404	0.07	0.06
0–25	108	0.42	0.57
25–50	232	0.53	0.58
50–75	64	0.65	0.71

Notes: Stock returns are measured for the twelve-month period extending from nine months prior to the fiscal year-end through three months after the fiscal year-end, earnings per share is scaled by the beginning-of-period stock price per share, and multinationality is equal to foreign sales/total sales. The sample of annual earnings reports is drawn from the 5-year period corresponding to the 1994–1998 calendar years. All correlations (Pearson) between annual accounting earnings per share and stock returns, the earnings coefficients from the regression of stock returns, and the earnings coefficients from the regression of stock returns on accounting earnings per share are significant at the 0.01 level or better.

Table 2B.4
Regression in Stock Return on Both Earnings and Earnings-Multinationality Interaction

$$(R_{i,t}) = \alpha_0 + \alpha_1 \cdot E_{i,t}/P_{i,t-1} + \alpha_2 E_{i,t} \, MULTY_i/P_{i,t-1} + \varepsilon_{i,t}$$

Parameter estimates

α_0	α_1	α_2	Sample Size	Adjusted R^2%	F-value (sig. level)
0.077	0.575	0.865	404	7.47	17.30
(18.57)*	(5.882)*	(5.57)*			(0.001)

Notes: Stock returns (R) are measured for the twelve-month period extending from nine months prior to the fiscal year-end through three months after the fiscal year-end. Earnings (E) are the accounting earnings per share, multinationality (MULTY) is equal to foreign sales/total sales, and price (P) is the stock price per share. Parameter estimates and t-statistics (in parentheses) are presented for the regression. A * designates statistical significance at the 0.01 level. The sample comprises firm-year observations from the 1994–1998 calendar years.

$$R_{i,t} = \alpha_0 + \alpha_1 \cdot E_{i,t}/P_{i,t-1} + \alpha_2 \, E_{i,t} \, MULTY_i/P_{i,t-1} \tag{2}$$
$$+ \alpha_3 \, E_{i,t} \, SIZE_i/P_{i,t-1} + \alpha_4 \, E_{i,t} \, GROWTH_i/P_{i,t-1}$$
$$+ \alpha_5 \, E_{i,t} \, RISK_i/P_{i,t-1} + \alpha_6 \, E_{i,t} \, DEBT_i/P_{i,t-1}$$
$$+ \alpha_7 \, E_{i,t} \, VAR_i/P_{i,t-1} + \alpha_8 \, E_{i,t} \, PERS + \varepsilon_{i,t}$$

The new variables are defined as follows: SIZE is the natural logarithm of a firm's market value of equity, RISK is a firm's systematic risk,[3] DEBT is the firm's ratio of total debt to total assets, GROWTH is measured as the market value of equity scaled by book value, VAR is the variability of earnings for all of the quarters of the period of analysis, PERS is persistence of earnings as measured by the first-order autocorrelation in earnings for the same period.

The results, shown in Table 2B.5, verify again the relation between multinationality and earnings' informativeness after the inclusion of these additional considerations. As expected, the market reaction to earnings was negatively related to systematic risk (α_5 [−0.532], significant at the 0.01 level), and to variability of earnings (α_7 [−0.338], significant at the 0.01 level). It is also positively related to firm size (α_3 [0.08], significant at the 0.01 level), growth opportunities (α_4 [0.351], significant at the 0.01 level), leverage (α_6 [0.199], significant at the 0.01 level), and earnings persistence (α_8 [0.057], significant at the 0.01 level).[4]

EARNINGS MANAGEMENT CONDITIONAL ON MULTINATIONALITY

The second hypothesis states that the magnitude of adjustments in managers' accounting choices is systematically related to multinationality. The higher the level of multinationality, the higher is managers' reliance on discretionary accruals, as measured by the magnitude of discretionary accrual adjustments.

An abnormal accruals research design is used to test the hypothesis of managers' accounting choices conditional on multinationality.[5] Basically, the abnormal accounting accrual (AAC) is computed as the current period accrual (AC) minus the expected normal accrual (E[AC]), and then standardized by beginning-of-year stock price (P):

$$AAC_{i,t} = [AC_{i,t} - E(AC)_{i,t}]/P_{i,t-1} \tag{3}$$

The accounting accrual (AC) is defined as the change in noncash working capital (i.e., change in noncash current assets less current liabilities) less depreciation expense.[6]

An accruals prediction model, suggested by Jones (1991), is used to estimate normal accruals. It is specified as:

$$AC_{i,t} = \beta_0/P_{i,t-1} + \beta_1 \cdot \Delta REV_{i,t}/P_{i,t-1} + \beta_2 \cdot PPE_{i,t}/ + \varepsilon_{it} \tag{4}$$

Table 2B.5

Regression of Returns on Earnings, Earnings-Multinationality Interaction, and Earnings Interaction with Other Determinants of Earnings Explanatory Power

$$(R_{i,t}) = \alpha_0 + \alpha_1 \cdot E_{i,t}/P_{i,t-1} + \alpha_2 E_{i,t} \cdot MULTY_i/P_{i,t-1} + \alpha_3 E_{i,t} \cdot SIZE_i/P_{i,t-1} + \alpha_4 E_{i,t} \cdot GROWTH_i/P_{i,t-1} + \alpha_5 E_{i,t} \cdot RISK_i/P_{i,t-1} + \alpha_6 E_{i,t} \cdot DEBT_i/P_{i,t-1} + \alpha_7 E_{i,t} \cdot VAR_i/P_{i,t-1} + \alpha_8 E_{i,t} \cdot PERS + \varepsilon_{i,t}^{(2)}$$

Parameter estimates

α_0	α_1	α_2	α_3	α_4	α_5	α_6	α_7	α_8	Sample Size	Adjusted R^2%	F
0.024	0.139	0.019	0.08	0.351	-0.532	0.199	-0.338	0.057	3.91	23.52	248.70*
(9.84)*	(5.09)*	(5.18)*	(2.73)*	(15.77)*	(-3.39)*	(3.48)*	(17.07)*	(4.20)*			

Notes: Stock returns (R) are measured for the twelve-month period from nine months prior to the fiscal year-end, earnings (E) is the accounting earnings per share, multinationality (MULTY) is the foreign sales/total sales, size (SIZE) is measured as the company's natural logarithm of the market value of equity, systematic risk (RISK) is measured by the market model beta, growth opportunities (GROWTH) are measured by the market-to-book ratio for common equity, leverage (DEBT) is measured by the ratio total debt to total assets, earnings variability (VAR) is measured by the standard deviation of earnings, earnings persistence (PERS) is the first-order autocorrelation in earnings, and price (P) is the stock price at the beginning of the period. The sample size comprises firm-year observations drawn from the 1994–1998 calendar years.

where the new variables are defined as follows:

$\Delta REV_{i,t}$ = changes in revenues from year t to $t-1$ for firm i

$PPE_{i,t}$ = gross property, plant, and equipment in year t

A time-series regression using available prior year data for seven years generated firm-specific and time-period-specific predictions of $E(AC_{i,t})$, which are then used in equation (3) to generate an estimate of abnormal accruals ($AAC_{i,t}$).

Because the interest in this study is with the magnitude of the accrual adjustments, rather than the direction of the accrual, the absolute value of the abnormal accrual (i.e., $/AAC_{i,t}/$) is used as a department variable in the following model:[7]

$$/AAC_{i,t}/ = \delta_0 + \delta_1 \cdot MULTY_i + \delta_2 \cdot SIZE_i + \delta_3 \cdot GROWTH_i \qquad (5)$$
$$+ \delta_4 \cdot RISK_i + \delta_5 \cdot DEBT_i + \delta_6 \cdot VAR_i + \delta_7 \cdot PERS_i + \varepsilon_{it}$$

Equation (5) is a multivariate-pooled cross-sectional regression model to be used to investigate the joint interaction of multinationality and the level of abnormal accounting accruals.

The model includes, in addition to the multinationality variable, other factors that have been shown in previous research to affect the magnitude of abnormal accruals (Warfield et al., 1997). These factors include size of the firm, growth, systematic risk, leverage, earnings variability, and earnings persistence. Consistent with the second hypothesis, a positive relation between the level of multinationality and the magnitude of abnormal accruals is predicted (i.e., $\delta_1 > 0$). The evidence in Table 2B.6 supports the hypothesis that the magnitude of abnormal accruals is positively related to the level of multinationality (i.e., δ_1 equals 0.00002, which is significantly greater than zero at the 0.01 level).[8]

SUMMARY AND CONCLUSIONS

This appendix presented two hypotheses linking the level of multinationality to both the informativeness of earnings and the magnitude of discretionary accounting accrual adjustments. The hypotheses draw on multinationality theories and exploits (1) the internalization and the international diversification opportunities provided by multinational firms and (2) managers' incentives in using discretionary accounting accrual adjustments. Based on both the internalization theory and the imperfect world capital markets theory, the first hypothesis postulates that the informativeness of earnings in explaining stock returns varies systematically with the level of multinationality in the corporation. Based on the managerial objectives theory, the second hypothesis postulates that the managers' accounting choices are systematically related to the level of multinationality. The results on a sample of U.S. multinational firms show a significantly greater

Table 2B.6

Regression of Absolute Abnormal Accruals on Multinationality and Other Determinants of the Magnitude of Discretionary Accruals

$$|AAC_{i,t}| = \delta_0 + \delta_1 \cdot MULTY_i + \delta_2 \cdot SIZE_i + \delta_3 \cdot GROWTH_i + \delta_4 \cdot RISK_i + \delta_5 \cdot DEBT_i + \delta_6 \cdot VAR_i + \delta_7 PERS_i + \varepsilon_{it}$$

Parameter estimates

δ_0	δ_1	δ_2	δ_3	δ_4	δ_5	δ_6	δ_7
-0.077	0.00002	0.0003	0.01	0.00001	0.08	0.008	-0.00001
(-1.13)	(8.52)*	(7.48)*	(7.39)*	(4.52)*	(5.62)*	(17.68)*	(0.51)*

Sample size	Adjusted	F-Value
368	28.55%	75.26*

Notes: Absolute abnormal accruals (*IAAC_{i,t}I*) is defined as the current-period accrual loss of the expected normal accruals, where the difference is standardized by the beginning-period stock price. All other variables are as defined in Table 2B.3. The sample comprises firm-year observations drawn from the 1994–1998 calendar years.

A * designates statistical significance at the 0.01 level, two-tailed tests.

earnings coefficient for firms with higher multinationality and a positive relation between the magnitude of discretionary accruals and the level of multinationality.

NOTES

1. The internalization theory is developed in Coase (1937), Caves (1974), Hymer (1976), Dunning (1980, 1988), Rugman (1980, 1981), Casson (1987), Buckley (1988), Morck and Yeung (1991, 1992), Mishra and Gobelli (1998).

2. See Agmon and Lessard (1977), Brewer (1981), Errunza and Senbet (1981), Adler and Dumas (1983), Fatemi (1984), Doukas and Travlos (1988), and others.

3. Systematic risk is measured by the market model beta using the most recent sixty months' stock returns prior to the test period.

4. To measure the degree of collinearity among the regression variables, condition indexes are calculated. The condition index shows that the regression was 23.6, considered by Belsley et al. (1980) as indicative of moderate to strong multicollinearity. Similarly, to assess the effect of cross-correlation in the residuals for the estimation of parameters, bootstrapping analysis was conducted. The results showed bootstrapping estimates qualitatively identical to the estimates reported in Table 2B.5.

5. The abnormal accruals research design was pioneered by Healey (1985), DeAngelo (1986, 1988), Liberty and Zimmerman (1986), and others.

6. Specifically, the accounting per share is calculated as follows (Compustat data item numbers are in parentheses):

$$AC_{i,t} = [\cap \text{ Accounts receivable}_{i,t} (2) + \cap \text{ Inventories}_{i,t} (3)$$
$$+ \cap \text{ Other Current Assets}_{i,t} (68)] - [\cap \text{ Current Liabilities}_{i,t} (5)]$$
$$- [\text{Depreciation and Amortization Expense}_{i,t}(14)]$$

where the change ($\cap$) is the difference between years (t and t$-$1). The Compustat data item numbers for stock price, $P_{i,t-1}$ is (24).

7. A similar methodology is used by Warfield et al. (1995).

8. Similar results were obtained when the Jones model (1991) was replaced by either the modified Jones model (Dechow et al., 1995) or the cross-sectional Jones model (Defond and Jiambalvo, 1994).

REFERENCES

Adler, M., and B. Dumas. 1983. International portfolio choice and corporation finance: A synthesis. *Journal of Finance* 38: 925–984.

Agmon, J., and D. Lessard. 1977. Investor recognition of corporate international diversification. *Journal of Finance* 32: 1049–1055.

Belsley, D.A., E. Kuh, and R.E. Welsh. 1980. *Regression Diagnostics: Identifying Influential Data and Sources of Collinearity.* New York: Wiley.

Bodnar, G.M., and J. Weintrop. 1997. The valuation of the foreign income of U.S. multinational firms: A growth opportunities perspective. *Journal of Accounting and Economics* 24: 69–97.

Brewer, H.L. 1981. Investor benefits from corporate international diversification. *Journal of Financial and Quantitative Analysis* 16: 113–126.

Buckley, P. 1988. The limits of explanation: Testing the internalization theory of the multinational enterprise. *Journal of International Business Studies* 19: 113–126.

Casson, M. 1987. *The Firm and the Market*. London: Basil Blackwell.

Caves, R.E. 1974. Causes of direct investment: Foreign firms' shares in Canadian and United Kingdom manufacturing industries. *Review of Economics and Statistics* 56: 273–293.

Coase, R.H. 1937. The nature of the firm. *Economica* 4: 386–405.

DeAngelo, L.E. 1986. Accounting numbers as market valuation substitutes: A study of management buyouts of public stockholders. *The Accounting Review* 41: 400–420.

———. 1988. Managerial competition, information costs, and corporate governance: The use of accounting performance measures in proxy contests. *Journal of Accounting and Economics* 10: 3–36.

Dechow, P.M., R.G. Sloan, and A.P. Sloan. 1995. Detecting earnings management. *The Accounting Review* 70: 193–225.

Defond, M.L., and J. Jiambalvo. 1994. Debt covenant violations and manipulation of accruals. *Journal of Accounting and Economics* 17: 145–176.

Doukas, J., and N.G. Travlos. 1988. The effect of corporate multinationalism on share-holders' wealth: Evidence from international acquisitions. *Journal of Finance* 43: 1161–1175.

Dunning, J.H. 1980. Toward an eclectic theory of international production: Some empirical tests. *Journal of International Business Studies* 11: 9–31.

———. 1988. The eclectic paradigm of international production: A restatement and some possible extensions. *Journal of International Business* 19: 1–31.

Errunza, V.R., and L.W. Senbet. 1981. The effects of international operations on the market values of the firm: Theory and evidence. *Journal of Finance* 36: 401–417.

Fatemi, A.M. 1984. Shareholders' benefits from corporate international diversification. *Journal of Finance* 39: 1325–1344.

Healey, P. 1985. The effects of bonus schemes on accounting decisions. *Journal of Accounting and Economics* 7: 85–107.

Hymer, S. 1976. *The International Operations of National Firms: A Study of Direct Foreign Investment*. Cambridge, MA: MIT Press.

Jones, J. 1991. Earnings management during import relief investigations. *Journal of Accounting Research* 29: 193–228.

Liberty, S.F., and J.I. Zimmerman. 1986. Labor union contract negotiations accounting choices. *The Accounting Review* 61: 692–712.

Mishra, C., and D.H. Gobelli. 1998. Managerial incentives, internalization, and market valuation of multinational firms. *Journal of International Business Studies* 29, 3: 583–598.

Morck, R., and B. Yeung. 1991. Why investors value multinationality. *Journal of Business* 64: 165–187.

Morck, R., and B. Yeung. 1992. Internationalization: An event study test. *Journal of International Economics* 33: 41–56.

Rugman, A.M. 1980. Internalization as a general theory of foreign direct investment: A reappraisal of the literature. *Journal of Economic Literature* 116: 365–375.

Rugman, A.M. 1981. *Inside the Multinationals: The Economics of Internal Markets*. New York: Columbia University Press.

Warfield, T.D., J.J. Wild, and K.L. Wild. 1997. Managerial ownership, accounting choices, and informativeness of earnings. *Journal of Accounting and Economics* 20, 61–91.

Appendix 2C. Growth Opportunities and Earnings Management

INTRODUCTION

This appendix develops and tests the hypothesis that managers of multinational firms with a high level of the investment opportunity set make accounting choices to reduce reported earnings compared to managers of multinational firms with a low level of the investment opportunity set. Unlike in other studies, we assume that earnings management is a present and continuous phenomenon rather than a behavior conditioned by an eventual crisis. While all firms potentially resort to earnings management, the level of growth opportunity, as measured by the level of the investment opportunity set, is assumed to affect the nature of earnings management for high-growth opportunities firms. These firms will then potentially resort to income-reducing accruals. We argue that a high level of the investment opportunity set causes higher actual and/or future profitability and thus higher reported accounting numbers. A result of the actual and/or potential higher reported accounting numbers is the possible perception of the accounting rates of return as "excessive" and indicative of monopolistic power on the part of the firm, thereby increasing both the political costs and the political risk. In such a case, managers' reporting of lower earnings may be expected to reduce both political costs and political risk.

Accrual analysis, similar to that of Jones (1991), is performed on a sample of high- and low-growth opportunities of multinational U.S. firms to determine the extent of earnings management. Our findings indicate that managers of high-growth opportunity multinational firms facing potentially high political costs and political risk report income-decreasing accruals compared to low-growth opportunity firms.

GROWTH OPPORTUNITIES AND EARNINGS MANAGEMENT

The firm is composed of the value of assets in place and the value of expected future investment options or growth opportunities. The lower the proportion of firm value represented by assets in place, the higher the growth opportunities for a given level of firm value. These potential investment opportunities are

Source: F. Alnajjar and A. Riahi-Belkaoui, "Growth Opportunities and Earnings Management," *Managerial Finance* 27, 2 (2001), pp. 72–81. Reprinted with the permission of the editor.

described by Myers (1977) as call options whose values depend on the likelihood that management will exercise them. Like call options, these growth opportunities represent real value to the firm (Kester, 1984). Growth options include such discretionary expenditures as capacity expansion prospects, product innovations, acquisitions of other firms, investment in brand name through advertising, and even maintenance and replacement of existing assets. A significant portion of the market value of equity is accounted for by growth opportunities (Pindyck, 1988). These benefits of growth opportunities are expected to result in higher profitability and realized growth (Kallapur and Trombley, 1999) and higher political risk (Monti-Belkaoui and Riahi-Belkaoui, 1999). Both increased profitability and political risk are expected to induce managers to resort to income-reducing accruals.

First, the increase in profitability of multinational firms with a high level of growth opportunities increases both their political visibility and political costs. The political cost hypothesis predicts that managers confronted with the possibility of politically imposed wealth transfers will resort to earnings management to reduce the likelihood and size of this transfer (Watts and Zimmerman, 1978). These multinational firms with high-growth opportunities, like high-income firms, which are particularly vulnerable to wealth-extorting political transfers in the form of legislation and/or regulation, have an incentive to resort to accruals or other means to reduce their reported income numbers compared to low-growth opportunity and low-income firms.

Second, political risk is a phenomenon that characterizes an unfriendly climate to multinational firms with visible profitability and high-growth opportunities (Monti-Belkaoui and Riahi-Belkaoui, 1999). It refers to the potential economic losses arising as a result of governmental measures or special situations that may limit or prohibit the operational and profitable activities of a multinational firm. One way to limit the potential emergence of political risk is to reduce the reported earnings number. Earnings management in high-growth-opportunities multinational firms may be a way of reducing the factors mitigating the emergence of political risk.

This study hypothesizes that high-growth-opportunities multinational firms make accounting choices to reduce income and net worth compared to low-growth-opportunities multinational firms.

RESEARCH DESIGN

The objective of the study is to examine the potential relationship between growth opportunities and the discretionary accruals of firms as those accruals reflect accounting choices made by management. The technique used by Jones (1991) and Cahan (1992) for the estimation of nondiscretionary accruals is adopted in this study. It estimates nondiscretionary accruals by regressing total accruals on the change in sales (a proxy for level of activity) and on the fixed asset balance. This approach leads to an estimate of discretionary accruals that

is less biased and less noisy than earlier models as well as eliminates the assumption that accruals remain stationary over time. The basic model is as follows:

$$A_{it} = b_0 + b_1 CHSALES_{it} + b_2 FIXASSETS_{it} + e_{it} \qquad (1)$$

where

A_{it} = total accruals in year t/total assets$_{it}$

$CHSALES_{it}$ = change in sales from year $t-1$ to year t, (Sales Revenues$_{it}$ − Sales Revenue$_{it-1}$) / Total Assets$_{it}$

$FIXASSETS_{it}$ = fixed assets at the end of year t (Fixed Assets$_{it}$ / Total Assets$_{it}$)

In the estimation process, Equation (1) is expanded to include an indicator variable to measure the discretionary accruals of high-growth firms. The expansion also includes total assets as a measure of size and dummy variables for each year of analysis.

The effect of multinationality is tested by estimating Equation (2).

$$A_{it} = B_0 + B_1 CHSALES_{it} + b_2 FIXASSETS_{it} + b_3 IOS_{it}$$
$$+ b_4 TA_{it} + b_5 YR_{it} \ldots + b_9 YR_{it} + e_{it} \qquad (2)$$

where TA is total assets, YR is a dummy variable for a year of analysis, and IOS is the investment opportunity set.

The expected sign of the coefficient for CHSALES is positive. It is expected to be negative for all the other explanatory variables. The coefficient of IOS will be negative if managers lower accruals for high-growth firms.

As in Hall and Stammerjohan (1997), a two-step generalized least square error components model is used in this study, as it is more efficient than the within-group estimator, fixed effects covariance model used by Cahan (1992).

DATA

Sample and Method

The sample consisted of all the firms included in Forbes' "most international" 100 American manufacturing and service firms for the 1987–1990 period. Financial data were collected from both the *Forbes* articles and Compustat. Total accruals are calculated for each firm as follows:

$$A_{it} = \frac{-DEP_{it} + (AR_{it} - AR_{it-1}) + (INV_{it} - INV_{it-1}) - (AP_{it}}{} $$
$$\frac{- AP_{it-1}) - (TP_{it} - TP_{it-1}) - DT_{it}}{TA_{it}}$$

where

DEP_{it} = depreciation expense and the depletion charge for firm i in year t

AR_{it} = accounts receivable balance for firm i at the end of year t

INV_{it} = inventory balance for firm i at the end of year t

AP_{it} = accounts payable for firm i at the end of year t

TP_{it} = taxes payable balance for firm i at the end of year t

DT_{it} = deferred tax expense for firm i at the end of year t

TA_{it} = total asset balance for firm i at the end of year t

The data are pooled over time and across firms, resulting in a sample of 339 firm-years. To test the effect of the investment opportunity set on discretionary accruals, a dichotomous indicator variable, IOS, is added to model (1). IOS takes on the value of 1 for the group firms classified as high-growth-opportunity firms and zero for firms classified as low-growth-opportunity firms. Model (1) is also expanded to include YR_{it}, dummy-coded variable as 1 for year t (t = 1987–1990), and TA_{it} for the total assets of the firm. The YR variables measure the time effect for each of the four years. The TA variable is added as a result of the size hypothesis whereby large firms are expected to make income-decreasing choices relative to small firms (Christie, 1990). The effect of size is important given the evidence presented later about the significant difference in size between the high-growth and the low-growth firms.

Measuring the Investment Opportunity Set

Because the investment opportunity set is not observable, there is no consensus on an appropriate proxy variable (Kallapur and Trombley, 1999). Similar to Smith and Watts (1992) and Gaver and Gaver (1993), we used an ensemble of variables to measure the investment opportunity set. The three measures of the investment opportunity set used are market-to-book assets (MASS), market-to-book equity (MV), and the earnings/price ratio (EP). These variables are defined as follows:

MASS = [Assets − Total Common Equity + Shares Outstanding * Share Closing Price] / Assets

MV = [Shares Outstanding * Share Closing Price / Total Common Equity]

EP = [Primary EPS before Extraordinary Items] / Share Closing Price

The results of a factor analysis of these measures of the investment opportunity set are shown in Table 2C.1. One common factor appears to explain the intercorrelations among the three individual measures. Based on these factor

Table 2C.1
Selected Statistics Related to a Common Factor Analysis of Three Measures of the Investment Opportunity Set for *Forbes'* "Most International 100 U.S. Firms"

1. **Eigenvalues of the Correlation Matrix: Total = 3, Average = 1**

Eigenvalue	1	2	3
	1.0540	0.9868	0.9592

2. **Factor Pattern**

FACTOR 1	MASS	MQV	EP
	0.62821	0.66411	0.46722

3. **Final Communality Estimates: Total = 1.053994**

MASS	MQV	EP
0.394651	0.441045	0.218299

4. **Standardized Scoring Coefficients**

FACTOR 1	MASS	MQV	EP
	0.59603	0.63009	0.43329

5. **Descriptive Statistics of the Common Factor Extracted from the Three Measures of the Investment Opportunity**

Maximum	Third Quartile	Median	First Quartile	Minimum	Mean
9.3593	3.2200	2.0450	1.5085	2.5209	1.9812

scores, high-growth firms are chosen from the top 25 percent of the distribution scores, while low-growth firms are chosen from the bottom 25 percent of the distribution factor scores.

TESTS AND RESULTS

Descriptive statistics are presented in Table 2C.2. The results for the error-components estimation of model (1) are reported in Table 2C.3. As expected, both CHSALES and FIXASSETS are statistically significant. The overall model is also significant with an F value of 30.818 and an adjusted R^2 of 16.73

Table 2C.2
Descriptive Statistics

A. High-Growth Sample

Variables	Mean	Standard Deviation	Maximum	Median	Minimum
Total Revenues (thousands)	3,624.6	2,8012.2	138,954	246,842	7,682
Total Assets (thousands)	54,186.5	50,397.7	261,860	35,475	8,462
Net Profit	1,812	1,320.65	8,132	1,608	0.4587

B. Low-Growth Sample

Variables	Mean	Standard Deviation	Maximum	Median	Minimum
Total Revenues (thousands)	6,556.19	3,696.6	18,805	5,835	2,816
Total Assets (thousands)	9.559.85	16,833.05	128,260	5,556	2,864
Net Profit	384.85	368.27	1,925.35	382.3	−618.2

percent. It appears that a significant portion of the variation in accruals of multinational firms can be explained by changes in sales and the fixed asset balance.

The error-components regression results for model (2) are reported in Table 2C.4. The results support the view that the variation in accruals can be explained by the change in sales, the fixed asset balance, and time-dependent effects. In addition, the variable of interest, IOS, is significant at the 0.01 level, with a one-tailed test, and its sign is negative. Because high growth was coded as 1, the positive sign of IOS indicates that discretionary accruals of high-growth firms were higher than for low-growth firms, which supports the political cost and political risk hypothesis.

SUMMARY AND CONCLUSIONS

This study examines, on a longitudinal basis, whether managers of multinational firms respond to the political costs associated with a high level of growth opportunities by adjusting their discretionary accruals. Discretionary accruals for the 100 largest U.S. multinationals were examined over the 1987–1990 period, using the residuals of a fixed effects covariance model that regressed total ac-

Table 2C.3
Results of Regression Estimation—Model (1)
$(A_{it} = b_0 + b_1 CHSALES_{it} + b_2 FIXASSETS_{it} + e_{it})$

Interdependent Variables	Expected Sign	Coefficient	t-value	One-tailed Probability
Intercept		-0.0326	7.538	0.0001
CHSALES	+	0.0180	4.059	0.0001
FIXASSETS	-	-0.1532	-7.885	0.0001
$n=$	339			
R^2		0.1723	F Statistic	Probability
Adjusted R^2		0.1673	30.818	0.0001

Variable definitions:

$$A_{it} = \frac{-DEP_{it} + (AR_{it} - AR_{it-1}) + (INV_{it} - INV_{it-1}) - (AP_{it} - AP_{it-1}) - (TP_{it} - TP_{it-1}) - DT_{it}}{TA_{it}}$$

Where

DEP_{it} = depreciation expense and the depletion charge for firm i in year t
AR_{it} = accounts receivable balance for firm i at the end of year t
INV_{it} = inventory balance for firm i at the end of year t
AP_{it} = accounts payable for firm i at the end of year t
TP_{it} = taxes payable balance for firm i at the end of year t
DT_{it} = deferred tax expense for firm i at the end of year t
TA_{it} = total asset balance for firm i at the end of year t
$CHSALES_{it}$ = (net sales$_{it}$ – net sales$_{it-1}$) / TA_{it}
$FIXASSETS_{it}$ = fixed assets$_{it}$ / TA_{it}

cruals on the change in sales, the fixed assets balance, and a dummy variable for each year of the study. The hypothesis is tested using a test designed with a dummy variable, coded 1 for high growth, included in the accrual model. This growth variable was significant with a positive sign, which indicates that the discretionary accruals were higher for high-growth firms. The results support the political cost and political risk hypothesis associated with multinationality and are consistent with the view that managers adjust earnings in response to a high level of growth.

The results, however, cannot be generalized, as the sample includes only the most multinational U.S. firms. This appendix identifies this area for future research. The longitudinal approach could be extended to explore response to a wider range of growth.

Table 2C.4
Results of Regression Estimation—Model (2)
$(A_{it} = B_0 B_1 CHSALES_{it} + b_2 FIXASSETS_{it} + b_3 IOS_{it} + b_4 TA_{it} + b_5 YR_{it} \ldots \ldots + b_9 YR_{it})$

Interdependent Variables	Expected Sign	Coefficient	t-value	One-tailed Probability
Intercept		-0.0158	-2.876	0.0156
CHSALES	+	0.0028	4.256	0.0001
FIXASSETS	-	-0.1818	-6.538	0.0002
IOS	+	0.0081	+2.656	0.0116
TA	-	-0.0000007	-2.588	0.0112
YR_1		-0.0031	-4.868	0.0001
YR_2		-0.0018	-4.062	0.0001
YR_3		-0.00132	-4.850	0.0001
R^2		0.3612	F Statistics	Probability
Adjusted R^2		0.3322	4.856	0.0001
n	166			

Variable definitions:

TA = Total Assets
TR = Year
IOS = 1 if growth opportunities are high; 0 if growth opportunities are low.

REFERENCES

Cahan, S. 1992. The effect of antitrust investigations on discretionary accruals: A refined test of the political-cost hypothesis. *The Accounting Review* 67 (January): 77–95.

Christie, A.A. 1990. Aggression of test statistics: An evaluation of the evidence on contracting and size hypotheses. *Journal of Accounting and Economics* 12 (January): 15–36.

Gaver, J.J., and K.M. Gaver. 1993. Additional evidence in the association between the investment opportunity set and corporate financing, dividend, and compensation policies. *Journal of Accounting and Economics* 16, 1/2/3: 125–140.

Hall, S.C., and W.W. Stammerjohan. 1997. Damage awards and earnings management in the oil industry. *The Accounting Review* (January): 47–65.

Jones, J. 1991. Earnings management during import relief investigations. *Journal of Accounting Research* 29 (Autumn): 193–228.

Kallapur, S., and M.A. Trombley. 1999. The association between investment opportunity set and realized growth. *Journal of Business, Finance, and Accounting* 96, 3 (December): 505–519.

Kester, W.C. 1984. Today's options for tomorrow's growth. *Harvard Business Review* 62, 2: 153–160.

Monti-Belkaoui, J., and A. Riahi-Belkaoui. 1999. *The Nature, Estimation, and Management of Political Risk.* Westport, CT: Greenwood.

Myers, S.C. 1977. Determinants of corporate borrowing. *Journal of Financial Economics* 5, 2: 147–175.

Pindyck, R.S. 1988. Irreversible investment, capacity choice and the value of the firm. *The American Economic Review* 78, 5: 969–985.

Smith, C.W., and R.L. Watts. 1992. The investment opportunity set and corporate financing, dividend, and compensation policies. *Journal of Financial Economics* 32, 3: 263–292.

Watts, R.L., and J.L. Zimmerman. 1978. Towards a positive theory of determination of accounting standards. *The Accounting Review* 53 (January): 112–134.

Appendix 2D. Contextual Accrual and Cash Flow Based Valuation Models: Impact of Multinationality and Reputation

INTRODUCTION

This appendix investigates the impact of the contextual factors of multinationality and reputation on accrual and cash flow based valuations. The nature and amount of information in cash flows and accruals were first examined by Wilson (1986) using stock behavior around the release of annual reports. He concluded that the market reacts more favorably the larger (smaller) are the cash flows (current accruals). Bernard and Stober (1989) were, however, unable to confirm Wilson's results over a longer period, and according to the state of the economy. This appendix extends the works of Wilson and Bernard and Stober in two ways. The first is to assess the generality and robustness of Wilson's results by using a total market value based valuation model rather than an excess-return based model. In situations where prices lead earnings, price level regressions are better specified than return/changes regressions for estimating the price earnings relation. The results confirm Wilson's results. The second is to examine two contextual models of the implications of cash and accruals. We argue that the preference of cash flows over accruals will arise under conditions of high multinationality and high reputation. Support for the hypotheses was found. In sum, we are able to identify the economic logic underlying how the market assimilates information about cash and accruals under the specific contextual environments of multinationality and corporate reputation.

Source: Reprinted from A. Riahi-Belkaoui, "Contextual Accrual and Cash Flow Based Valuation Models: Impact of Multinationality and Reputation," *Advances in Financial Planning and Forecasting* 2001, pp. 25–35. Copyright 2001. Reprinted with permission from Elsevier Science.

MARKET VALUATION MODELS

A Simplified Model

A simplified model relates market value of equity at the end of a period to the corresponding accruals and cash flows as follows:

$$MV_{it} = a_0 + A_{it} + a_{2i} CF_{it} + e_{it} \tag{1}$$

where

MV_{it} = Market value of equity of firm i at the end of year t
AT_{it} = Total accruals of firm i at the end of year t
CF_{it} = Cash flows of firm i at the end of year t

All variables are deflated by total assets at the end of year t.

Impact of Multinationality

Investors recognize the enhancement of firm value through internationalization. The evidence shows that investors recognize multinationality given that multinational firms show lower systematic risk and unsystematic risk compared to securities of purely domestic firms (Errunza and Senbet, 1981; Yang et al., 1985; Agmon and Lessard, 1977). To test the incremental association between market value of equity and multinationality, after controlling for accruals and cash flows, equation (1) is adjusted as follows:

$$MV_{it} = a_0 + a_{1i}A_{it} + a_{2i} CF_{it} + a_{3i} MULTY_{it} + e_{it}^1 \tag{2}$$

where

$MULTY_{it}$ = Level of multinationality of firm i at the end of year t

Impact of Reputation

To create the right impression or reputation, firms signal their key characteristics to constituents to maximize their social status (Spence, 1974). Basically, corporate audiences were found to construct reputation on the basis of accounting and market information or signals regarding firm performance (Fombrum and Shanley, 1990; Riahi-Belkaoui and Pavlik, 1991; Belkaoui, 1992). Then reputations have become established and constitute signals that may affect actions of firms' stakeholders, including their shareholders. Specifically, a good reputation can be construed as a competitive advantage within an industry (Fom-

brum and Shanley, 1990). This implies that investors use corporate reputation in determining firm value. To test for incremental association between the market value equity and reputation after controlling for accruals, cash flows, and multinationality, equation (2) is adjusted as follows:

$$MV_{it} = a_0 = a_1 A_{it} + a_{2i} CF_{it} + a_{3i} MULTY_{it} + a_{4i} REP_{it} + e_{it}^2 \qquad (3)$$

where

REP_{it} = Corporate reputation score for firm i at the end of year t

RESEARCH METHOD

In this study, incremental associations between market value and cash flow from operations, multinationality, and corporate reputation, after controlling for accruals, are presented as evidence of the relevance of the contextual environment of cash flow based valuation models. To describe and assess the significance of these relationships, we use three linear regression approaches (Equations 1–3) that relate market value of equity to the accounting and non-accounting variables mentioned earlier.

Data and Sample Selection

The population consists of firms included in both *Forbes'* most international 100 American manufacturing and service firms and *Fortune*'s surveys of corporate reputation from 1987 to 1990. The security data are collected from the CSRP Return files. The accounting variables are collected from Compustat. Cash flows from operations are reported under SFAS No. 95 (Compustat item 308). The derivation of the total accruals, multinationality, and corporate reputation variables are explained later. The final sample included 360 firm-year observations that have all the accounting and nonaccounting variables.

Measuring Total Accruals

Total accruals are calculated for each firm as follows (Healy, 1985):

$$A_{it} = \frac{DEP_{it} + (AR_{it} - AR_{it-1}) + (INV_{it} - INV_{it-1}) - (AP_{it} - AP_{it-1}) - (TP_{it} - TP_{it-1}) - DT_{it}}{TA_{it}}$$

where

DEP_{it} = Depreciation expense and the depletion charge for firm i in year t
AR_{it} = Accounts receivable balance for firm i at the end of year t

INV_{it} = Inventory balance for firm i at the end of year t

AP_{it} = Accounts payable for firm i at the end of year t

TP_{it} = Taxes payable balance for firm i at the end of year t

DT_{it} = Deferred tax expense for firm i in year t

TA_{it} = Total asset balance for firm i at the end of year t

Measuring Multinationality

Previous research has attempted to measure three attributes of multinationality:

1. *Performance*—in terms of what goes on overseas (Dunning 1995).
2. *Structure*—in terms of how resources are used overseas (Stopford and Wells 1972).
3. *Attitude or Conduct*—in terms of what is top management orientation (Perlmutter, 1969).

Sullivan (1994) developed nine measures, of which five were shown to have a high reliability in the construction of a homogeneous measure of multinationality: (1) foreign sales as a percentage of total sales (FSTS), (2) foreign assets over total assets (FATA), (3) overseas subsidiaries as a percentage of total subsidiaries (OSTS), (4) top management's international experience (TMIE), and (5) psychic dispersion of international operations (PDIO).

In this study we follow a similar approach by measuring multinationality through three measures: (1) foreign sales/total sales (FSTS), (2) foreign profit/total profits (FPTP), and (3) foreign assets/total assets (FATA). As shown in Table 2D.1, one common factor appears to explain the intercorrelations among the three variables, as the first eigenvalue alone exceeds the sum of commonalities. The common factor is significantly and positively correlated with the three measures. The factor scores were used to measure the degree of multinationality of firms in the sample.

Measuring Corporate Reputation

A multiple-constituency view of effectiveness is used in this study, where organizational effectiveness measures the extent to which an organization meets the needs, expectations, and demands of important external constituencies beyond those directly associated with the company's products and markets (Riahi-Belkaoui and Pavlik, 1992). A good example of the multiple constituency view is the annual reputational index of corporations disclosed by *Fortune* magazine.

The *Fortune* survey covers every industry group comprising four or more companies. The industry groups are based on categories established by the U.S. Office of Management and Budget (OMB). The survey asked executives, directors, and analysts in particular to rate a company on the following eight key attributes of reputation:

Table 2D.1
Selected Statistics Related to a Common Factor Analysis of Three Measures of Multinationality for *Forbes'* "Most International 100 U.S. Firms" for the 1987– 1990 Period

1.　Eigenvalues of the Correlation Matrix:

Eigenvalues	1	2	3
	1.8963	0.9169	0.1868

2.　Factor Pattern
FACTOR 1

FS/TS	0.93853
FP/TP	0.40913
FA/TA	0.92089

3.　Final Communality Estimates: Total = 1.389626

FS/TS	FP/TP	FA/TA
0.8808	0.16738	0.84804

4.　Standardized Scoring Coefficients
FACTOR 1

FS/TS	0.49494
FP/TP	0.21575
FA/TA	0.48563

5.　Descriptive Statistics of the Common Factor Extracted from the Three Measures of Multinationality

Maximum	201.051
Third Quartile	52.231
Median	41.501
First Quartile	30.648
Minimum	5.198
Mean	43.062

Variable definitions:
FS/TS: Foreign sales/ Total sales.
FP/TP: Foreign profits/Total profits.
FA/TA: Foreign assets/Total assets.

1. Quality of management

2. Quality of products/services offered

3. Innovativeness

4. Value as long-term investment

5. Soundness of financial position

6. Ability to attract/develop/keep talented people

7. Responsibility to the community/environment

8. Wise use of corporate assets

Table 2D.2
Selected Statistics Related to a Common Factor Analysis of Measures of Reputation

1.   Eigenvalues of the Correlation Matrix:
Eigenvalues

1	2	3	4	5	6	7	8
6.7805	0.5562	0.3835	0.1343	0.1808	0.0544	0.0476	0.0331

2.   Factor Pattern*
FACTOR 1

R_1 0.9537	R_4 0.9650	R_7 0.8080
R_2 0.9184	R_5 0.8987	R_8 0.9484
R_3 0.8796	R_6 0.9809	

3.   Final Communality Estimates: Total = 1.389626

R_1	R_2	R_3	R_4	R_5	R_6	R_7	R_8
0.9096	0.8435	0.7737	0.9312	0.8077	0.9621	0.6520	0.8996

4.   Standardized Scoring Coefficients
FACTOR 1

R_1 0.1406	R_4 0.1423	R_7 0.1191
R_2 0.1354	R_5 0.1325	R_8 0.1398
R_3 0.1279	R_6 0.1446	

Descriptive Statistics of the Common Factor Extracted from the Eight Measures of Reputation

Maximum	9.001
Third Quartile	7.274
Median	6.604
First Quartile	6.076
Minimum	3.154
Mean	6.592

* R_1 = Quality of management.
  R_2 = Quality of products/services.
  R_3 = Innovativeness.
  R_4 = Value as long-term investment.
  R_5 = Soundness of financial position.
  R_6 = Ability to attract, develop and keep talented people.
  R_7 = Responsibility to the community and environment.
  R_8 = Wise use of corporate assets.

Ratings were on a scale of 0 (poor) to 10 (excellent). The score met the multiple-constituency ecological model view of organizational effectiveness. For purposes of this study, the 1987 to 1990 *Fortune* magazine surveys were used. To obtain a unique configuration, a factor analysis is used to isolate the factor common to the eight measures of reputation. All the observations were subjected to factor analysis, and one common factor was found to explain the intercorrelations among the eight individual measures. Table 2D.2 reports the results of

the common factor analysis. One common factor appears to explain the inter-correlations among the eight variables, as the first eigenvalue alone exceeds the sum of the commonalities. The common factor is significantly and positively correlated with the eight measures. As pointed out earlier, based on the factor scores, high-reputation firms were chosen from the top 24 percent of the distri-bution factor scores while low-reputation firms were chosen from the bottom 25 percent of the distribution factor scores.

RESULTS

Panel A of Table 2D.3 reports descriptive statistics for the variables used in our tests and panel B shows correlations among variables. The correlations re-ported in panel B of Table 2D.3 show that all correlations between MV_{it}, A_{it}, CF_{it}, $MULTY_{it}$, and REP_{it} are significant at the 0.01 level. The significant as-sociation among these variables indicates some degree of collinearity among the independent variables in the regression analyses. However, the maximum con-dition index in all subsequent regressions with earnings and both cash flow variables is only 4.45. As suggested by Belsey et al. (1980), mild collinearity is diagnosed for maximum condition indices between 5 and 10, and severe collinearity for an index over 30. Thus, collinearity does not seem to influence results.

For each of the multivariate regressions to be reported, we perform additional specification tests, including checks for normality and consideration of various scatter plots. A null hypothesis of normality could not be rejected at the 0.01 level in all cases, and the plots revealed some heteroskedasticity but no other obvious problems. Therefore, we calculated the *t*-statistics after correcting for heteroskedasticity.

Table 2D.3 presents the regression results for equations (1) to (3). Equation (1) relates the total market value deflated by total assets to the accruals and cash flows from operations, also deflated by total assets. As shown in Table 2D.4, the coefficient for total accruals is significantly negative, while the coefficient for cash flows is significantly positive. As expected, the total market value is negatively related to the total accruals and positively related to cash flows. As in Wilson (1986), these results show that the market reacts favorably the larger (smaller) are the cash flows (current accruals). At the same time, the results show that accruals and cash flows from operations provide incremental value-relevance beyond one another in explaining market value.

Equation (2) relates the total market value to multinationality in addition to accruals and cash flows from operations. As shown in Table 2D.4 the coefficient of multinationality is significantly positive at the 0.01 level. In addition, R^2 increased from 62.96 percent in equation (1) to 73.28 percent in equation (2). The evidence suggests that multinationality provides incremental value-relevance beyond accruals and cash flows in explaining market value.

Table 2D.3
Descriptive Statistics and Correlations

Panel A: Descriptive Correlations

Variables	Mean	Standard Deviation	Minimum	25%	Median	75%	Maximum
MV_{it}	0.894	0.791	0.018	0.381	0.665	1.132	5
A_t	0.047	0.024	0.010	0.031	0.047	0.062	0.175
CF_{it}	0.104	0.062	0.052	0.065	0.112	0.143	0.254
$MULTY_{it}$	43.062	19.682	5.198	30.648	41.503	52.231	201.059
REP_{it}	6.592	0.974	3.154	6.076	6.604	7.264	9.001

Panel B: Correlations

	MV_{it}	A_t	CF_I	$MULTY_{it}$	REP_{it}
MV_{it}	1.000				
A_t	0.061*	1.000			
CF_I	0.717*	0.454*	1.000		
$MULTY_{it}$	0.096*	0.023	-0.012	1.000	
REP_{it}	0.512*	0.070	0.495*	0.009	1.000

MV_{it} = Market value of equity for firm i in period t.
A_{it} = Total accruals for firm i in period t.
CF_{it} = Cash flows from operations for firm i in period t.
$MULTY_{it}$ = Index of multinationality for firm i in period t.
REP_{it} = Index of reputation for firm i in period t.
*Significant at $\alpha = 0.01$.

Equation (3) relates the market value to the accounting variables of accruals and cash flows and the nonaccounting variables of multinationality and corporate reputation. As shown in Table 2D.4, the coefficient for corporate reputation (0.0821) is significantly positive at the 0.01 level. This evidence suggests that corporate reputation provides incremental value relevance beyond accruals, cash flows, and multinationality in explaining market value.

To rule out the possibility that the total accruals and cash flows are proxying for cross-sectional differences in industry membership, the regressions were also run with a dummy variable representing twenty-two industries. The industry dummy variable was found to be insignificant.

Table 2D.4
Regression Results of Linear Models[1]

	Model 1	Model 2	Model 3
Intercept	0.1703 (2.737)*	-0.1082 (-1.36)	-0.6129 (-2.870)
A_{it}	-11.2791 (-9.521)*	-16.7071 (-14.621)*	-16.2253 (-12.406)*
CF_{it}	11.8366 (24.703)*	14.6982 (30.106)*	13.8484 (22.240)*
$MULTY_{it}$		0.0043 (3.3347)*	0.0047 (3.253)
REP_{it}			0.0821 (2.534)*
Adjusted R^2	0.6296	0.7328	0.7588
N	360		

Notes:
1. Model 1: $MV_{it} = a_0 + a_{1t} A_{it} + a_{2i} CF_{it} + e_{it}$.
Model 2: $MV_{it} = a_0 + a_{1t} A_{it} + a_{2i} CF_{it} + a_{3i} MULTY_{it} + e^1_{it}$.
Model 3: $MV_{it} = a_0 + a_{1t} A_{it} + a_{2i} CF_{it} + a_{3i} MULTY_{it} + REP_{it} + e^2_{it}$.
2. MV = Market value of equity of firm i at the end of year t.
A_{it} = Total accruals of firm i at the end of year t.
CF_{it} = Cash flows of firm i at the end of year t.
$MULTY_{it}$ = Level of multinationality of firm i at the end of year t.
REP_{it} = Corporate reputation score for firm i at the end of year t.
*Significant at 0.001 level.
**Significant at 0.05 level.

SUMMARY AND CONCLUSIONS

This appendix examined the generality and robustness of an accrual and cash flow based model that includes the contextual factors of multinationality and corporate reputation. The evidence confirms previous results presented by Wilson (1986) using total market value as a dependent variable and a price level rather than a return/changes regression. Basically, the larger (smaller) the market value, the larger (smaller) the cash flows (current accruals). In addition, the preference of cash flows over accruals arises under conditions of high multinationality and high corporate reputation. The results verify the economic logic

underlying how the market assimilates information about cash and accruals under the specific contexts of multinationality and reputation. First, a price level regression seems to provide a better specification of this economic logic. Second, contextual factors play a fundamental role in the same economic logic. Future research needs to examine the role of other contextual factors in the determination of the relationship between the market value and accruals and cash flows.

REFERENCES

Agmon, T., and D. Lessard. (1977). Investor Recognition of Corporate International Diversification. *Journal of Finance* 32, 1049–1055.

Belkaoui, A. (1992). Organizational Effectiveness, Social Performance and Economic Performance. *Research in Corporate Social Performance and Policy* 12, 143–155.

Belsey, D., E. Kuh, and R. Welsch. (1980). *Regression Diagnostics*. New York: John Wiley & Sons.

Bernard, V., and T. Stober. (1989). The Nature and Amount of Information in Cash Flows and Accruals. *The Accounting Review* (October), 624–652.

Dunning, J.H. (1995). Reappraising the Eclectic Paradigm in an Age of Alliance Capitalism. *Journal of International Business Studies* 26, 461–492.

Errunza, V., and L. Senbet. (1981). The Effects of International Corporate Diversification, Market Valuation and Size Adjusted Evidence. *Journal of Finance* 11, 717–743.

Fombrum, C., and M. Shanley. (1990). What's in a Name? Reputational Building and Corporate Strategy. *Academy of Management Journal* 33, 233–258.

Healy, P.M. (1985). The Effect of Bonus Schemes on Accounting Decisions. *Journal of Accounting and Economics* 7, 85–107.

Perlmutter, H.V. (1969). The Tortuous Evaluation of the Multinational Corporation. *Columbia Journal of World Business* 7, 9–18.

Riahi-Belkaoui, A., and E. Pavlik. (1991). Asset Management Performance and Reputation Building for Large U.S. Firms. *British Journal of Management* 2, 231–238.

Riahi-Belkaoui, A., and E. Pavlik. (1992). *Accounting for Corporate Reputation*. Westport, CT: Quorum Books.

Spence, A.M. (1974). *Market Signaling: Information Transfer in Hiring and Related Screening Process*. Cambridge, MA: Harvard University Press.

Stopford, J.M., and L.T. Wells. (1972). *Managing the Multinational Enterprise*. New York: Basic Books.

Sullivan, D. (1994). Measuring the Degree of Internationalization of a Firm. *Journal of International Business Studies* 25, 325–342.

Wilson, P. (1986). The Relative Information Content of Accruals and Cash Flows: Combined Evidence at the Earnings Announcement and Annual Report Release Date. *Journal of Accounting Research* (September), 165–200.

Yang, H., J. Wansley, and W. Lane. (1985). Stock Market Recognition of Multinationality of a Firm and International Events. *Journal of Business, Finance, and Accounting* 2, 263–274.

Chapter 3

Creativity in Accounting

INTRODUCTION

Creativity in accounting implies a liberal interpretation of accounting rules, allowing choices that may result in a depiction of financial situations that are more or less optimistic than the real situations. The creativity in accounting may take different forms depending on the objectives of the preparers of the accounting reports. These forms of creativity in accounting are generally known in practice and in the literature as (1) the selective financial misrepresentation hypothesis, (2) big bath accounting, and (3) creative accounting. Each of these forms is explicated and illustrated in this chapter as evidence of this general thesis of "designed" versus "principle" accounting.

THE SELECTIVE FINANCIAL MISREPRESENTATION HYPOTHESIS

Accounting information is basically the accounting surrogate used by decision makers who can't rely on directly observed events. A manipulation of these surrogates provides decision makers with the opportunity of sending signals that shape people's perceptions of managerial performance, which is made possible by arbitrary, complicated, and misleading rules. The selective financial misrepresentation hypothesis as advanced by Revsine[1] maintains, "The problem is not accidental, but instead results from contrived and flexible reporting rules promulgated by standard setters who have been 'captured' by the intended regulatees and others involved in the financial reporting process."[2] The "capturing" refers to the process where the main objective of regulation, which is the protection of consumers, is reversed to make the regulatees the beneficiaries.[3] The

selective financial representation hypothesis is assumed to be across both public and private sectors "since participation in both sectors is motivated to support standards that selectively misrepresent economic reality when it suits their purpose."[4] It applies to managers, shareholders, auditors, and standard setters.

1. Managers prefer "loose" reporting standards over tight standards because they allow (1) a shifting of income between years more favorable to bonus attainment, (2) impressing the shareholders, and (3) protecting their jobs by forestalling takeovers.[5]

2. Shareholders benefit also from the loose standards given that the smoothing of reporting earnings by managers lowers the volatility of reported earnings, lowering the market's perception of default risk and increasing firm value.

3. Auditors may prefer the same reporting rules that distort economic reality for client *harmony* or rigid rules when they present a convenient shield to hide behind.[6]

4. Standard setters may favor the self-misrepresentation hypothesis for both self-protection and altruism.

5. Academics may favor the selective misrepresentation hypothesis as it provides them with the opportunity of providing theories and proposals in exchange for more remuneration and prestige.

The situation calls for a change by insulating the standard-setting process from regulatory capture. Revsine suggests the following four-step process:

1. educating the public,

2. improving the process for selecting and monitoring standard setters,

3. establishing new funding arrangements, and

4. creating independence for the standard setters.[7]

SEC Chairman Levitt proposed a six-part action plan to address these issues and improve the "reliability and transparency" of financial statements:

• Public companies will be required to make detailed disclosures about the impact of changes in accounting assumptions so that the market can "better understand the nature and effects of the restructuring liabilities and other loss accruals."

• New SEC guidance will emphasize "the need to consider qualitative, not just quantitative factors" when judging materiality.

• The American Institute of Certified Public Accountants (AICPA) will clarify the rules for auditing purchased research and development and "argue for existing guidance on restructuring, large acquisition write-offs, and revenue recognition practices."

• Additional SEC guidance on revenue recognition may be published. This project will consider the applicability of recently adopted software revenue recognition standards to other industries.

• The FASB will accelerate certain projects that relate to the definition of constructive liability.

• The SEC's Divisions of Enforcement and Corporation Finance will review companies that announce "restructuring liability reserves, major write-offs, or other practices that appear to manage earnings."[8]

"BIG BATH" ACCOUNTING

"Big bath" accounting refers generally to the steps taken by management to drastically reduce current earnings per share in order to increase future earnings per share. The situation is akin to a choice of income-decreasing procedures that increase the probability of meeting future earnings' targets. As stated by Healy,

[I]f earnings are so low that no matter which accounting procedures are selected target earnings will not be met, managers have incentives to further reduce current earnings by deferring revenues on accelerating write-offs, a strategy known as "taking a bath."[9]

The big bath procedure may generally follow a change in the management, giving an opportunity to new managers to develop a lower income anchor against which they will be evaluated in the future, guaranteeing themselves an initial good performance.[10]

A good description of "big bath" follows:

Companies are most likely to take a big bath during particular periods. First, when new managers take over, they are tempted to write off the old projects and assets of their predecessors to show strong improvements during the coming years. Second, when a company has a large nonrecurring gain, it might search for expenses to charge against it. And third, when earnings are particularly weak, management sees an opportunity to shift additional expenses (which will most likely not even be noticed) to the current period. The benefit, naturally, is that the additional current changes mean fewer changes in the future.[11]

Another good definition of "big bath" follows:

The bath is described as a "clean up" of balance sheet accounts. Assets are written down or written off, and provisions are made for estimated losses and expenses which may be incurred in the future. These actions decrease income or increase losses for the current period while relieving future income of expenses, which it would otherwise have had to absorb. In simple terms taking a bath tends to inflate future income by depressing current income.[12]

Most of the evidence in "big bath" accounting is anecdotal and of a journalistic nature.

The following three stories give good examples of how "big bath" accounting is used.

1. In December 1990, the Financial Accounting Standards Board (FASB) issued Statement No. 106, "Employers' Accounting for Post Retirement Benefits

Other than Pensions" to account for health care and other welfare benefits provided to retirees, their spouses, dependents, and beneficiaries. These other welfare benefits refer to life insurance offered outside a pension plan, dental care as well as medical care, eye care, legal and tax services, tuition assistance, day care, and housing assistance. At the time of the adoption of FASB Statement No. 106, a transitional amount is computed. It is equal to the difference between (1) the accumulated postretirement benefit obligation (APBO) and (2) the fair value of the plan assets, plus any accrued obligation or less any prepaid cost (asset). Given that most plans were unfunded and most employees were accruing benefits costs for the first time, the transition amounts were material. The choices were either (1) an immediate charge to expense for unrecognized past costs as well as recognition of the total unrecognized liability, which will create a major drain on the reported earnings in the year of change, or (2) deferral and amortization of the expense, as well as the recognition of a rapidly increasing liability, which will create a major drain on the earnings for many years.[13] The choice of the first option will constitute a good example of a "big bath" choice. In fact, the adoption of FASB No. 106 led (1) IBM to declare a $2.3 billion change, resulting in IBM's first-ever quarterly loss in March 1991, (2) General Electric Co. to declare a $2.7 billion change, and (3) AT&T to absorb a $2.1 billion pretax hit for postretirement benefits in the fourth quarter of 1993.[14]

2. In March 2001, Procter & Gamble announced that it would take a $1.4 billion change to reduce its workforce by 9 percent or 9,600 employees. These changes followed a $2.1 billion restructuring effort that started in 1999. Then, in June 2001 the company announced that it would take another change of $900 million to write off underperforming assets. This is a good example of a "big bath" approach that seems unending, stretching the definition of onetime expense too liberally.

3. Nortel Networks, a company that stood in the year 2000 as a glamour stock, declared a $19.2 billion loss in the second quarter of the year 2001. The $19.2 billion loss exceeded the annual gross domestic product of El Salvador and approaches that of Bolivia. In a year the market value of the company shrank by one-quarter trillion dollars. Of this $19.2 billion loss, $12.3 billion was a write-off that Nortel was taking in goodwill on recent acquisitions. The story unfolds as follows. In the year 2000 Nortel went on an acquisition spree, acquiring eleven technology concerns at a time when its own tangible assets were just $167 million. This did not stop Nortel from paying an exorbitant $19.7 billion, mostly in shares for the acquisitions, which was equivalent to 118 times the value of these acquired companies. For example, in 2000 Nortel paid Xros $3.2 billion in stock at a time when Xros' tangible assets were $3 million. This "big bath" story is a good example of a management making blundering buys and then trying to start again from scratch.

CREATIVE ACCOUNTING

Creative accounting is a term generally used in the popular press to refer to what journalists suspect that accountants do to make financial results look much better than they should. This suspicion is prevalent in most countries. It is most acknowledged in the United States by Schilit,[15] in the United Kingdom by Griffiths,[16] in France by Stolowy,[17] and in Australia by Rennie[18] and Craig and Walsh.[19] As a result of this international evidence in the phenomenon, creative accounting has acquired various characterizations and definitions. Descriptions of creative accounting follow:

1. Creative accounting represents the means by which is achieved a deviation between accounts that are anything other than an approximation and that have their basis in the transactions and events of the year under review and the original starting point.[20]

2. Creative accounting involves manipulation, deceit, and misrepresentation.[21]

3. Creative accounting involves an accounting sleight of hand.[22]

4. Creative accounting include activities such as "fiddling the books," "cosmetic reporting," and "window dressing."[23]

5. Creative accounting is the "transformation of financial accounting figures from what they actually are to what preparers desire by taking advantage of the existing rules and/or ignoring some or all of them."[24] It involves both "window dressing" and "off-balance sheet financing." Window dressing is defined as the arrangement of affairs so that the financial statements give a misleading or unrepresentative impression of their financial position.[25] Off-balance sheet financing is defined as "the funding or refunding of a company's operations in such a way that, under legal requirements and existing accounting conventions, some or all of the finance may not be shown on its balance sheet."[26]

6. Creative accounting was also referred to as the use of accounting gimmicks to boost anemic earnings or to smooth out erratic earnings.[27] This is accomplished by the use of seven major shenanigans defined as follows:

   a. Recording revenue before it is earned

   b. Creating fictitious revenue

   c. Boosting profits with nonrecurring transactions

   d. Shifting current expenses to a later period

   e. Failing to record or disclose liabilities

   f. Shifting current income to a later period

   g. Shifting future expenses to an earlier period.[28]

Shenanigans are defined as follows:

Unlike obscenity, financial shenanigans are easy to define but more difficult to detect in practice. Financial shenanigans are actions or omissions intended to hide or distort the real financial performance or financial condition of an entity. They range from minor

deceptions (such as failing to clearly segregate operating from non-operating gains and losses) to more serious misapplications of accounting principles (such as failing to write off worthless assets; they also include fraudulent behavior, such as the recording of fictitious revenue to overstate the real financial performance).[29]

EXAMPLES OF CREATIVE ACCOUNTING

Examples of creative accounting from different countries have been documented in the literature. In France, the titles of professional and academic articles give a clear appreciation of the magnitude and the gravity of the problem. The terms and/or titles include[30] (1) the "art of cooking the books,"[31] (2) "the art of computing its profits,"[32] (3) "the art of presenting a balance sheet,"[33] (4) "the provisions or the art of saving money,"[34] (5) "a fine art."[35] Like human beings, French accounts are "made up,"[36] with "their book unproved,"[37] getting a "face lift"[38] with "depreciation muscled and provisions plumped,"[39] "dressed,"[40] and "cleaned."[41] Stolowy[42] goes one step further by identifying the options available within French generally accepted accounting principles that can be used to generate creative accounting solutions; similar categories were also offered by Bonnet.[43]

Evidence for creative accounting was also noticed for Spain.[44] But, the United States and the United Kingdom seem to provide a more favorable terrain for the creative accounting process. The U.K. evidence on creative accounting is provided by Griffiths,[45] Naser,[46] and Smith.[47] Smith's book identifies specific cases of creative accounting in the use of accounting techniques on acquisition and disposal, extraordinary and exceptional items, off-balance-sheet finance, contingent liabilities, capitalization of costs, brand accounting, changes in depreciation policy, convertibles with put options, pension fund accounting, and currency mismatching.[48] The following clever explanation is provided for the choice of the title of the book:

The title *Accounting for Growth* was a deliberate pun. We feel that much of the apparent growth in profits which had occurred in the 1980's was the result of accounting sleight of hand rather than genuine economic growth, and we set out to expose the main techniques involved, and to give live examples of companies using those techniques.[49]

Naser defined creative accounting as

1) the process of manipulating accounting figures by taking advantage of the loopholes in accounting rules and the choices of measurement and disclosure practices in them to transform financial statements from what they should be, to what preparers would prefer to see reported, and 2) the process by which transactions are structured so as to produce the required accounting results rather than reporting transactions in a neutral and consistent way.[50]

From a review of the literature he identified the following factors that may motivate managers to adopt creative accounting schemes:

1. *Misinformation, signaling, and financial motives.* This argument is derived from Peasnell and Yaansah's[51] distinction between the misinformation and signaling motives and financial motives to establish creative accounting schemes.[52]

2. *The agency and the political cost incentives.* This argument is derived from the argument that the choice of accounting techniques depends on the political process of cash flow effects and contracting.

3. *Poor management.* This argument is derived from the thesis that poor management, by neglecting the system of accounting information and failing to respond to change, resorts to creative accounting to reduce the predictive nature of certain ratios.[53]

4. *Reducing the uncertainty and risk.* This is derived from an argument made by Goodfellow[54] that creative accounting schemes are used as a result of increased volatility in the related market elements, interest, inflation and exchange rates.

5. *The weakness of the current accounting concepts, particularly under inflation.* This is derived from arguments made that off-balance-sheet financing schemes are the result of the lack of authoritative accounting guidance in the subject,[55] and as a result of the failure of historical cost accounting to deal effectively with inflation.[56]

Naser[57] also illustrated schemes of creative accounting associated with short-term investment, accounting for stock, accounting for tangible fixed assets, accounting for intangible assets, accounting for long-term liabilities, and accounting for shareholders' contributed capital. Griffiths[58] illustrated similar schemes associated with income and expenses, foreign currencies, pensions, stock, current assets, share capital, fixed assets, cash and borrowings, off-balance-sheet financing, acquisitions and mergers, brands and goodwill, and deferred taxation. Despite the Accounting Standards Board's (ASB) effort to outflow the most flagrant abuses, creative accounting goes on in the United Kingdom. Griffiths offers the following explanation:

The biggest problem it [the ASB] faces is the unwitting conspiracy between the city and the industry which ensures that the black and white which so many appear to demand will be condemned always to a murky grey. While much is made of the tension between companies and their investors there is a remarkable overlap in their interests. Both would like to see a steady increase in a business's earnings growth profile. In reality it is rarely achievable. However, that does nothing to diminish the zealous pursuit of this elusive holy grail.[59]

In the U.S. context, various books presented flagrant cases of creative accounting.[60] The most recent example by Schilit identified seven so-called shenanigans. They are discussed as follows:

1. The first shenanigan consists of recording revenue too soon, either before the earnings process has been completed or before an exchange has occurred. It is generally done by

   a. shipping goods before a sale is finalized.

   b. Recording revenue when important uncertainties exist as in the cases where (1) the risks and the benefit of ownership have not been transferred to the buyer, (2) the buyer may return the goods, and (3) the buyer may not pay for the goods.

   c. Recording revenue when future services are still due, especially in the case of hasty recognition of franchise revenue.

2. The second shenanigan consists of recording bogus revenues. It is generally done by:

   a. Recording income on exchange of similar assets.

   b. Recording refunds from suppliers as revenue.

   c. Using bogus estimates of interim financial reports.[61]

3. The third shenanigan consists of boosting income with onetime gains. It is generally done by:

   a. Boosting profits by selling undervalued assets where the undervaluation was a result of one of the following situations:

     • "A Company acquired assets in a business combination that was accounted for as a pooling of interest.

     • A Company uses the LIFO [last in, first out] inventory method (especially with many inventory pools).

     • A Company acquired real estate (or other investments) years ago that has appreciated considerably in value."[62]

   b. Boosting profits by retiring debt.

   c. Failing to segregate unusual and nonrecurring gains or losses from recurring income.

   d. Burying losses under noncontinuing operations.

4. The fourth shenanigan consists of shifting current expenses to a later permit. It is generally done by:

   a. Improperly capitalizing costs, notably start-up costs.

   b. Depreciating or amortizing costs too slowly by choosing long amortization periods for intangibles and leasehold improvements and by increasing the depreciation or amortization period.

   c. Failing to write off worthless assets by not writing off bad loans and other uncollectibles and by keeping worthless investments on the books.[63]

5. The fifth shenanigan consists of failing to record or disclose all liabilities. It is generally done by:

   a. Reporting revenue rather than a liability when cash is received.

   b. Failing to accrue expected or contingent liabilities.

   c. Failing to disclose commitments and contingencies.

   d. Engaging in transactions to keep debt off the books.[64]

6. The sixth shenanigan consists of shifting current income to a later period by creating reserves to shift sales revenue to a later period.

7. The seventh shenanigan consists of shifting future expenses to the current period. It is done by:

a. Accelerating discretionary expenses into the current period by prepaying operating expenses or decreasing the depreciation or amortization period.

b. Writing off future years' depreciation or amortization.[65]

FLEXIBILITY AND CREATIVE ACCOUNTING

The U.S. generally accepted accounting principles have tended to shy away from rigid positions in accounting problems and provided flexibility allowing judgment and choices among various options. What resulted from this flexibility and the need to exercise judgment is a move toward creativity in the judgment, leading potentially to creative accounting schemes. In short, there is a continuum of thinking going from flexibility to creativity to creative accounting.

As stated by Jameson:

Creative accounting is not against the law. It operates within the letter both of the law and of accounting standards but it is quite clearly against the spirit of both. . . . It is essentially a process of using the rules, the flexibility provided by them and the omissions within them, to make financial statements look somewhat different from what was intended by the rule. It consists of rule-bending and loophole-seeking.[66]

In what follows, some of the options available under U.S. GAAP that may lead to creativity and creative accounting are presented.

The Balance Sheet

1. The balance sheet is supposed to be a reflection of the financial structure of the firm. Unfortunately, historical cost is the common valuation basis of most assets and liabilities. What's missing are the current values of the assets and liabilities as well as significant nonquantitative information. Basically, the historical cost basis is a "creative accounting" device used for the sake of practicality and verifiability to avoid showing the fair value of the firm.

2. The assets are segregated in current and noncurrent assets where the rule of thumb is that if an asset is to be turned into cash or to be used to pay a current liability within a year of the operating cycle, whichever is longer, that asset is considered a current asset. The classification scheme is arbitrary and can easily be used as a form of creative accounting classification.

3. Each type of assets and liabilities can be classified or measured according to different options and refinements available within generally accepted accounting principles and therefore is an ideal tool for creative accounting. They are illustrated in the next sections of this chapter.

4. The balance sheet is a stock concept, reflecting the so-called financial structure at one time, which is the end of the fiscal year. Between the end of the year and issuance of the balance sheet, subsequent events or post–balance sheet events need to be disclosed in the notes. These events generally provide

evidence about conditions that (1) either existed at the balance sheet, affect the estimates used in preparing financial statements, and call for additional adjustments or (2) existed after the balance sheet date and call for additional disclosure. Examples of subsequent events that require disclosure include:

a. Sale of bonds or capital stock; stock splits or stock dividends.

b. Business combination pending or effected.

c. Settlement of litigation when the event giving rise to the claim took place subsequent to the balance sheet date.

d. Loss of plant or inventories from fire or flood.

e. Losses on receivables resulting from conditions (such as customer's major casualty) arising subsequent to the balance sheet date.

f. Gains or losses on certain marketable securities.[67]

A form of creative accounting is the failure to adjust and/or disclose these events.

Income Statement

1. The bottom figure of net income for the year does not reveal the real picture. More useful insights are revealed from a segregation of results from regular continuing operations from the results of nonrecurring activities. For example, an $18.6 million income reported by National Patent Development, a maker of soft contact lenses, is a markup of (1) $7.5 million of income from gain on the sale of stock by a subsidiary, (2) $2.4 million gain in the exchange of stock, (3) $ 3.6 million from gain on the sale of stock in its investment portfolio, and (4) $3.2 million from the settlement of lawsuits related to patent infringements. These nonoperating or nonrecurring gains are not sustainable.[68]

2. The income figures are much affected by the type of accounting methods in general and allocation methods in particular. One can just imagine the surprise of those actors, writers, and producers who signed "net profit contracts" in highly successful movies to find out later that, thanks to big studios' ability to allocate overhead costs creatively, the movies declared a loss.

3. Revenues consist generally of sales, fees, interest, dividends, and rents while gains and losses consist of many types resulting from the sale of investments, sale of plant assets, settlement of liabilities, write-off of assets due to obsolescence or casualty, and theft; expenses consists of cost of goods sold, depreciation, interest, rent, salaries and wages, and taxes. Creative accounting blurs the distinction between revenues and gains and between expenses and losses to highlight a different performance[69] between operating activities and nonoperating activities. For example, loss-reporting Internet firms may want to highlight a positive gross margin by shifting some product costs to period costs or to unusual activities.

4. Most firms have adopted a "modified, all-inclusive concept" with irregular items classified in the following five general categories:

a. Discontinued operations
b. Extraordinary items
c. Unusual gains and losses
d. Changes in accounting principle
e. Changes in estimate

Each of these categories leads to good potential for creative accounting. Let's examine each:

Discontinued operation. The profession requires that the results of operations of a segment that will be disposed of be reported in conjunction with the gain and loss on disposal, separately from continuing operations. However, the disposal of a part of a business, the shifting of activities from one time of a business to another, and the phasing out of a product line and the changes due to technological improvement, which all contribute to disposal of assets, are not considered disposals of a segment or a business and are not classified as discontinued operations. In addition, if a loss is expected on disposal, the estimated loss is reported at the measurement date, while an expected gain is reported when realized, which is ordinarily the disposal date. The conservative position creates an opportunity for immediate recognition of losses and a deferring of gains until realized.

Extraordinary items. APB opinion No. 30 gives the following definitions:

"Extraordinary items are events and transactions that are distinguished by their unusual nature and by the infrequency of their occurrence." Both of the following criteria must be met to classify an event or transaction as an extraordinary item:

a. Unusual Nature. The underlying event or transaction should possess a high degree of abnormality and be of a type clearly unrelated to, or only incidentally related to, the ordinary and typical activities of the entity, taking into account the environment in which the entity operates.
b. Infrequency of Occurrence. The underlying event or transaction should be of a type that would not reasonably be expected to recur in the foreseeable future, taking into account the environment in which the entity operates.[70]

In addition, the APB indicated that the following gains and losses are not extraordinary items:

a. Write-down or write-off of receivables, inventories, equipment leased to others, deferred research and development costs, or other intangible assets.
b. Gains or losses from exchange or translation of foreign currencies, including those relating to major devaluations and revaluations.

c. Gains or losses on disposal of a segment of a business.

d. Other gains or losses from sale or abandonment of property, plant, or equipment used in the business.

e. Effects of strikes, including those against competitors and major suppliers.

f. Adjustment of accruals on long-term contracts.[71]

This definition makes it difficult to classify an item as extraordinary. At the same time it allows the exercise of a lot of judgment in determining whether an item should be reported as extraordinary. A firm may consider a write-down or write-off of receivables or inventory an extraordinary item if it can prove that they are the result of an "unusual" and "infrequent" event such as an earthquake. The creative accounting part resides in finding the good excuse of "unusual" and "infrequent" nature of the activity. This situation is helped by the inconsistent professional position that considers (1) the disposal of a business segment at a gain or loss not as an extraordinary item and (2) the material gains or losses from extinguishment of debt as an extraordinary item.

Unusual gains and losses. These are unusual or infrequent items that are disclosed separately from extraordinary items. The most frequent and abused item, a sign of creative accounting, is the well-known and well-used restructuring change relating to major reorganization of a company's affairs, such as costs incurred for employee layoffs, plant closings, write offs of assets, and so on. Some firms tend to exaggerate with this form of creative accounting, such as when restructuring changes were taken six years in a row between 1988 and 1993 by Citicorp, five out of six years in 1988–1994 by Eastman Kodak Co., and seven out of ten years from 1985 to 1994 by Westinghouse Electric. These known "first cousins" to extraordinary gains and losses are the most flagrant form of creative accounting in the income statement.

Changes in accounting principle. The adoption of an accounting principle different from the one previously used is recognized by the inclusion of the cumulative effect net of tax in the current year's income statement. The change of inventory method or depreciation method may be dictated by either economic circumstances or purely creative accounting purposes to affect the level of profit.

Changes in estimates. They are normal, nonrecurring corrections and adjustments, such as changes in the realizability of receivables and inventories, changes in estimated lives of equipment, intangible assets, changes in estimated liability for warranty costs, income taxes and salary payments that change the income statement only in the account affected. They provide ideal options for creative accounting.

5. While the income contains all the revenues, expenses, gains, and losses recognized during a period, many items bypass income and are "dumped" directly in the equity section as "comprehensive income." Examples of these items include gains and losses in available-for-sale securities.

Cash

1. Cash consists of coin, currency, available funds on deposits at the bank, and negotiable instruments such as money orders, certified checks, cashier's checks, personal checks, and bank drafts. Money market funds are generally classified as temporary investments. If they provide checking account privileges, they are classified as cash. Checking account privileges can increase cash and decrease temporary investments.

2. Lending institutions may require firms to maintain a minimum cash balance in checking or saving accounts, known as compensating balances. These legally restructured deposits need to be disclosed separately among the "cash and cash equivalent items" in current assets. Similarly, restricted cash for specific purposes such as petty cash, payroll, and dividend funds also deserves a separate classification. The separate classification applies also to bank overdraft.

3. Short-term paper needs to be classified as temporary investments. Similarly, postdated checks and IOUs should be classified as receivables, while postage in hand should be classified as prepaid expenses. Any misclassification of accounts cited in the previous paragraphs is merely an attempt at creative accounting.

Receivables

1. A distinction should be made between trade receivables and nontrade receivables. Examples of nontrade receivables include (1) advances to employees and subsidiaries, (2) dividends and interest receivable, (3) deposits to cover potential damages and losses, (4) deposits as guarantee of performance in payments, and (5) claims. These nontrade receivables may be classified as accounts receivable or notes receivable.

2. Short-term receivables are valued and reported at then net realizable value, which is what is expected to be received in cash. This requires the estimation of both uncollectible receivables and any returns and allowances to be granted. Recording the uncollectibles may be either through the direct write-off method or the allowance method. The allowance method allows either the use of percentage-of-sales (income statement) approach, the percentage-of-receivable (balance sheet) approach, or the aging schedule approach. While the percentage-of-receivable approach provides a more accurate valuation of receivables in the balance sheet, the percentage-of-sales approach provides better matching in the income statement.

3. More creative accounting is possible in the creation of two other contra accounts to the accounts receivable, namely, the allowance for sales returns and allowances and the allowance for collection expenses.

4. Accounts or notes receivables may be transferred to another company for cash. Depending on meeting specific conditions, the transfer may be accounted for as a secured borrowing or a sale of receivables, with a different impact in

the balance sheet. A sale occurs if these conditions are met: (1) the transferred assets are isolated from the transferer, (2) the transferee has the right to pledge or sell the assets, and (3) the transferer does not maintain control through a repurchase agreement. If the conditions are not met, it is accounted for as a secured borrowing.

5. Creative accounting is possible in the classification of receivables if there are "failures" in (1) the segregation of different types of receivables, (2) ensuring that the valuation accounts are appropriately offset against the proper receivable accounts, (3) the disclosure of any loss contingencies on receivables, (4) the disclosure of receivables pledged as collateral, and (5) the disclosure of significant concentration of risks arising from receivables.

6. Because the numerical guidelines exist for concentration risk, three items need to be disclosed: (1) information on the characteristic that determines the concentration, (2) amount of loss that could occur upon nonperformance, and (3) information on any collateral related to the receivable.

Inventory

1. For a manufacturing concern, inventories refer to finished goods inventory, goods-in-process inventories, and raw materials inventory. A separate manufacturing or factory supplies inventory may also be included. Proper segregation of the firm items would be more informative than the disclosure of a single amount for inventories.

2. Another useful segregation would include goods in transit, consigned goods, and special sales arrangements such as (1) sales with buyback agreement, (2) sales with high rates of return, and (3) sales on installment.

3. In sales with buyback arrangements, the firm may finance its inventory and not show an inventory or a liability on its balance sheet. Basically, it involves a product financing arrangement whereby Firm X sells an inventory to Firm Y and agrees at the same time to repurchase it later at a set price. Firm Y uses the inventory as a collateral to get a loan and to pay Firm X. Firm X eventually repurchases the inventory in the future, allowing Firm Y to use the proceeds to repay the loan. This allows Firm X to avoid personal property taxes in some states, remove current liability from its balance sheet, and affect its income.

4. In the case of sales with a high rate of return as in publishing, music, toys, and sporting goods, the firm may record the sales and estimate sales returns and allowance amount or wait until it has indications of the amount of inventory that will be returned. Creative accounting may be needed to determine when the inventory is sold and removed from the balance sheet.

5. In the case of sales in installment, the question is whether to withhold the legal title to the merchandise until all the payments have been made or record the sale after an estimation of the bad debt.

6. Product costs are "attached" to the inventory while the selling and administrative expenses are charged as period costs. While it is easy to consider

direct material and direct labor as product costs, the manufacturing overhead costs are allocated. Some of these costs may be "improperly" treated as period costs in an effort to "boost" the level of gross margin.

7. Interest costs related to assets constructed for internal use on assets produced as discrete projects (such as ships or real estate projects) for lease or sale are capitalized. Creative accounting may lead to the capitalization of interest costs for projects that are routine and repetitive.

8. The use of absorption costing for GAAP reporting and tax purposes leads to a profit that is more a function of production rather than sales strategy (i.e., it leads to the creation of "inventory" profits).

9. Costs such as bidding, warehousing, purchasing, officer salaries, and administrative and selling expenses may be capitalized for tax purposes. Creative accounting may lead to efforts to capitalize some of these costs for GAAP reporting.

10. Cost-flow assumptions include (1) the specific identification method, (2) the average cost method, (3) the first in, first out method (FIFO), and (4) the last in, first out method (LIFO). The cost-flow assumptions are not necessarily consistent with the flow of goods. While the choice of a cost-flow assumption should be to best reflect periodic income, other considerations may prevail.

11. Firms may use LIFO for tax and GAAP reporting and use other cost-flow techniques for internal reporting. As a result, a LIFO reserve is created and is equal to the difference between (1) inventory at the lower of LIFO cost or market and (2) inventory at replacement cost or at the lower of cost determined by some acceptable inventory accounting method or market. Either the LIFO reserve or the replacement cost of the inventory should be disclosed.

12. The use of LIFO has many benefits. However, LIFO liquidation, resulting from the erosion of LIFO inventory, can lead to distortions in net income and heavy tax payments.

13. Dollar-value FIFO techniques are generally used to protect LIFO layers from erosion. Subjectivity may enter in the selection of the items to be put in a pool. In addition, the firm may set up pools that are easy to liquidate, thereby increasing income by decreasing inventory and matching lower cost inventory to revenues. Creative accounting may become a matter of setting an adequate number of pools.

14. Inventories are valued on the basis of the lower of cost or market. The market is determined by the middle value of (1) net realizable value, (2) replacement cost, and (3) net realizable value less a normal profit margin and depends on judgments pertaining to (1) the sales price, (2) the normal profit margin, and (3) the replacement cost.

Property, Plant, and Equipment

1. Property, plant, and equipment or plant assets or fixed assets are valued at historical cost, which fails to account for changes in specific and general price levels.

2. Self-constructed assets either do not include fixed overhead or include an allocated portion. Creative accounting may enter into the allocation process. In addition, actual interest capitalized is a result of judgment in (1) the qualifying assets, (2) the capitalization period, and (3) the amount to capitalize.

3. Judgment and creativity may be required for the capitalization of costs subsequent to acquisition, such as additions, improvements and replacements, rearrangement and reinstallation, and repairs. As an example, if the judgment about repairs is that it is ordinary, the change is expensed; however, if the judgment is that it is major, it is capitalized.

Depreciation

1. Depreciation is a way of allocating the cost of a tangible asset over an estimated life of the asset. It requires a judgment on (1) the appropriate systematic and rational way of allocation and (2) an estimate of the useful life of the asset.

2. While the estimation of the useful life is supposed to consider physical factors (such as casualty or expiration of physical life) and economic factors (such as obsolescence), arbitraries in the estimation of the useful life may be a result of the use of creative accounting.

3. Depreciation techniques include the (1) activity method, the (2) straight line method, (3) decreasing change accelerated methods such as sum-of-the-year's digits and declining-balance method, and (4) special depreciation methods such as group and composite methods and hybrid combination methods. The selection of a technique is supposed to be based on securing the best matching of revenues and expenses. Other considerations such as practicality, lowering of taxes, and creative accounting may predominate.

4. In addition to the judgments about depreciation, firms may elect to make judgments about the need to recognize impairments of long-lived assets. Examples of events and circumstances that may lead to an impairment follow:

A significant decrease in the market value of an asset

A significant change in the extent or manner in which an asset is used

A significant adverse change in legal factors or in the business climate that affects the value of an asset

An accumulation of costs significantly in excess of the amount originally expected to acquire or construct an asset

A projection or forecast that demonstrates continuing losses associated with an asset.[72]

The impairment decision rests on a recoverability test comparing the sum of the expected future net cash flows (undiscounted) to carrying amount of the asset. The events and circumstances leading to impairment as well as the recoverability tests may rest on judgment based on creative accounting considerations.

5. Either the full cost concept or the successful efforts concept may be used for the accounting for exploration costs in the oil and gas industry. One may early guess that big oil companies will rely on the successful efforts method while small, exploration-oriented companies will rely on full cost accounting. A large oil company using full cost accounting will show a material increase in income.

6. Knowledgeable guesses, at best, are used for the estimation of recoverable reserves and disposal value.

Intangible Assets

1. Intangibles, such as patents, copyrights, franchises, goodwill, organization costs, and trademarks or trade means, are characterized by both the lack of physical evidence and the degree of uncertainty concerning future benefits. In the cases of both specifically identifiable intangibles and goodwill-type intangibles, they are capitalized if purchased and expensed if created internally. If capitalized, they are amortized over a period not exceeding forty years. The flexibility and the judgment entering into the determination of the useful life of the intangibles lead to possible creative accounting scenarios.

2. Both product patents and process patents are amortized over the legal life or the useful life, whichever is shorter. In addition, the legal fees are capitalized as part of the patents. Both the determination of the useful life and legal fees are left to judgments conducive to creative accounting solutions. For example, the value of a patent on a balance sheet may just increase because of the mounting costs in successfully defending a patent suit. The higher the legal fees, the higher the value of the patents.

3. The legal life of copyrights (life of the creator plus fifty years) is not a guarantee that the firm may choose a shorter period of time for the amortization of copyrights.

4. Even though the firm is allowed up to forty years to amortize a trademark or trade name, it may choose a shorter period.

5. A totally arbitrary period may also be chosen for the amortization of organization cost, even though the maximum period is forty years.

6. The operating losses incurred in the early years by a developing-stage firm can be capitalized by some firms, although expensing makes more sense.

7. Franchises with limited life are expenses, while franchises with an indefinite life or a perpetual franchise should be capitalized and amortized over a period not exceeding forty years. The definition of the life of the franchise is left to contractual arrangements that may be defined with creative accounting scenarios in mind.

8. Goodwill is the difference between the purchase price and the fair market value of the assets. It is generally amortized over a period not exceeding forty years. Both the valuation of assets and the choice of the amortization period

create various scenarios for creative accounting. The amortization of negative goodwill, or bad will, will create the unusual situation of increasing earnings.

9. Both specifically intangible and goodwill types of intangibles may be subject to loss or impairment if it is judged that the undiscounted sum of future net
cash flows is less than the carrying value of the intangible.

10. The costs of research and development activities are expensed when incurred. The judgment of activities that are considered as R&D activities and the
activities not considered R&D are a matter of judgment and therefore susceptible
to creative accounting scenarios.

11. Software costs for software created internally are expensed until technological feasibility has been established. Then, they are capitalized and amortized over future periods. Software costs, if purchased to be sold, leased, or
marketed to third parties, are capitalized and amortized over a future period.

Current Liabilities

1. Current liabilities are obligations whose liquidation is reasonably expected
to require use of existing resources properly classified as current assets or the
creation of other current liabilities and that have a maturity within one year of
the operating cycle, whichever is longer. The account will not be comparable
from one industry to another given the different operating cycles adopted.

2. Both the maturing portion of long-term debt and a liability that is due
within a year (or operating cycle) should be classified as a current liability. Any
other long-term debt classified as current liabilities is a form of creative accounting.

3. Property taxes payable can be changed in (1) the year in which paid, (2)
the year ending on assessment (or lien) date, (3) the year beginning on assessment (or lien) date, (4) calendar or fiscal year of taxpayer including assessment
(or lien) date, (5) calendar or fiscal year of taxpayer prior to the payment date,
(6) fiscal year of governing body levying the tax, and (7) year appearing on the
tax bill.

4. While gain contingencies are recognized only in the notes, loss contingencies are recognized by a charge to expense and a liability if the event is probable
and the loss can be reasonably estimated. Whether an event is probable, reasonably probable, or remote is left to the exercise of judgment and hence creativity.

5. Both litigation, claims, and assessments as well as unfilled suits and un-
asserted claims whose outcomes can be predicted need to be recognized by a
liability. Failure to do so is clearly a manifestation of creative accounting.

6. A contingent liability that is generally not recorded or infrequently recorded by a lot of firms is environmental liability in spite of the staggering costs
that could be incurred for the cleaning of toxic waste sites. A range for the
liability needs to be determined, and a best estimate within the range is to be

reported. Failure to find a best estimate results in the reporting of the lower end of the range and the disclosure of the higher end of the range.

Long-Term Debt

1. Long-term debt is issued with specific covenants and restrictions stated in the bond indenture or note agreement. To the extent that some of these stipulations are important, they should be disclosed in the notes. Failure to do so defeats the full disclosure principle.

2. Because of differences between the stated rate or coupon rate and the market or effective rate, bonds are issued at either a premium or a discount. The amortization of the discount or premium may be based on either the effective interest method or the straight-line method.

3. The debt issue costs are generally capitalized, then amortized.

4. While debt may be extinguished through cash payments, a lot of firms resort to in-substance defeasance, which requires the firm to set up an irrecoverable trust of securities whose principal and interest are pledged to pay off debt.

5. Firms may try to acquire debt and avoid recording the obligations on the balance sheet through various forms of off-balance-sheet financing. This may be easily accomplished by two entities, X and Y, forming a new entity, W, that borrows funds that are guaranteed by the firms X and Y. In this case X and Y have incurred more debt that does not appear on the balance sheets. The agreement with the new entity may include either a take-or-pay contract or a throughput agreement. These off-balance-sheet financing schemes are good examples of creative accounting schemes.

6. It is interesting to note that in case of trouble debt restructuring whose terms are modified, the official accounting positions that (1) the creditor's loss is based on cash flows discounted at the historical effective rate of interest and (2) the debtor's gain are computed on the basis of undiscounted amounts.

Stockholders' Equity

1. Subscriptions receivable, which indicate the amount yet to be collected before subscribed stock will be issued, may be accounted for as subscriptions receivable on the balance sheet (a current asset account) or a deduction from stockholders' equity (a contra equity account). The contra equity account is favored by the SEC.

2. Stock issued for services or property other than cash is valued at the more clearly determinable fair value of the stock issued or fair market value of the noncash considerations received. A choice of the fair market value of the noncash considerations received may lead to judgments that cause either an overvaluation of the assets, resulting in "watered stock," or an undervaluation of the assets, resulting in "secret reserves."

3. The costs of issuing stocks may be (1) debited to paid-in-capital in excess of par or stated value, as a reduction of the amounts paid-in, or (2) capitalized as an organization cost and expensed over an arbitrary time not exceeding forty years.

4. Although treasury stock is subtracted from the total common stock, some firms may find an "unusual" explanation for classifying it as an asset on the balance sheet.

5. Treasury stock may be accounted for at the cost method or the par value method or a method required by a state law.

6. In the case of "greenmail payments" to repurchase shares to avert a hostile takeover, the premium is debited to treasury stock rather than charged as an expense.

7. A separable disclosure is needed for redeemable preferred stock, nonredeemable preferred stock, and common stock. The SEC requires that redeemable preferred stock not be included in stockholders' equity.

8. Transient preferred, which is preferred stocks to be redeemed over short periods, is just "thinly" disguised debt.

Retained Earnings

1. Restrictions on payment of dividends and other distributions to owners may exist for (1) firms operating in states using the 1950 Model Business Corporation Acts, (2) firms operating in states using the 1984 Revised Model Business Corporation Act, and (3) firms using hybrid restrictions. Adequate disclosures about these restrictions and the legality of dividends are required.

2. Information on dividend policy warrants disclosure.

3. Property dividends should be based on the fair value of the property to be distributed, and gains or losses resulting from the reevaluation should be recognized.

4. Whenever appropriation of retained earnings takes place, the firm should offer an adequate explanation for the action taken.

Investments

1. Various classification schemes are needed to account for investments creating opportunities for creative accounting.

2. Debt securities can be classified as (1) held-to-maturity, (2) trading securities, or c) available-for-sale. The unrealized gains and losses are recognized in net income for trading securities and in other comprehensive income and as a separate component of stockholders' equity for available-for-sale securities. As such, the classification judgment has an impact on the level of income reported.

3. Equity securities for holding less than 20 percent are also classified as

either available-for-sale or trading securities. The unrealized gains and losses are also recognized in net income for trading equity securities and in other comprehensive income for available-for-sale securities.

4. Firms may elect to transfer securities from one classification group to another, thereby affecting the level of income or the level of comprehensive income.

Revenue Recognition

1. Revenue recognition means that the revenues have been both realized and earned. The timing of recognition is (1) the date of sale for the sale of product from an inventory, (2) services performed and billable for rendering a service, (3) as time passes or assets are used for the use of an asset, and (4) date of sale for the sale of asset other than inventory. However, departures from the sales basis are frequent and need to be justified.

2. For revenue recognized at a point of sales, creative accounting may take place in three cases of (1) sales with buyback agreements, (2) sales when right of return exists, and (3) trade loafing and channel surfing.

3. Is a sale with buyback agreements a sale or creative accounting?

4. When should sales with right of return be recorded? Should they be recorded when the return privileges have expired?

5. Are the techniques of trade loafing and channel surfing legitimate sales or a form of creative accounting? Offering deep discounts to generate "phony sales" is a form of profit distortion and creative accounting.

6. For long-term construction contracts, revenue is recognized before delivery using either (1) the percentage-of-completion method or (2) the completed-contract method. When using the percentage-of-completion method, the determination of the progress toward completion is based on judgmental techniques such as (1) cost-to-cost method, (2) the "efforts expended methods," and (3) "units of work performed method."

7. When revenue is deferred until cash is received, two techniques may be used, either (1) the installment sales method or (2) the cost recovery method.

Income Taxes

1. Deferred tax assets and deferred tax liabilities are recognized as a result of the differences between pretax, financial income and taxable income. Judgment is needed for the portion of deferred tax asset that will not be realized and that needs to be recognized by a valuation allowance.

2. The deferred tax accounts need to be classified as either net current amount or net noncurrent amount based on a judgment of the expected reversal date of the temporary difference (if not related to a specific asset or liability).

Leases

4. One or more of four criteria need to be met before a lease is recorded as a capital lease resulting in capitalization on the balance sheet. Not meeting any of the four criteria results in classifying and accounting for the lease as an operating lease. The lease contract may be written in such a way as to fail to meet any of the four criteria. This is a form of "creative contracting" resulting in "creative accounting."

CONCLUSIONS

Good evidence of designed or managed accounting is the amount of creativity in accounting practice. The creativity is generally a by-product of the flexibility and the variety of options available within GAAP as well as the result of very "liberal" reading of the accounting rules. This creativity is manifest in the inside use of (1) selective financial misrepresentation, (2) big bath accounting, and (3) creative accounting.

NOTES

1. L. Revsine, "The Selective Financial Misrepresentation Hypothesis," *Accounting Horizons* (December 1991), pp. 16–27.

2. Ibid., p. 16.

3. G.J. Stigler, "The Theory of Economic Regulation," *Bell Journal of Economics and Management Science* (Spring 1971), pp. 3–21.

4. Revsine, "The Selective Financial Misrepresentation Hypothesis," p. 17.

5. Ibid.

6. Ibid., p. 19.

7. Ibid., p. 24.

8. "SEC Chairman Discusses Earnings Management," *Deloitte & Touche Review* (October 12, 1998), p. 1.

9. P.N. Healy, "The Effect of Bonus Schemes on Accounting Decisions," *Journal of Accounting and Economics* 7 (1985), p. 86.

10. N.L. Moore, "Management Changes and Discretionary Accounting Decisions," *Journal of Accounting Research* (Spring 1973), pp. 100–107.

11. H.M. Schilit, *Financial Shenanigans* (New York: McGraw-Hill, 1993), p. 121.

12. R.M. Copeland and M.L. Moore, "The Financial Bath: Is It Common?" *MSU Business Topics* (Autumn 1972), p. 63.

13. R.E. Kieso and J.J. Weygandt, *Intermediate Accounting*, 9th ed. (New York: John Wiley & Sons, 1998), p. 1126.

14. Ibid., p. 1126.

15. Schilit, *Financial Shenanigans*.

16. I. Griffiths, *Creative Accounting* (London: Irwin, 1986); I. Griffiths, *New Creative Accounting* (London: Macmillan, 1995).

17. S. Herve, "Comptali Creative," in Bernard Colasse (ed.), *Encyclopedie de Comptabilite, Controle de bestion et audit* (Paris: Economica, 2000), pp. 157–158.

18. P. Revsine, "The Corporate AIDS—Funny Financing and Creative Accounting," *Rydges* (November 1989), pp. 18–20.

19. R. Craig and P. Walsh, "Adjustments for Extraordinary Items, in Smoothing Reported Profit of Listed Australian Companies: Some Empirical Evidence," *Journal of Business Finance and Accounting* (Spring 1989), pp. 229–245.

20. Griffiths, *New Creative Accounting*, pp. vii–viii.

21. M. Jameson, *A Practical Guide to Creative Accounting* (London: Kogan Page, 1988).

22. Pijper, T., *Creative Accounting: The Effectiveness of Financial Reporting in the U.K.* (London: Macmillan, 1994).

23. M.R. Mathews and M.H.B. Perera, *Accounting Theory and Development* (Melbourne: Nelson, 1996), p. 228.

24. K.H.M. Naser, *Creative Financial Accounting: Its Nature and Use* (New York: Prentice-Hall, 1993), p. 2.

25. Ibid., p. 2.

26. Ibid.

27. Schilit, *Financial Shenanigans*, p. ix.

28. Ibid., p. x.

29. Ibid., p. 1.

30. H. Stolowy and G. Breton, "A Framework for the Classification of Accounts Manipulations," Working paper, HEC, Paris, 2001.

31. J.J. Bertolus, "L' Art de Truquez Un Bilan," *Science & Vie Economie* (June 1988), pp. 17–23.

32. M. Lignor, "L'Art de Calculer Ses Benefices," *L'Enterprise* 50 (1989), pp. 17–18, 20.

33. I. Goumin, "L'Art de Presenter Un Bilan," *La Tribune* (March 28, 1991), p. 11.

34. D. Pourquery, "Les Provisions on L' Art de Mettre de l'Argent de Cote," *Science & Vie Economie* 73 (1991), pp. 72–75.

35. D. Le double, "La Creative en Comptabilite," *Semaine Juridique* 25 (1993), p. 224.

36. P. Agede, "Haliller Ses Comptes," *L'Enterprise* 106 (1994), pp. 82–85.

37. P. Lonliere, "Pour Embellir ses Comptes, Teromson Cede Ses Pnetes," *Liberation* (May 5, 1992), pp. 20–32.

38. Agede, "Haliller Ses Comptes," p. 83.

39. Ibid., p. 84.

40. J. Audas, "Le Window-Dressing un L' Halillage des Bilans," *Option Finance* (January 18, 1993), p. 29.

41. A. Feity, "La BIMP Innove pour Nettoyer son Bilan," *Option Finance* (May 30, 1994); N. Sibbert, "Club Mediterrannee—le Nettoyage des Computes," *La Vie Francaise* (February 1–7, 1994), p. 11; J.F. Polo, "Elf Toilette ses Computes avant la Privatisation," *Les Echos* (January 19, 1994), p. 11.

42. Stolowy, "Comptabilite Creative," pp. 157–178.

43. F. Bonnet, *Pieges (et Delices) de la Comptabilite (Creative)* (Paris: Economica, 1995).

44. J. Blake and O. Amat, "Creative Accounting Is Not Just an English Disease," *Management Accounting* (October 1996), p. 54.

45. Griffiths, *Creative Accounting*; Griffiths, *New Creative Accounting*.

46. Naser, *Creative Financial Accounting*.

47. T. Smith, *Accounting for Growth* (London: Century Business, 1996).

48. Ibid.

49. Ibid., p. 4.

50. Naser, *Creative Financial Accounting*, p. 59.

51. Ibid., p. 59.

52. K.V. Peasnell and R.A. Yaasnah, "Off-Balance Sheet Financing," *Certified Research Report 10* (London: Chartered Association of Certified Accountants, 1998).

53. J. Argenti, *Corporate Collapse: The Cause and Symptoms* (New York: McGraw-Hill, 1976).

54. J.M. Goodfellow, "Now You See Thru, Now You Don't," *CA Magazine* (December 1988), pp. 16–23.

55. R. Dieter and J. Watt, "Get off the Balance Sheet," *Financial Executive* (January 1980), pp. 42–49; J.E. Stewart and B.S. Neuhausen, "Financial Instruments and Transactions: The CPA's New Challenge," *Journal of Accounting* (August 1986), pp. 102–112; J. Samuels, C. Rickwood, and A. Piper, *Advanced Financial Accounting* (London: McGraw-Hill, 1989).

56. Argenti, *Corporate Collapse*.

57. Naser, *Creative Financial Accounting*.

58. Griffiths, *New Creative Accounting*.

59. Ibid., p. xi.

60. A.J. Briloff, *Unaccountable Accounting* (New York: Harper & Row, 1972); A.J. Briloff, *More Debits than Credits* (New York: Harper & Row, 1972); Schilit, *Financial Shenanigans*.

61. Ibid., pp. 43–45.

62. Ibid., p. 61.

63. Ibid., p. 79.

64. Ibid., p. 107.

65. Ibid., p. 119.

66. Jameson, *A Practical Guide to Creative Accounting*, p. 20.

67. Kieso and Weygandt, *Intermediate Accounting*, p. 219.

68. Ibid., p. 147.

69. Ibid.

70. "Reporting the Results of Operations," *Opinions of the Accounting Principles Board No. 30* (New York: AICPA, 1973).

71. Ibid.

72. Kieso and Weygandt, *Intermediate Accounting*, p. 557.

SELECTED REFERENCES

Griffiths, I. *Creative Accounting*. London: Irwin, 1986.

Griffiths, I. *New Creative Accounting*. London: Macmillan, 1995.

Jameson, M. *A Practical Guide to Creative Accounting*. London: Kogan Page, 1988.

Naser, K.H.M. *Creative Financial Accounting: Its Nature and Use*. New York: Prentice-Hall, 1993.

Pijper, T. *Creative Accounting: The Effectiveness of Financial Reporting in the U.K.* London: Macmillan, 1994.

Priloff, A.J. *Unaccountable Accounting*. New York: Harper & Row, 1972.

Priloff, A.J. *More Debits than Credits.* New York: Harper & Row, 1976.

Revsine, L. "The Selective Financial Misrepresentation Hypothesis." *Accounting Horizons* (December 1991), pp. 16–27.

Schilit, H.M. *Financial Shenanigans: How to Detect Accounting Criminals and Fraud in Financial Reports.* New York: McGraw-Hill, 1993.

Smith, T. *Accounting for Growth.* London: Century Business, 1996.

Appendix 3A. The Context of the Contemporary Accounting Profession

INTRODUCTION

Standard setting, the practice of the auditing and accounting craft, and accounting research are practiced in a shifting and conflictual terrain as new environmental conditions emerge. These environmental changes may be characterized by three new trends: (1) technical and ideological proletarianization of accountants in public and private practices, (2) the institutional capitalism of the new governing class, and (3) the assimilation of academic accountants into a flawed universal class. This defines a new social order where a diverse group of protagonists from different contradictory classes take, define, and defend their view and the scope of the discipline. This appendix describes the elements of this new order as it bears on conflict in the field of accounting and contributes to the malaise, inadequacies, issues, and unresolved problems facing the accounting world (Belkaoui, 1985b).

GENESIS OF EMERGING STRUCTURAL CHANGES

Most countries in the world are facing economic, social, political, and cultural crises, whether they are developing or developed countries. These crises, which defeat the idea of the stability of monopoly capitalism, emanate from the organization of production at the world level, not just within the U.S. economy. At the world level there is no monopoly capitalism, but there are a large number of firms competing in an overall, anarchistic situation of global production (Bergesen, 1983, p. 11). Despite the efforts to solve these crises, the prospects of immediate relief seem dim. In effect, regarding the most pressing problems of inflation, unemployment, inequality, imbalances in international trade, and Third World debt, governments have resorted to the politics of short-term situations without a clear vision of the desired evolution of societies and economies (Touraine, 1977, p. 3).

Source: Reprinted from A. Riahi-Belkaoui, "The Context of the Contemporary Accounting Profession," *Advances in Public Interest Accounting* 4, 1991, pp. 83–97. Copyright 1991. Reprinted with permission from Elsevier Science.

These crises persist, leaving a trail of failures in the economic and political relations of capitalist reproduction. This should not be surprising, as it is in the nature of capitalistic production to be constantly exposed to a variety of internally and externally generated disturbances setting off general crises.

A Marxist view of these crises stems from the position that "though capitalism is capable of self-expansion, the accumulation process deepens the internal contradictions on which it is based, until they erupt in a crisis: the limits to capitalism are *internal* to it" (Shaikh, 1978, p. 220). These contradictions originate in the needed class structure in which the continued existence of one dominating class requires the continued existence of a subordinate class. Societies are now constituted by groups of protagonists competing for economic and social power and political authority. Dominant modes of interaction, however, consistently favor one category of actors and result in the systematic exploitation of others (Offe, 1985, p. 2). At every societal level, groups of protagonists face each other over the contradictions that separate them. As an example, in the debt crises, financial capital and industrial capital find themselves in conflict; management and shareholders are in disagreement in management buyouts; and employees and management dispute each other's claims to pension funds.

Accounting is not immune to these contradictions. The management of certified public accountant (CPA) firms ally themselves with the managers of institutional capitalism, while the working accountants in CPA firms are proletarianized. Because of these contradictory interests within the profession, management attempts to create a "manufactured consciousness" of the users through a domination of information. Accounting academics strive to develop a consciousness that can help accountants to function as a universal class. Instead, they create a flawed universal class, motivated by self-interest and the need to monopolize their special brand of "cultural" capital.

The emerging structural changes in the accounting environment (i.e., contradictory classes in the accounting profession and academic accountants as a flawed universal class) are contradictions created by the global conflicts and the emergence of new protagonists in the accounting environment as well as in other environments. They lead to class differences and conflicts over the role and conduct of the discipline. They are examined next.

TECHNICAL AND IDEOLOGICAL PROLETARIANIZATION OF ACCOUNTANTS

The first element in the new era of conflict is the emergence of new class differences among accountants. Accountants as professional employees in accounting or nonaccounting organizations are considered members of the new class of salaried professionals. They are identified by Bell and other "postindustrial" theorists as major protagonists of the new coming postindustrial society or as members of the "new working class," "professional-managerial class,"

"new petty bourgeoisie," or "new class" and are identified by Marxist theorists as major new actors in contemporary capitalism (Bell, 1961; Ehrenreich and Ehrenreich, 1976; Poulantzas, 1975; Touraine, 1977).[1] There was a tremendous growth of accountants in the labor force from 22,916 in 1900 (0.08 percent of the labor force) to 1,047,000 in 1980 (1.08 percent of the labor force), a percentage increase from 1900 to 1980 of 4,468.86 percent (Derber, 1983). It is the highest increase among professionals, surpassing that of physicians (224.01 percent), lawyers (408.27 percent), architects (750.58 percent), dentists (371.94 percent), engineers (3,717.26 percent), and natural scientists (2,399.17 percent).[2] The U.S. Bureau of Labor Statistics reports that in 1986 there were 1.3 million accountants and auditors, up from 1.1 million in 1983 (Kleiman, 1987).

This growth of accountants followed the need for more advanced accounting technologies to deal with requirements of a more sophisticated production apparatus. The use of these advanced technologies requires accountants to pool their efforts in small and/or large CPA firms, leading to a decline in opportunities for self-employment in the field and to their dependence on the financial and institutional resources of corporations and the state.

Accountants were reluctant to abandon the idea of an independent economic position; however, increasingly, they joined accounting and nonaccounting firms, small and large, corporate or state bureaucracies. In the process they became subject to the authority and control of heteronomous management and suffered a slow degradation of status and reward.[3] What really resulted from these developments is a proletarianization of accountants, working according to a division of labor conceived and monitored by management, following procedural rules and repertoires created by administrative processes and/or fiat. While they still maintain control over their own knowledge base, which gives them some negotiating powers, their contractual employment totally subordinates them to a heteronomous management that appropriated the power over the total labor process.

The proletarianization of accountants reflected a shift of control toward employers or management and a loss of the creative freedom that accountants enjoyed as self-employed professionals. Thus, the change in accounting technology forced a change in the structure of the accounting labor process and put the accountants in a new form of "proletarian class," subordinated, like the craftspeople before them, to capitalist management. In the process, as theorized by Marx, they lost control of both the *means* and *ends* of labor, a phenomenon labeled *technical* proletarianization (Baran and Sweezy, 1966; Braverman, 1966). It has been speeded up and made easier by the higher degree of specialization and fragmentation imposed on accounting practice, a process of "deskilling," that is, of rationalizing previously professional tasks into a number of routinized functions requiring little training. An AICPA task force lists forty-one activities that describe the six general work categories performed by CPAs in public accounting practice: engagement management and administration, au-

diting, tax practice, management advisory services, other professional services, and office and firm administration (AICPA, 1983). A challenge facing accounting firms over the coming decade will be the need for even more *specialization* in auditing, tax, and consulting.

In addition to technical proletarianization, the emergence of the "new working class" or "professional managerial class" led also to an *ideological proletarianization*, which refers to the appropriation of control by management for capital, over the goals and social purposes to which work is put (Marglin, 1975). Ideological proletarianization may be more pronounced in accounting due to the general inability of accountants to control organizational policy and the specific goals and purposes of work. The accountant, bound by the specialized tasks, has lost control of the nature of the total product and may be indifferent to the outcome of the activities in which he or she was involved. This loss of vision of the total product and its use and disposition allows the direct management of labor (i.e., the technical proletarianization). In this way, technical and ideological proletarianization feed on each other.

The technical proletarianization of the accountant may lead to the accountant's losing the knowledge base as "capital" restructures through management the specification of the product and management restructures the organization of work.[4]

Proletarianization renders the accountant a mere technician of functionaries, separate from the major social, moral, and technological issues of his or her profession.[5] The end and social use of the accountant's labor is institutionally channeled with little provision made for his or her interest as a professional and the interest of the clients.[6] Marx discusses a similar transition from independent professional "craftsman" to de-skilled worker as the transition from formal subsumption to real subsumption.

These changes have led to the decrease in the number and quality of people going into accounting programs. The accounting profession lacks "glamour," and survey results suggest that accountants come from poorer socioeconomic backgrounds than do attorneys and physicians (Estes, 1984). The director of personnel at one of the Big Eight firms explains as follows: "Part of it is that a number of people find investment banking sexier, more exiting. You can make a big buck a lot quicker" (Kleiman, 1987). The lack of glamour may force the profession to offer high entry-level salaries. For now, in answer to the technical and ideological proletarianization, the accountant as well as other members of the "new working class" may respond by either *ideological desensitization*, a denial or separation of the self from the ideological control of the job, disclaiming either interest or responsibility for the social issues to which their work is put, or *ideological cooperation*, a redefinition of one's goals to make them consistent with institutional imperatives (Derber, 1983, p. 335).

In either case—ideological desensitization or ideological cooperation—there is high likelihood of alienation of accountants from their work, evidenced by the high level of turnover. About 85 percent of the accounting graduates joining

the big CPA firms will leave within ten years for positions in government, industry, education, or smaller CPA firms (Kollaritsch, 1968). Benke and Rhode (1984) estimated the replacement cost of each entry-level staff accountant to exceed $20,000, and for one large CPA firm with a turnover of 10,000 employees over a recent ten-year period (Healy, 1976), that price would be $200 million in replacement costs. Other studies reported an increase in the level of turnover (Benke, 1978; Konstans and Ferris, 1981). Variables explaining this high turnover were found to be (1) the work environment in the audit department, (2) the coworkers and uncompensated overtime (in the tax department), and (3) professional challenge in the management services department (Benke and Rhode, 1984).

Alienation in the domain of work has a fourfold aspect: a person is alienated from the object that he or she produces, from the process of production, from himself or herself, and from the community of his or her fellows.

In their alienated condition, the mind-set of accountants, their consciousness, is to a large extent only the reflection of the conditions in which they find themselves and of the position in the process of production. This situation is particularly serious for female accountants. The percentage of female accounting graduates with bachelor's and master's degrees increased from 28 percent in 1976–1977 to 49 percent in 1985–1986. Yet, they feel that they do not have the same chance for promotion as men (Jayson and Williams, 1986) and that they do not earn as much (Olson and Frieze, 1986).

INSTITUTIONAL CAPITALISM AND CLASSWIDE RATIONALITY

The second element in the new conflictual order concerns the nature of the governing class in corporations and accounting firms. The social organization of the corporate community is composed of enduring informal and formal networks among large corporations, senior managers and directors of these companies, and the associations that represent them to the public (Useem, 1982, 1983). The policies espoused by business are the product of this social organization. While the results are not very conclusive, there is still the generally accepted notion that the corporate community is socially unified, cognizant of its classwide interest, and politically active. It is characterized by a socially cohesive national upper class, composed chiefly of corporate executives, primary owners, and their descendants, who constitute "the governing class of America" (Domhoff, 1974, p. 109). The same conclusion is drawn for Britain with the argument that

elite pluralism does not . . . prevent elites in capitalist society from constituting a dominant economic class, possessed of a high degree of cohesion and solidarity, with common interest and common purposes which far transcend their specific differences and disagreements. (Miliband, 1969, p. 47)

This governing class is composed of

those who own and those who control capital on a larger scale: whether top business executives or rentiers make no difference in this context. Whatever divergences of interest there may be among them on this score and others, latent as well as manifest, they have a common stake in one overriding cause: to keep the working rule of the society capitalist. (Westergaard and Resler, 1975, p. 346)

From this common cause stemmed the need for them to have common background and patterns of socialization, generally articulated in a new class awareness (Scott, 1979, pp. 125–126). This new class entered the political arena, with an unusual force and coherence, ensuring the success of the likes of Reagan and Thatcher and influencing their policies (Useem, 1983, p. 285). This situation precipitated the shift from "managerial capitalism" to "institutional capitalism." With managerial capitalism replacing family capitalism, managers and professional management found themselves in charge. Institutional capitalism, spurred by the rise of the new governing class, emerged to give to corporations a new power and class orientation. As stated by Useem,

[C]ompany management is now less than fully in charge; classwide issues intrude into company decisions; and competition is less pitched. Management decisions to underwrite political candidates, devote company resources to charitable causes, give advertising space to matters of public movement, and assume more socially responsible attitudes derive in part from company calculus, but also from a classwide calculus. (Useem, 1983, p. 305)

A *classwide rationality*, replacing the former assumption of *corporate rationality*, assumes that the corporate elite is largely capable of identifying and promoting its common political objectives. This classwide principle, replacing both the *upper class principle* and its successor, the corporate principle, and asserting that membership in the corporate elite is primarily determined in a set of interrelated networks transecting virtually all corporations, is also present in the accounting firms. Although corporate rationality still characterizes much of the internal organization of accounting firms, classwide rationality now characterizes its highest circles. Old school ties and kindred signs of proper breeding facilitate the access to the highest circles of the CPA firms.[7] The classwide principle espoused by the managerial elite of the CPA firms led them to espouse the broader need of big business and to oppose public regulation of their trade[8] (Previts, 1978; Arthur Andersen & Co., 1979; Elliott and Schultze, 1979; Chetkovich, 1980; Flegm, 1984). While not limited to the elite accounting firms, the political interest of the new corporate elite has been shown to transcend individual firms and to possess an internal cohesion that facilitates expression of those interests in the political process (Useem, 1982). In fact, challenges to the position of accounting firms, whether from Congress or the SEC, have further consolidated the political capacities of the new corporate elite of accounting

firms, as they were able to weather the storms of various congressional investigations, the findings of special task forces, and SEC interventions. The classwide rationality of the high circles of the CPA firms, the social cohesion of its members, and their commitment to special interests have proven to be a formidable weapon to any attempts to regulate them (Olson, 1982, chap. 3; Belkaoui, 1989).

For example, in 1986 a bill was introduced in the House of Representatives of the U.S. Congress requiring auditors to report immediately to federal authorities any suspicions of fraud that are detected in auditing a company's books. It also called for the signing of the financial statements by the individual auditor, not just the firm. As a result of the pressures put forth by the accounting profession, the bill did not pass.

In addition to their role in the profession, accountants and other financial specialists are prominently represented in the managerial hierarchies of corporations (Armstrong, 1987, p. 415). In the United Kingdom company directors with backgrounds in banking or accountancy outnumber those with any form of technical training (BIM, 1972). An emphasis on financial as opposed to alternative means of control, especially at the higher level, was introduced by the same accountants in key positions (Granick, 1971, p. 56). As a result of this trend, Armstrong argued that organized professions are competitively engaged in "collective mobility projects" (cf. Larson, 1977), aimed at securing access to key positions of command in management hierarchies (Armstrong, 1985). Their goal is seen as complete control by a competitive use of their techniques.

The means of competition is the monopolization of a body of knowledge and expertise which offers, or appears to offer, a solution to a key problem within the functions of capital. To the extent that professions succeed by these means in attaining command positions, they are then in a position to sponsor characteristic means of controlling the rest of the management hierarchy and, ultimately, the labor process itself (if indeed this was not the crisis which enabled them to achieve dominance in the first place). (Armstrong, 1987, pp. 416–425)

ACADEMIC ACCOUNTANTS: A FLAWED UNIVERSAL CLASS

The third element in the new conflictual order is a new class of academic accountants. The proletariat as a universal class was best expressed by Marx and Engels' theory of the "universal class of the proletariat" in the *Holy Family* (Engels and Marx, [1844] 1975), refuting Bruno Bauer's criticisms and doubts that the proletariat could develop consciousness that would be necessary to perform its function as a universal class (Engels and Marx, 1975, p. 86). Gouldner joins the critical group, arguing that the lowliest class never came to power and that throughout the world during the twentieth century, a new class of intellectuals emerged, looking like the universal class defined by Hegel (Hegel, 1942,

pp. 131–134, 197–200), but not representing a universal class (Gouldner, 1979). *The new class is thus a flawed universal class.*

Gouldner advanced two major propositions: first, the rise of a "new class" of humanistic intellectuals and technical intelligentsia, whose universalism is badly flawed; and second, the growing dominance of this class, as a cultural bourgeoisie having monopoly over cultural capital and professionalism from which it gains its power.

This new class includes both technical and human intellectuals. It forms one "speech community" sharing a "culture of critical discourse" (CCD). The CCD is a concept derived from the different linguistic repertoires identified in sociolinguistics (Berstein, 1974). Its definition is similar. The culture of critical discourse (CCD) is a historically evolved set of rules, a grammar of discourse, which (1) is conceived to justify its assertions, (2) whose mode of justification does not proceed by involving authorities and (3) prefers to elicit the *voluntary* consent of those addressed solely on the basis of arguments addressed. This is a culture of discourse in which there is nothing that speakers will on principle permanently refuse to discuss or make problematic; indeed, they are even willing to talk about the value of talk itself and its possible inferiority to silence or to practice.

This grammar is the deep structure of the common ideology shared by the new class. *The shared ideology of the intellectuals and intelligentsia is thus an ideology about discourse.* Apart from the underlying technical languages (or sociolects) spoken by specialized professions, intellectuals and intelligentsia are commonly committed to a culture of critical discourse. CCD is the latent but mobilizable infrastructure of modern "technical language" (Gouldner, 1978, pp. 176–177) as well as of modern intellectuals and their linguistic culture.

This new class is flawed because it is considered elitist and self-seeking and uses its special knowledge to advance its own interests and power.[9] It does not represent the universal interest. The new class is dominant because of its monopolistic access to cultural capital. Borrowing from Pierre Bourdieu's theory of cultural reproduction (Bourdieu, 1977), Gouldner suggests that the new class uses cultural reproduction to maintain its interest and power just as economic reproduction is used to serve the interests of the holders of economic capital. Therefore, members of the new class will develop within the process of "cultural capital accumulation" to further their particular interests and the interests of those who share their culture of critical discourse.

The new class relies on credentials in capitalizing culture and monitoring the supply of specifically trained labor.

Culture is transmitted through education and socialization. Generally, it is known that those with more formal education have life-time earnings in excess of those with less. This increased income reflects the capital value of increased education. (Gouldner, 1979, p. 26)

This gives them a privileged position in the labor market and the potential for a new dominant class position. The trend has started with the new class developing a high level of status consciousness to defend their privileges (e.g., academic freedom to publish, to review, to recruit, etc.).

Whether the supply of accounting research by academic accountants is in response to the demand for value-free knowledge (Peasnell and Williams, 1986), or to the demands of the markets for excuses (Watts and Zimmerman, 1979), academic accountants are also motivated by self-interest and the pressing need to publish (Orleans, 1962). They have gained a power associated with their monopoly over the cultural accounting capital. The research findings have given them consulting and policy-making powers to advance their own interests rather than the universal interest. For a culture of critical discourse, they have developed their linguistic repertoires, which differentiate them from other accounting speech communities (Belkaoui, 1978, 1980; Haried, 1980). As a new class, academic accountants also rely on credentials as criteria for membership, including Ph.D. degrees and publications in the "right" journals.[10]

According to Gouldner,

[P]rofessionalism is one of the public ideologies of the New Class. [P]rofessionalism is a tacit claim of the New Class to technical and moral superiority over the old class . . . professionalism tacitly deauthorized the old class. (Gouldner, 1979, p. 19)

Through the new professional role, the academic accountants claim their own cultural research domain and in the process receive a higher compensation from the market system for accepting the professional role (Lewis et al., 1984).

Intellectuals who are willing to behave like professionals are allowed to form a relatively autonomous stratum with particularistic interest. They can use the mechanisms of licensing and the professional associations to establish monopolies with their markets. (Szelenyi, 1982)

The fragmentation of the American Accounting Association with separate "cultural" sections evidences this phenomenon (Belkaoui and Chan, 1987).

The same fragmentation orients the accounting researcher more toward immediate political actions (policy) than toward "theoretical" formulations of problems with general significance. This new close relationship to the policymaker, whether it is the FASB, the SEC, the AAA, or any other institution, makes him or her a "bureaucratic" intellectual who exercises advisory and technical functions within a bureaucracy as opposed to those intellectuals who elect to stay unattached to a bureaucracy (Nettl, 1969, pp. 15–32; Merton, 1968, pp. 265–266).

The bureaucratic intellectual is reduced to being an "ideologue" because he or she subordinates or abandons the search for a universally comprehensive understanding of social, cultural, and physical reality in favor of an immediately

instrumental arbitration of competing policies or courses of action (Barrow, 1987, p. 423). Such a role is unfortunate if one subscribes to the prevailing assumption that a "particularization" of intellectual activity that links or constrains academic inquiry to specific social interests or needs leads to a fall from the "sacred" and a descent into the dishonorable realm of "ideology" (Mannheim, 1971, pp. 116–131; 1986, pp. 265–266; Ashcraft, 1980).

In addition to the role of teachers involved in the process of creating formal knowledge as opposed to its mere transmission (Aron, 1962; Lipset and Dobson, 1972; Shils, 1972a, pp. 206–209; Berger, 1976, p. 5), the intellectuals moved to a role of "rationalization." As Shils suggests, in all modern societies (both liberal and totalitarian) "the trend of the present century" has been to increase pressures toward internal homogeneity due to the "incorporation of intellectuals in organized societies" (1972b, p. 191). Intellectuals serve to elaborate the underlying "laws" of national and social organization relevant to the routing development and application of scientific knowledge to economic production and its social organization (Machlup, 1962; Price, 1965; Bell, 1973, pp. 165–166; Galbraith, 1978, pp. 292–306). The call came mostly from the state to assist in reorienting the underlying mass population and in developing policies to ameliorate and prevent disturbances (Habermas, 1970, pp. 62–80; Galbraith, 1978, pp. 206–220; Gouldner, 1979, pp. 24–25).[11] As a result, intellectuals have typically labored under the patronage of ruling classes or in institutions controlled by them (Aron, 1962, p. 204; Parsons, 1970, p. 14]. The accounting intellectuals fit the described scenarios as they strive to provide the right excuses (Watts and Zimmerman, 1979) and create a new but flawed universal class.

CONCLUSIONS

A new order is appearing in the field of accounting in which a diverse group of protagonists from different contradictory classes define and defend their view of the scope and the conduct of the discipline. First, accountants as members of the new class of salaried professionals have lost control of the labor process, resulting in a technical and ideological proletarianization of the accountants. Second, a new governing class inbred by classwide rationality and internal cohesion has given rise to an institutional capitalism that supplants the interest of individual firms. Finally, the academic accountants, as part of the flawed universal class, are motivated by their subjectified interests and the need to monopolize their special brand of "cultural" capital. What results is a new class-based conflict in accounting characterized by the contradictions and antinomies inherent in the predicament of the new "socialized" accounting workforce.

NOTES

1. A Marxist definition includes this professional-managerial class of "salaried mental workers who do not own the means of production and whose major function in the

social division of labor may be described broadly as the reproduction of capitalist culture and capitalist class relations" (Ehrenreich and Ehrenreich, 1976, p. 13).

2. The data are taken from the Bureau of Labor Statistics and the Bureau of Census.

3. The starting salaries of accounting undergraduates joining the big CPA firms declined in real terms in the 1980s, hovering in 1987 around $22,000.

4. The growth of management advisory services activities, the increased specialization in the profession, the emerging conflict between professionalism and commercialism in accounting, and the call for non-CPA associate membership for non-CPAs point in that direction (Belkaoui, 1985b).

5. The *Report* of the National Commission on Fraudulent Financial Reporting (1987) noticed a breakdown in the financial reporting system and revealed that fraudulent financial reporting usually occurs as the result of certain environmental, institutional, or individual forces and opportunities.

6. The managing partner of the Grant Thornton accounting firm, who had a crucial role in the fraud at E.S.M. Government Securities Inc., gave this account of the same conflict: "I often wondered what I would do if somebody walked in and said, 'Look what I've found.' But it never happened. I gave them [his team of auditors] the same baloney answer that I had been given back in '78. It never dawned on them that it just didn't make sense" (Branningan, 1987, p. 29).

7. Marx refers to the opportunistic and pragmatic alliance described in *The Eighteenth Brumaire of Louis Napoleon* (1852), involving a conservative peasantry and Louis Napolean. Following Marx's analysis in the *Eighteenth Brumaire*, both corporations and accounting firms live under economic conditions of existence that separate their model of life, their interest, and their culture from those of other classes and puts them in hostile opposition to the latter; they form a class.

8. Arthur Andersen & Co., basing its computations on company-supplied data, estimated the annual cost of governmental regulation (1977 impact of six general regulatory agencies and programs on forty-eight large companies, all members of the Business Roundtable) at $2.6 billion. Throughout the report, Arthur Andersen did not bother to provide an estimate of the benefits of regulation (Comptroller General, 1977; DeFina, 1977; Weidenbaum, 1978; Arthur Andersen, 1979; Data Resources, 1979; Green and Waitzman, 1980).

9. Burnam saw the emergence of the new class as necessary to fulfill the basic functional requirements of modern society (Burnam, 1962, pp. 256–266).

10. Konrad and Szelenyi go one step further by arguing that the knowledge of the intellectuals reflects their own interests, and when they become a class, their knowledge is subordinated to those interests (Konrad and Szelenyi, 1979, p. 9).

11. As a result the legitimacy of contemporary universities is more and more dependent on their ability to adopt national economic and political goals as part of their traditional historical mission (Price, 1984/1985).

REFERENCES

American Institute of Certified Public Accountants (AICPA), Practice Analysis Task Force. *AICA Report of the Practice Analysis Task Force.* New York: AICPA, 1983, pp. 119–125.

Armstrong, P. "Changing Management Control Strategies: The Role of Competition be-

tween Accounting and Other Organizational Professions." *Accounting, Organizations and Society* (May 1985), pp. 129–148.

———. "The Rise of Accounting Controls in British Capitalist Enterprises." *Accounting, Organizations and Society* (October 1987), pp. 415–436.

Aron, R. *The Opinion of the Intellectuals.* New York: W.W. Norton, 1962.

Arthur Andersen & Co. *Cost of Government Regulation Study.* Washington, DC: Business Roundtable, 1979.

Ashcraft, R. "Political Theory and the Problem of Ideology." *Journal of Politics* (August 1980), pp. 687–705.

Baran, P., and P.M. Sweezy. *Monopoly Capital.* New York: Monthly Review Press, 1966.

Barrow, C.W. "Intellectuals in Contemporary Social Theory: A Radical Critique." *Sociological Inquiry* (Fall 1987), pp. 415–430.

Belkaoui, A. "Linguistic Relativity in Accounting." *Accounting, Organizations and Society* (October 1978), pp. 97–100.

———. "The Interprofessional Linguistic Communication of Accounting Concepts: An Experiment in Sociolinguistics." *Journal of Accounting Research* (Autumn 1980), pp. 362–374.

———. *Accounting Theory.* San Diego: Harcourt, 1985a.

———. *Public Policy and the Practice and Problems of Accounting.* Westport, CT: Quorum Books, 1985b.

———. *The Coming Crisis in Accounting.* Westport, CT: Quorum Books, 1989.

Belkaoui, A., and J. Chan. "Professional Value System of Academic Accountants." *Advances in Public Interest Accounting* 2 (1987).

Bell, D. *The End of Ideology.* New York: Free Press, 1973.

Benke, R.L. "A Multivariate Analysis of Job Satisfaction of Professional Employees in Big Eight Public Accounting Firms." Unpublished D.B.A. diss., Florida State University, 1978.

Benke, R.L., Jr., and J.G. Rhode. "Intent to Turnover among Higher Level Employees in Large CPA Firms." *Advances in Accounting* 1 (1984), pp. 157–174.

Berger, P.L. "The Socialist Myth." *Public Interest* 44 (Summer 1976), pp. 3–16.

Bergesen, A. *Crisis in the World Systems.* Beverly Hills, CA: Sage, 1983.

Berstein, S. "Social Class, Language and Socialization." In F.A. Sebeok (ed.), *Current Trends in Linguistics.* The Hague: Mouton, 1974.

BIM. "The Board of Directors: A Survey of Its Structure, Composition and Role." Management Survey Report No. 10. BIM, 1972.

Bourdieu, P. *Reproduction in Education, Society and Culture.* Beverly Hills, CA: Sage, 1977.

Branningan, M. "Auditor's Downfall Shows a Man Caught in Trap of His Own Making." *Wall Street Journal* (March 4, 1987), p. 29.

Braverman, H. *Labor and Monopoly Capital.* New York: Monthly Review Press, 1966.

Burnam, J. *The Managerial Revolution.* Bloomington: Indiana University Press, 1962.

Chetkovich, M.N. "The Accounting Profession Responds to the Challenge of Regulation." In J.W. Buckley and J.F. Weston (eds.), *Regulation and the Accounting Profession.* Belmont, CA: Lifetime Learning Publications, 1980.

Comptroller General, Government Regulatory Activity. *Justification, Processes, Impacts, and Alternatives.* Washington, DC: General Accounting Office, 1977.

Data Resources. *The Macroeconomic Impact of Federal Pollution Control Program, 1978 Assessment.* Washington, DC: Council on Environmental Quality, 1979.

Defina, R. *Public and Private Expenditures for Federal Regulation of Business.* St. Louis: Washington University, Center for the Study of American Business, 1977.

Derber, C. "Managing Professionals." *Theory and Society* 12 (1983), pp. 309–341.

Domhoff, G.W. *The Bohemian Grove and Other Retreats.* New York: Harper & Row, 1974.

Ehrenreich, B., and J. Ehrenreich. "The Professional Managerial Class." *Radical America* 11 (1976), pp. 7–31.

Elliott, R.X., and W. Schultze. "Regulation of Accounting: Practitioner's Viewpoint." In A.R. Abdel-Khalik (ed.), *Government Regulations of Accounting and Information.* Tallahassee: University Presses of Florida, 1979.

Engels, F., and K. Marx. *The Holy Family.* In F. Naun and F. Engels, *Collected Works,* Vol. 4. New York: International Publishers, 1975.

Estes, R. "An Intergenerational Comparison of Socioeconomic Status among CPAs, Attorneys, Engineers and Physicians." In B. Schwartz (ed.), *Advances in Accounting,* Vol. 1. Greenwich, CT: JAI Press, 1984, pp. 1–18.

Flegm, E.H. *Accounting: How to Meet the Challenges of Relevance and Regulation.* New York: John Wiley & Sons, 1984.

Galbraith, J.K. *The New Industrial State.* Boston: Houghton Mifflin, 1978.

Gouldner, A. "The New Class Project, I." *Theory and Society* 6 (1978), pp. 153–203.

Gouldner, A.W. *The Future of the Intellectuals and the New Class.* New York: Continuum Publishing, 1979.

Granick, D. *Managerial Comparisons of Four Developed Countries: France, Britain, the United States and Russia.* Cambridge, MA: MIT Press, 1971.

Green, M., and N. Waitzman. "Cost, Benefit and Class." *Working Payers for a New Society* 7 (May/June 1980), pp. 39–51.

Habermas, J. *Toward a Rational Society.* Boston: Beacon Press, 1970.

Haried, A.A. "The Semantic Dimensions of Financial Statements." *Journal of Accounting Research* (Autumn 1980), pp. 632–674.

Hegel, G.W.F. *Hegel's Philosophy of the Right,* translated by T.M. Knot. Oxford: Clarendon Press, 1942.

Healy, J. "The Drudge Is Dead." *MBA* (November 1976), pp. 48–56.

Jayson, S., and K. Williams. "Women in Management Accounting: Moving Up . . . Slowly." *Management Accounting* (July 1986), pp. 20–26.

Kleiman, C. "Scrutiny Hasn't Put Crimp in Auditing." *Chicago Tribune* (November 29, 1987), Section 8, p. 1.

Kollaritsch, F.P. "Job Migration Patterns of Accountancy." *Management Accounting* (September 1968), pp. 52–55.

Konrad, G., and I. Szelenyi. *The Intellectuals on the Road to Class Power.* New York: Harcourt Brace Jovanovich, 1979.

Konstans, C., and K. Ferris. "Female Turnover in Professional Accounting Firms: Some Preliminary Findings." *Michigan CPA* (Winter 1981), pp. 11–15.

Larson, M.S. *The Rise of Professionalism: A Sociological Analysis.* Berkeley: University of California Press, 1977.

Lewis, M.T., W.T. Lin, and D.Z. Williams. "The Economic Status of Accounting Educators: An Empirical Study." In B. Schwartz (ed.), *Advances in Accounting,* Vol. 1. Greenwich, CT: JAI Press, 1984, pp. 127–144.

Lipset, S.M., and R.B. Dobson. "The Intellectual as Critic and Rebel." *Daedalus* 101 (Summer 1972), pp. 137–198.

Machlup, F. *The Production and Distribution of Knowledge in the United States.* Princeton, NJ: Princeton University Press, 1962.

Mannheim, K. "The Ideological and Sociological Interpretation of Intellectual Phenomena." In K.H. Wolff (ed.), *From Karl Mannheim.* New York: Oxford University Press, 1971.

———. *Ideology and Utopia.* San Diego: Harcourt Brace Jovanovich, 1986.

Marglin, S. "What Do Bosses Do?" *Review of Radical and Political Economics* 6 (Summer 1975), pp. 60–112, and 7 (Spring 1975), pp. 20–37.

Marx, K. *Early Writings,* translated and edited by T.B. Bottomore. New York: McGraw-Hill, 1964.

Merton, R.K. *Social Theory and Social Structure.* New York: Free Press, 1968.

Miliband, R. *The State in Capitalist Society.* New York: Basic Books, 1969.

National Commission on Fradulent Financial Reporting. *Report of the National Commission on Fraudulent Reporting.* New York: AICPA, 1987.

Nettl, J.P. "Power and the Intellectuals." In C.C. O'Brien and W.D. Vanech (eds.), *Power and Consciousness.* New York: New York University Press, 1969, pp. 53–124.

Offe, C. *Disorganized Capitalism.* Cambridge, MA: MIT Press, 1985.

Olson, J., and L. Friez. "Women Accountants—Do They Earn As Much As Men?" *Management Accounting* (July 1986), pp. 27–31.

Olson, W.E. *The Accounting Profession, Years of Trial—1969–1980.* New York: AICPA, 1982.

Orleans, H. *The Effects of Federal Programs on Higher Education.* Washington, DC: Brookings Institution, 1962.

Parsons, T. "The Intellectual: A Social Role Category." In P. Reiff (ed.), *On Intellectuals.* New York: Doubleday, 1970.

Peasnell, K.V., and D.J. Williams. "Ersatz Academics and Scholar-Saints: The Supply of Financial Accounting Research." *Abacus* (September 1986), pp. 121–135.

Poulantzas, N. *Classes in Contemporary Capitalism.* London: Verso, 1975.

Previts, G.J. "The SEC and Its Chief Accountants: Historical Impressions." *The Journal of Accountancy* (August 1978), pp. 13–22.

Price, D.K. *The Scientific Estate.* Cambridge, MA: Harvard University Press, 1965.

Price, G. "Universities Today: Between the Corporate State and the Market." *Culture, Education and Society* 39 (Winter 1984/1985), pp. 43–58.

Scott, J. *Corporations, Classes and Capitalism.* London: Hutchinson, 1979.

Shaikh, A. "An Introduction to the History of Crisis Theories." In *U.S. Capitalism in Crisis.* New York: Union for Radical Political Economists, 1978, pp. 219–241.

Shils, E. *The Constitution of Society.* Chicago: University of Chicago Press, 1972a.

———. *The Intellectuals and the Powers.* Chicago: University of Chicago Press, 1972b.

Szelenyi, I. "Gouldner's Theory of Intellectuals as a Flawed Universal Class." *Theory and Society* 11 (1982), pp. 779–798.

Touraine, A. "An Introduction." In N. Brisbaum (ed.), *Beyond the Crisis.* New York: Oxford University Press, 1977, pp. 3–13.

Useem, M. "Classwide Rationality in the Politics of Managers and Directors of Large Corporations in the United States and Great Britain." *Administrative Science Quarterly* 27 (1982), pp. 199–226.

———. "Business and Politics in the United States and United Kingdom." *Theory and Society* (1983), pp. 281–307.

Watts, R.L., and J.L. Zimmerman. "The Demand for and Supply of Accounting Theories: The Market for Excuses." *The Accounting Review* (April 1979), pp. 273–305.

Weidenbaum, M.L. *Business, Government and the Public*. Englewood Cliffs, NJ: Prentice-Hall, 1978.

Westergaard, J., and H. Resler. *Class in a Capitalist Society*. London: Heinemann, 1975.

Williams, P.F. "The Legitimate Concern with Fairness." *Accounting, Organizations and Society* (March 1987), pp. 169–192.

Chapter 4

Fraud in Accounting

Fraud in the accounting environment is on the increase, causing enormous losses to firms, individuals, and society and creating a morale problem in the workplace. It takes place as corporate fraud, fraudulent financial reporting, white-collar crime, or audit failures. This chapter explicates the nature of fraud in the accounting environment, provides some theoretical explanations of the phenomenon from the field of criminology, and explores some outcome situations arising from corporate fraud.

NATURE OF FRAUD IN THE ACCOUNTING ENVIRONMENT

Fraud has many definitions. It is a crime. The Michigan criminal law states:

Fraud is a generic term, and embraces all the multifarious means which human ingenuity can devise, which are resorted to by one individual to get advantage over another by false representations. No definite and invariable rule can be laid down as a general proposition in defining fraud, as it includes surprise, trick, cunning and unfair ways by which another is cheated. The only boundaries defining it are those that limit human knavery.[1]

Fraud is the intentional deception of another person by lying and cheating for the purpose of deriving an unjust, personal, social, political, or economic advantage over that person.[2] It is definitively immoral.

Within a business organization fraud can be perpetrated for or against the firm. It is then *corporate fraud*. Management or a person in a position of trust can perpetrate it. It is then *management fraud* or *white-collar crime*. It may

involve the use of an accounting system to portray a false image of the firm. It is then a form of *fraudulent financial reporting*. It may also involve a failure of the auditor to detect errors or misstatements. It is then an *audit failure*. In all these cases—corporate fraud, management fraud, white-collar crime, fraudulent financial reporting, audit failure—the accountant as preparer, auditor, or user stands to suffer heavy losses.

Corporate Fraud

Corporate fraud or economic crimes are perpetrated generally by officers, executives, and/or profit center managers of public companies to satisfy their short-term economic needs. In fact, the short term-oriented management style may create the need for corporate fraud, given the pressure to increase current profitability in the face of few opportunities and the need to take unwise risks with the firm's resources. As confirmed by Jack Bologna:

Rarely is compensation based on the longer term growth and development of the firm. As a consequence of this myopic view of performance criteria, the executives and officers of many public companies have a built-in incentive or motivation to play fast and loose with their firm's assets and financial data.[3]

In fact, more than the pressure for short-term profitability, economic greed and avarice blot social values and lead to corporate fraud. Evidence from the Federal Bureau of Investigation shows that arrests from two categories of corporate fraud have climbed: fraud jumped 75 percent between 1976 and 1986, and embezzlement rose 26 percent.[4] In fact, corporate fraud goes beyond mere fraud and embezzlement. The situation points to a myriad of activities that may result in corporate fraud. The increase in corporate fraud in the United States and elsewhere is the result of the erosion in business ethics.

Fraudulent Financial Reporting

Fraudulent financial reporting is so rampant that a special commission was created to investigate it: the National Commission on Fraudulent Financial Reporting. The commission defined fraudulent financial reporting as "intentional or reckless conduct, whether act or omission, that results in materially misleading financial statements." Such reporting undermines the integrity of financial information and can affect a range of victims: shareholders, creditors, employees, auditors, and even competitors. It is used by firms that are facing economic crises as well as by those motivated by misguided opportunism.

Common types of fraudulent financial reporting include

1. the manipulation, falsification, or altering of records or documents
2. the suppression or omission of the effects of completed transactions from records or documents

3. the recording of transactions without substance

4. the misapplication of accounting policies, and

5. the failure to disclose significant information

There is a deliberate strategy to deceive by distorting the information and the information records. This results from a number of documented dysfunctional behaviors: smoothing, biasing, focusing, gaming, filtering, and illegal acts. Such behaviors generally occur when managers have a low belief both in the analyzability of information and in the measurability and verifiability of data.[5] Of all these documented dysfunctional behaviors, the one most likely to result in fraudulent financial reporting is the occurrence of illegal acts by violation of a private or public law through various types of fraud. One type of fraud is within the accounting system. Examples include the following:

1. False input scams (creating fake debits)

   a. False or inflated claims from vendors, suppliers, benefits claimants, and employees or false refund or allowance claims by customers

   b. Lagging on receivable payments or customer bank deposits

   c. Check kiting

   d. Inventory manipulation and reclassification

      (1) Arbitrary write-ups and write-downs

      (2) Reclassification to lower value-obsolete, damaged, or "sample" status

   e. Intentional misclassification of expenditures

      (1) Operational expense versus capital expenditures

      (2) Personal expense versus business expense

   f. Fabrication of sales and cost of sales data

   g. Misapplication and misappropriation of funds and other corporate assets (theft and embezzlement)

   h. Computerized input and fraudulent access scams

      (1) Data diddling and manipulation

      (2) Impersonation and impostor terminal

      (3) Scavenging

      (4) Piggybacking

      (5) Wiretapping

      (6) Interception and destruction of input and source documents

      (7) Fabrication of batch or hash totals

      (8) Simulation and modeling fraud (fraudulent parallel systems)

   i. Forgery, counterfeiting, or altering of source documents, authorizations, computer program documentation, or loan collateral

   j. Overstating revenues and assets

   k. Understating expenses and liabilities

      l. Creating off-line reserves

      m. Related party transactions

      n. Spurious assets and hidden liabilities

      o. "Smoothing" profits

      p. Destruction, obliteration, and alteration of supporting documents

      q. Exceeding limits of authority

2. False throughput scams

      a. Salami slicing, trapdoors, Trojan horse, logic

      b. Designed random error during processing cycle

3. Output scams

      a. Scavenging through output

      b. Output destruction, obliteration

      c. Theft of output reports and logs

      d. Theft of programs, data files, and systems programming and operations documentation[6]

Fraud does not always start with an illegal act. Managers are known to choose accounting methods in terms of their economic consequences. Various studies have argued that managerial preferences for accounting methods and procedures may vary, depending on the expected economic consequences of those methods and procedures. It has been well established that the manager's choice of accounting methods may depend on the effect on reported income,[7] the degree of owner versus manager control of the company,[8] and methods of determining managerial bonuses.[9] This effort to use accounting methods to show a good picture of the company becomes more pressing on managers who are facing some form of financial distress and are in need of showing the economic events in the most optimistic way. This may lead to suppressing or delaying the dissemination of negative information.[10] The next natural step for these managers is to use fraudulent financial reporting. To hide difficulties and to deceive investors, declining and failing companies have resorted to the following fraudulent reporting practices: (1) prematurely recognizing income, (2) improperly treated operating leases as sales, (3) inflating inventory by improper application of the last in, first out (LIFO) inventory method, (4) fictitious amounts in inventories, (5) failure to recognize losses through write-offs and allowances, (6) improperly capitalized or deferred costs and expenses, (7) unusual gains in operating income, (8) overvalued marketable securities, (9) "sham" year-end transactions to boost reported earnings and (10) changing their accounting practices to increase earnings without disclosing the changes.[11]

One factor in the increase of fraudulent financial reporting that has escaped scrutiny is the failure of accounting educational institutions to teach ways of detecting fraud and the importance of its detection to the entire financial reporting system. The emphasis in the university and the CPA examinations is

with financial auditing rather than with forensic, fraud, or investigative reporting. J.C. Threadway Jr., chairman of the National Commission on Fraudulent Financial Reporting, sees it this way:

If you go back to the accounting literature of the 1920s or earlier, you'll find the detection of fraud mentioned as the objective of an audit much more prominently. Our work to date in looking at the way accounting and auditing are taught today in colleges and business schools indicates that fraud detection is largely ignored. In fact, there are texts currently in use that do not even talk about the detection of fraud.[12]

Because the Securities and Exchange Commission is dedicated to the protection of the interests of investors and the integrity of capital markets, it is concerned that adequate disclosures are provided for the public to allow a better judgment of the situation. One financial disclosure fraud enforcement program called for disclosures in four areas:

1. Liquidity problems, such as (1) decreased inflow of collections from sales to customers, (2) the lack of availability of credit from suppliers, bankers, and others, and (3) the inability to meet maturing obligations when they fall due.
2. Operating trends and factors affecting profits and losses, such as (1) curtailment of operations, (2) decline of orders, (3) increased competition, or (4) cost overruns on major contracts.
3. Material increases in problem loans must be reported by financial institutions.
4. Corporations cannot avoid their disclosure obligations when they approach business decline or failure.

Corporations need to adopt measures to reduce exposure on causes of fraudulent and questionable financial reporting practices. Examples of suggestions for the reduction of exposure include:

1. The formulation of desired behavior
2. The maintenance of effective system of internal control
3. The maintenance of effective financial organization with acknowledged responsibility for maintaining good financial reporting practices
4. The maintenance of effective internal audit function
5. Having the board of directors play an active role in reviewing financial reporting policies and practices
6. The monitoring of capabilities and circumstances of individuals in positions affecting the financial reporting
7. The promise and use of strong penalties for the violation of guidelines
8. Making sure that the performance targets are realistic
9. Being aware of high emphasis on short-term financial performance[13]

White-Collar Crime

White-collar crime was a concern for Durkheim, who was convinced that the "anomie state" of "occupational ethics" was the cause "of the incessant recurrent conflicts, and the multifarious disorders of which the economic world exhibits so sad a spectacle."[14] At the same time, Ross noticed the rise in vulnerability created by the increasingly complex forms of interdependence in society and the exploitations of these vulnerabilities by a new class that he called "criminaloid."[15] He argued that a new criminal was at large, one

> who picks pockets with a railway rebate, murders with an adulterant instead of a bludgeon, burglarizes with a "rake-off" instead of a jimmy, cheats with a company prospectus instead of a deck of cards, or scuttles his town instead of his ship.[16]

The phrase "white-collar crime" was originated in Edwin Sutherland's presidential address to the American Sociological Society in December 1939.[17] He defined it as "a crime committed by a person of respectability and high social status in the course of his occupation."[18] A debate followed, with Clinard and Reier's defining white-collar crime as restricted only to "illegal activities among business and professional men,"[19] and Harting's defining it as "a violation of law regulating business, which is committed for a firm by the firm or its agents in the conduct of its business."[20] Basically, one view of white-collar crime focused on occupation, and the other focused on the organization, but in fact the world of both occupation and organization is the world of white-collar crime and constitutes what the knife and gun are to street crime.[21] White-collar crimes have not been condemned as vehemently as other common crimes. One reason is that their crime is not to cause physical injury but to further organizational goals. In fact, individuals were found to consider organizational crimes far less serious than those with physical impact.[22] Another reason for the indifference to white-collar crime may be the possibility that members of the general public are themselves committing white-collar crimes on a smaller scale.[23] In addition, the white-collar criminal generally finds support for his or her behavior in group norms, which place him or her in a different position from the common criminal. As Aubert explains:

> But what distinguishes the white-collar criminal in this aspect is that his group often has an elaborate and widely accepted ideological rationalization for the offenses, and is a group of great social significance outside the sphere of criminal activity—usually a group with considerable economic and political power.[24]

The white-collar criminal is motivated by social norms, accepted and enforced by groups that indirectly give support to the illegal activity. In many cases the organization itself is committing the white-collar crime, sometimes because it may be the only response to economic demands.

White-collar crime may be characterized by five principal components: (1) intent to commit the crime, (2) disguise of purpose, (3) reliance on the naïveté of the victim(s), (4) voluntary victim action to assist the offender, and (5) concealment of the violation.[25] Unlike traditional crime, its objective is to steal kingly sums rather than small sums of money, and its modus operandi is to use technology and mass communications rather than brute force and crude tools. In addition, white-collar crime relies on the ignorance and greed of its victim.[26] It inflicts economic harm and physical harm and damages the social fabric.

Audit Failure

Auditors are expected to detect and correct or reveal any material omissions or misstatements of financial information. When auditors fail to meet these expectations, an audit failure is the inevitable result. The level of audit quality can avoid the incurrence of audit failures. Audit quality has been defined as the probability that financial statements contain no material omission or misstatements.[27] It has also been defined in terms of audit risk, with high-quality services reflecting lower audit risk.[28] Audit risk was defined as the risk that "the auditor may unknowingly fail to appropriately modify his opinion on financial statements that are materially misstated."[29]

Audit failures do, however, occur and, as a consequence, bring audit firms face-to-face with costly litigation and loss of reputation, not to mention court-imposed judgments and out-of-court settlements. The client's or user's losses lead to the litigation situation and the potential of payments to the plaintiff. Litigation can be used as an indirect measure of audit quality using an inverse relation—auditors with relatively low (high) litigation offer higher- (lower-) quality audits. This relation was verified in a study that indicated, as expected, that non-Big Eight firms as a group had higher litigation occurrence rates than the Big Eight and that supported the Big Eight as quality-differentiated auditors.[30]

But not all litigations follow directly from audit failures. In a study that described the role of business failures and management fraud in both legal actions brought against auditors and the settlement of such actions, Palmrose found that (1) nearly half of the cases that alleged audit failures involved business failures or clients with severe financial difficulties, and (2) most lawsuits that involved bankrupt clients also involved management fraud.[31] These findings point to the fact that business failures and management fraud play a great role in the occurrence of audit failures, which calls for the auditor to take a responsible attitude in the detection of fraud, as it may affect the audit quality, the audit risk, and the potential for costly litigations. As stated by Connor:

Establishing the requirement to identify the conditions underlying fraudulent reporting as an independent objective of the audit process would help to clarify auditor responsibility and increase auditor awareness of this responsibility. Performance of the recom-

mended procedures of management control review and evaluation and fraud risk evaluation would improve the probability of detecting conditions leading to misstated financial statements. The required focus on financial condition would help identify more effectively those entities that would qualify as business failure candidates in the near term.[32]

Although management fraud and business failure may play a great role in audit failures, there are other reasons for such failures. For example, St. Pierre and Anderson's extended analysis of documented audit failures identified three other reasons: (1) error centering on the auditor's interpretation of generally accepted accounting principles; (2) error centering on the auditor's interpretation of generally accepted auditing standards or implementation of generally accepted auditing standards; and (3) error centering on fraud of the auditor.[33]

FRAMEWORK FOR FRAUD IN THE ACCOUNTING ENVIRONMENT

We have established that fraud is rampant in the accounting environment, taking the shape of corporate fraud, fraudulent financial reporting, white-collar crime, and audit failures. The main issue is to determine the causes and, above all, provide an explanation for the situation. Descriptive characteristics of the person or the situation that may lead to fraud in the accounting environment abound. For example, there is a need to watch for "red flags," which do not necessarily prove management fraud, but when enough of them exist, there is the potential for corporate fraud. Red flag characteristics to be wary of in the course of an audit include the following:

• A person who is a wheeler-dealer
• A person without a well-defined code of ethics
• A person who is neurotic, manic-depressive, or emotionally unstable
• A person who is arrogant or egocentric
• A person with a psychopathic personality

Financial pressures lead to the following possible red flags within the industry

1. Unfavorable economic conditions within that industry
2. Heavy investments or losses
3. Lack of sufficient working capital
4. Success of the company dependent on one or two products, customers, or transactions
5. Excess capacity
6. Severe obsolescence
7. Extremely high debt

8. Extremely rapid expansion through new business or product lines

9. Tight credit, high interest rates, and reduced ability to acquire credit

10. Pressure to finance expansion through current earnings rather than through debt or equity

11. Profit squeeze (costs and expenses rising higher and faster than sales and revenues)

12. Difficulty in collecting receivables

13. Unusually heavy competition (including low-priced imports)

14. Existing loan agreements with little flexibility and tough restrictions

15. Progressive deterioration in quality earnings

16. Significant tax adjustments by the IRS

17. Long-term financial losses

18. Unusually high profits with a cash shortage

19. Urgent need for favorable earnings to support high price of stock, meet earnings forecast, and so on

20. Need to gloss over a temporary bad situation and maintain management position and prestige

21. Significant litigation, especially between stockholders and management

22. Unmarketable collateral

23. Significant reduction in sales backlog indicating future sales decline

24. Long business cycle

25. Existence of revocable and possibly imperiled licenses necessary for continuation of business

26. Suspension or delisting from a stock exchange[34]

27. Fear of a merger

Merchant cites as causes of fraudulent financial reporting organizational factors and personal circumstances:

By providing incentives for deception, by failing to persuade managers and employees that chances of detection are higher and penalties severe, and by failing to provide adequate moral guidance and leadership, corporations increase the use of illegal and unethical practices.[35]

Although these descriptive characteristics may be useful for detecting the potential for fraud in the corporate environment, they do not provide an adequate normative explanation of why fraud happens. The field of criminology offers various models and theories that are very much applicable to fraud in the accounting environment and may offer alternative explanations for the phenomenon.

The Conflict Approach

The consensus approach and the conflict approach are two major views that hypothesize about law and society.[36] Influenced by anthropological and sociological studies of primitive law, the consensus approach sees laws developing out of public opinion as a reflection of popular will. The conflict approach sees laws as originating in a political context in which influential interest groups pass laws that are beneficial to them. A third view argues for an integrated approach that focuses on the different functions of the consensus and conflict approaches, with the conflict approach ideal to explain the creation of criminal law and the consensus perspective, the operation of the law.

In the case of the accountant and fraud it can be argued, using the conflict approach, that accounting interest groups presented a favorable picture of their problematic situation by insisting that they can control for fraud and worked to get their view of the situation more widely recognized. The process led to less stringent regulation enacted for fraudulent reporting cases and white-collar crime. Basically, it fits with the notion that the criminal law that emerges after the creation of the state is designed to protect the interests of those who control the machinery of the state, including the accounting profession.

The consensus approach refers instead to the widespread consensus about the community's reaction to accounting fraud and to the legislation enacted. The consensus approach to accounting fraud may have resulted from either the ignorance or the indifference of the general public to the situation. Another explanation is the idea of differential consensus related to the support of criminal laws.[37] While serious crimes receive strong support for vigorous actions, crimes relating to the conduct of business and professional activities generate an apathetic response.

If one adopts a conflict model of crime, then the origin of the fraudulent practices in accounting may be linked to a society's political and economic development. As society's political and economic development reaches higher stages, institutions are created to accommodate new needs and to check aggressive impulses. In the process these restraining institutions create a system of inequality and spur the aggressive and acquisitive impulses that the consensus model of crime mistakes for part of human nature. The powerful elites rather than the general will arise to label the fraudulent practices in accounting as criminal because these crimes affect these elites as they are related to property and its possession and control. At the same time, members of that same elite constitute a major component of those participating in the fraudulent practices in accounting. Their motivation to engage in the practices remains the question. The conflict model of crime would attribute the practices to a system of inequality that values certain kinds of aggressive behavior. Basically, those engaging in fraudulent practices in accounting are reacting to the life conditions of their own social class: acquisitive behavior of the powerful, on the hand, and the high-risk property crimes of the powerless, on the other. One would conclude

that the focus of the attack on the fraudulent practices should be toward the societal institutions that led to the isolation of the individuals. It implies a re-organization of these institutions to eliminate the illegal possession of rights, privileges, and position.[38]

The Ecological Theory

An examination of some of the notorious accounting frauds, white-collar crimes, and audit failures may suggest that some criminal types are attracted to business in general and to accounting in particular. Therefore, the criminal cases are not indicative of a general phenomenon in the field but the result of the criminal actions of the minority of criminal types that have been attracted to the discipline of accounting. This approach is known as the "Lombrosian" view of criminology. But with the Lombrosian theory of a physical "criminal type" los-ing its appeal, the ecological theory appears as a more viable and better alter-native to an explanation of the fraud phenomenon in accounting. It adopts as a basis of explanation of corporate fraud the concept of social disorganization, which is generally defined as the decrease in influence of existing rules of be-havior on individual members of the group. Criminal behavior in the accounting field is to be taken as an indicator of a basic social disorganization. First, weak social organization of the discipline of accounting leads to criminal behavior. Second, with the social control of the discipline waning because of the general public indifference, some accountants are freed from moral sensitivities and are predisposed to corporate fraud, white-collar crime, and audit failure. Then the general public's failure to function effectively as an agency of social control is the immediate cause of corporate fraud, white-collar crime, fraudulent financial reporting, and audit failure. Basically, some accountants are freed from moral sensitivities when social control breaks down or fails to function properly.

The Cultural Transmission Theory

Unlike the ecological theory, which assumes that criminal behavior is a prod-uct of common values incapable of realization because of social disorganization, the cultural transmission theory attempts to identify the mechanisms that relate social structure to criminal behavior. One mechanism is the conception of dif-ferential association, which maintains that a person commits a crime because he or she perceives more favorable than unfavorable definitions of law violation. A person learns to become a criminal. As explained by Sutherland:

As part of the process of learning practical business, a young man with idealism and thoughtfulness for others is inducted into white-collar crime. In many cases he is ordered by a manager to do things, which he regards as unethical or illegal, while in other cases he learns from those who have the same rank as his own how they make a success. He

learns specific techniques for violating the law, together with definitions of situations in which those techniques may be used. Also he develops a general ideology.[39]

This mechanism assumes, then, that delinquents have different values from those of nondelinquents. Criminal behavior is the result of values that condone crime. Criminals have been socialized into the values that condone crime. They were transmitted into a culture of crime. Their behavior is an expression of specific values.[40]

Basically, what is implied is that fraudulent behavior in accounting is learned; it is learned indirectly or by indirect association with those who practice the illegal behavior. An accountant engages in fraud because of the intimacy of his or her contact with fraudulent behavior. This is called the process of "differential association." Sutherland explains:

It is a genetic explanation of both white-collar criminals and lower-class criminality. Those who become white-collar criminals generally start their careers in good neighborhoods and good homes, graduate from colleges with some idealism, and with little selection on their part, get into particular business situations in which criminality is practically a folk way. The lower-class criminals generally start their careers in deteriorated neighborhoods and families, find delinquents at hand from whom they acquire the attitudes toward, and the techniques of, crime through association with delinquents and through partial segregation from law-abiding people. The essentials of the process are the same for the two classes of criminals.[41]

Anomie Theories

Anomie, as introduced by Durkheim, is a state of normlessness or lack of regulation, a disordered relation between the individual and the social order, which can explain various forms of deviant behavior.[42] Merton's formulation of anomie focuses not on the discontinuity in the life experiences of an individual but on the lack of fit between values and norms that confuses the individual.[43] As an example in achieving the American Dream, a person may find himself or herself in a dilemma between cultural goals and the means specified to achieve them. The ways adopted include conformity, innovation, ritualism, retreatism, and rebellion.[44]

Conformity to the norms and use of legitimate means to attain success do not lead to deviance. Innovation refers to the use of illicit means to attain success and may explain white-collar crime in general and fraudulent accounting and auditing practices in particular. Merton states: "On the top economic levels, the pressures toward innovation not infrequently erase the distinction between business-like stirrings this side of the mores and sharp practices beyond the mores."[45]

Ritualism refers to an abandoning of the success goal. "Though one draws in one's horizons, one continues to abide almost compulsively by institutional

norms."[46] Retreatism is basically a tacit withdrawal from the race, a way of escaping from it all.

Finally, rebellion is a revolutionary rejection of the goals of success and the means of reaching it. Those adaptations are a result of the emphasis in our society on economic success and on the difficulty of achieving it.

Only when a system of cultural values extols, virtually above all else, certain common success-goals for the population at large while the social structure rigorously restricts or completely closes access to approved modes of reaching these goals *for a considerable part of the same population* does deviant behavior ensue on a large scale.[47] Interestingly enough, Merton goes as far as suggesting that deviance develops among scientists because of the emphasis on originality. Given limited opportunity and short supply, scientists would resort to devices such as reporting only data that support one's hypothesis, secrecy, stealing ideas, and fabricating data.[48]

Unlike Durkheim, Merton believes that anomie is a permanent feature of all modern industrial societies. Their emphasis on achievement and the pressures that result lead to deviance. The anomie thesis is further explored in the work of Cohen[49] and Cloward and Ohlin.[50] Cohen attributes the origins of criminal behavior to the impact of ambition across those social positions for which the possibilities of achievement are limited. What results is a nonutilitarian delinquent subculture.[51] Individuals placed in low social positions accept societal values of ambition but are unable to realize them because of lack of legitimate opportunities to do so. Cloward and Ohlin suggest that the resulting delinquent behavior is, however, conditioned by the presence or absence of appropriate illegitimate means.[52]

Corporate fraud, fraudulent reporting practices, white-collar crime, and audit failures are a result of anomie in modern societies. Basically, delinquent accountants emerge among those whose status, power, and security of income are relatively low but whose level of aspiration is high, so that they strive to emerge from the bottom using even illegal ways. Fraudulent behavior among accountants is then the solution to status anxiety. It results from the discrepancy between the generally accepted values of ambition and achievement and the inability to realize them and the availability of appropriate illegitimate means.

A Framework for Fraud in Accounting

The various theories from the field of criminology offer alternative explanations for corporate fraud, white-collar crime, fraudulent financial reporting, and audit failures. They can be integrated in a framework to be used for identifying the situations most conducive to those phenomena (see Figure 4.1). Basically, the framework postulates that corporate fraud, white-collar crime, fraudulent financial reporting, and audit failures occur most often in the following situations:

In which accounting and business groups have presented a favorable picture

Figure 4.1
A Framework for Fraud in Accounting

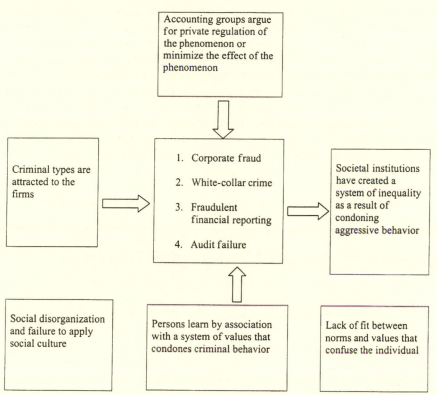

of their problematic situation by insisting that they can control for fraud and worked to get their view of the situation more widely recognized. What may exist is a situation in which the accountants and/or businessmen have stated that they are taking private actions to avoid public regulation of the phenomena, whereas in fact their actions were mere cosmetic changes or camouflage of serious problems in the profession. There have been many examples of situations in which the accounting profession has argued for private regulation of various problems that affect the profession, the discipline, and standard setting and has thwarted the actions of legislators who were trying to put a stop to the abuses. One has only to recall the failure of various congressional committees investigating the profession to enact any fundamental regulations to change the nature, character, structure, and behaviors of the profession to illustrate the point. From a conflict approach, this is clearly a situation in which the interests of those who control the machinery of the state, including the power of the accounting profession, are protected from stringent regulation.

In which societal institutions have accumulated power, privileges, and posi-

tion, creating a perception of inequality in those who are not members of these institutions. Basically, the situation may lead to an isolation of individuals in a situation in which the acquisitive behavior of the powerful is evident in their daily lives. The lower-level accountant may react to this situation of powerlessness, inferiority, and exclusion by resorting to the various types of illegal activities covered in this chapter. It would be a mere reaction to a system of inequality that values aggressive behavior as explained by the conflict model.

In which firms in general have attracted some criminal types. This Lombrosian view of the phenomenon applies to various accounting frauds.

In which social disorganization in general and failure to apply social control exist. Basically, weak social organization of the discipline and failure of the general public to be concerned creates a climate conducive to fraud.

In which people are placed in a system of values that condones corporate fraud, white-collar crime, fraudulent financial reporting, and audit failures.

In which there is a lack of fit between values and norms that compose the person.

OUTCOME SITUATIONS THAT ARISE FROM CORPORATE FRAUD

Away from RICO to ADR

There is definitely a dramatic increase in the number of claims against certified public accountants (CPAs) and in the amounts sought by claimants as a result of the expanding scope of accountants' liability and the Racketeer-Influenced and Corrupt Organization (RICO) Act liability. RICO, originally used by people victimized by a "pattern of racketeering activity" to sue for treble damages and attorney fees, has been used more and more in commercial litigation growing out of fraudulent securities offerings, corporate failures, and investment disappointments. A situation in which codefendent auditors (sometimes in alleged conspiracy with their client and its management) had violated the federal mail and securities fraud statutes by improperly auditing and issuing audit opinions on their client's financial statements on two or more specified occasions and by employing in the operations of their firms (in or affecting interstate commerce) the fees received for those audits, by reason of which plaintiffs were injured in their business or property, is claimed to allege a violation of statutory provisions of RICO.[53] Efforts were made in 1987 to reform the civil provisions of RICO. In fact, a Senate bill introduced by Senator Howard Metzenbaum continues to permit plaintiffs to seek multiple damages in cases otherwise punishable under the securities laws if the plaintiffs are small investors. The definition of small investor includes more than 50 percent of the more than 45 million investors in securities in the United States. This spells bad news for the accounting profession. Witness the following statement made by B.Z. Lee, the AICPA's choice for testifying to the need to reform RICO:

Of greatest concern to the accounting profession . . . is the fact that RICO continues to be used to evade the standards of the securities laws and to raise the stakes in ordinary litigation arising from securities transactions.[54]

For now, fraudulent cases that involve auditors will continue to be prosecuted with RICO liability in mind. In these fraudulent cases accountants have found themselves named as codefendants. The rationale behind the courts' proneness to hold auditors liable for losses associated with business failures results from the belief that auditors "(1) can best prevent the losses associated with business failures and (2) are able to spread their liability through insurance."[55] What auditors face is a dangerous gamble that is trial by jury, especially with the risk of RICO-treble damage judgments. Not only may the average juror not understand the complexities of the cases, but the CPA may face the situation of claims without merit because his or her factual and legal positions may be misunderstood or rejected by the same jurors. The trial by jury may also be an expensive alternative even if the CPA's position prevailed. Witness the following assessment of the situation:

Even if the accountant ultimately prevails at trial, the costs of protracted litigation, including attorneys' fees and deposition costs, can be prohibitively high. Thus, even a win before a jury often translates into great pecuniary loss. Litigation costs and exposure aside, an additional substantial burden is placed on an accountant defendant who is called away from practice—losing both time and fees—and required to produce and review records, study claimants' documents and testimony, appear as a witness on deposition, attend depositions of others and be in attendance at trials.[56]

The trial by jury can also be detrimental to accountants because of the several often repeated arguments that are increasingly persuasive in courts. These arguments include the perceptions (1) that auditors are equipped to prevent the losses associated with business failures, (b) that accountants have deep pockets that can use their insurance to spread the losses, and (c) that equity calls for placing the blame for losses resulting from business failures on auditors.[57] What appear to be more beneficial options for resolving claims against CPAs are the alternative dispute resolution (ADR) methods: arbitration, court-assessed arbitration, mediation, and mistrial.

The AICPA's special committee on accountants' legal liability prepared in 1987 a paper on ADR as a flexible approach to resolving litigation with a client by transforming the typical confrontational position into one of cooperation to reach a mutually advantageous solution.[58] One suggestion made is for the accountant and his or her client to agree on some element of an engagement letter or on a separate agreement that any disputes between them will be determined by ADR procedures. The following two model paragraphs are offered for an engagement letter, one specifically for arbitration and the other for general procedure:

Model Arbitration Paragraph

Any controversy or claim arising out of or relating to our engagement to [describe service, e.g., audit the company's financial statements] shall be resolved by arbitration in accordance with the Commercial Arbitration Rules of the American Arbitration Association, and judgment on the award rendered by the Arbitrator(s) may be rendered in any Court having proper jurisdiction.

Model General ADR Paragraph

In the event of any dispute between us relating to our engagement to [describe engagement, e.g., audit the company's financial statements; prepare the company's tax returns], we mutually agree to try in good faith to resolve the dispute through negotiation or alternative dispute resolution techniques before pursuing full-scale litigation.[59]

Arbitration is now appearing as the more viable option. The pros for arbitration include (1) its informal nature, (2) the choice of knowledgeable professionals as arbitrators, (3) its low cost, (4) its avoidance of the wrong judgments by an unsophisticated jury, (5) the neutralizing of the hostility factor to professionals and sympathy factor to alleged victims prevalent in a jury trial, and (6) the elimination of the risk of a runaway jury's returning a verdict that far exceeds actual losses. These features are summed up as follows.

In arbitration, extensive and time-consuming discovery, which has become standard practice in litigation, is generally not permitted. During the preparatory stages of arbitration, lengthy depositions usually aren't allowed, and limited documentation is exchanged on an informal basis. At arbitration hearings, the rules of evidence are more relaxed. Because of the expertise of the members of the panel, the need for experts to make detailed explanations to unsophisticated jurors is substantially reduced. Fewer witnesses need to be called to testify, fewer technical requirements need to be met, and fewer technical evidentiary objections and arguments need to be made.[60]

Naturally, there are limitations to arbitration. The major limitations are the absence of judicial review and the loss of the court's requirement that evidence be legally admissible and weighed in accordance with legal principles. Other limitations are expressed as follows.

While the American Institute of CPAs' accountants' legal liability special committee has submitted proposed alternative dispute resolution and arbitration clauses, the inclusion of these clauses in the initial engagement letter may subject a member to a coverage defense in any subsequent litigation. . . . Arbitration includes numerous negative points such as limited discovery, limited appeal and a difficulty in confining the arbitrators' decision to case and statutory law. This is particularly true when a defense may involve a question of privity. These negative points severely affect the insurer's ability to defend an insured in a malpractice claim. It seems to me that a CPA may subject himself to an

insurance coverage dispute by including an arbitration clause in the initial engagement letter, since the clause binds the CPA and his insurer to submit to future arbitration.[61]

The Liability Exposure Expands

With the number of lawsuits filed in 1987 reaching one private lawsuit for every fifteen Americans, accountants were not immune to the epidemic of lawsuits. The consequences include escalating judgments and legal costs and astronomical increases in the premiums for professional liability. Even the AICPA professional liability insurance plan increased the premium to 200 percent by the end of 1985, along with a coupling of deductibles and reduction in the maximum coverage available from $20 million in 1984 to $5 million in 1985. The situation is explained as follows: As a result of the premium increase, some medium-sized firms previously paying about $3,400 for $5 million in coverage saw their bills jump to $10,250. In addition, the deductible per claim doubled from $3,500 to $7,000.[62]

To make things worse, megasuits are now being filed against the eight largest accounting firms. Examples include (1) the $260 million damage suit filed in 1985 by the British government for alleged negligence against the auditors of the Delorean Motor Co. in Northern Ireland and (2) the $100 million judgment brought against an Australian accounting partnership in *Cambridge Credit Corporation Ltd. v. Hutcheson.*[63]

The nature of accounting liability has changed since the first English lawsuit against an auditor in 1887.[64] Two major suits had a profound effect: Judge (later Justice) Benjamin N. Cardozo's opinion in *Ultramares Corp. v. Touche* in 1931[65] and the McKesson & Robbins business fraud and settlement with accountants in 1938.[66] The *Ultramares Corp. v. Touche* decision was that accountants are liable for negligence to their clients and to those who they know will be using their work product. More precisely, Judge Cardozo held that accountants could not be held liable to third parties because it might

expose accountants to a liability in an indeterminate amount for an indeterminate time to an indeterminate class. The hazards of business conducted on these terms are so extreme as to enkindle doubt whether a flaw may not exist in the implication of a duty that exposes to these consequences.[67]

The doctrine known as the "privity defense" has recently been eroded with a dramatic expansion in the scope of an auditor's availability for negligence. As Minow states: "The new theory seems to be that the accountant should be held responsible for a business that doesn't function properly."[68] The new *doctrine of indeterminate liability* extends the accountants' liability to any investor or creditor who can convince the court or a jury that the accountant, in hindsight, could have prevented a business failure or fraud by disclosing it. Another new doctrine known as the *fraud-on-the-market theory* allows investors to recover

from defendants for alleged misrepresentations of which the investors were completely unaware as long as reliance on the statements by the market affected the price of the security bought or sold by the plaintiff. An example of the new doctrines came in 1983, when the New Jersey Supreme Court, in *Rosenblaum v. Adler*, held that the accountants can be held of negligence to any reasonable "third parties" relying on that information, especially that which the accountants are able to use and misuse:

Independent auditors have apparently been able to obtain liability insurance covering these risks or otherwise to satisfy their financial obligation. We have no reason to believe they may not purchase malpractice insurance policies that cover their negligence leading to misstatements relied upon by persons who received the audit from the company pursuant to a proper business purpose. Much of the additional costs incurred either because of more thorough auditing review or increased insurance premiums would be borne by the business entity and its stockholders or its customers.[69]

There is definitely a misperception of the accounting profession and its work product. Victor Earle, general counsel of Peat, Marwick, Main & Co., stated this misperception with prescience a decade ago:

The misconceptions in the public mind are at least fivefold: first, as to scope—that auditors make a 100% examination of the company's records, which can be depended upon to recover all errors or misconduct; second, as to evaluation—that auditors test the wisdom and legality of a company's multitudinous business decisions; third, as to precision—that the numbers set forth in a company's audited financial statements are immutable absolutes; fourth, as to reducibility—that the audited results of a company's operations for a year can be synthesized into a single number; and fifth, as to approval—that by expressing an option on a company's financial statement, the auditors "certify" its health and attractiveness for investment purposes.[70]

The liability exposure of U.S. accounting firms doing audits of overseas subsidiaries of American companies also increased tremendously in March 1988, when a federal judge ruled that United States-based accounting firms can be sued in U.S. courts for allegedly shoddy audits in other nations. The decision came after the Court denied a motion by Arthur Andersen & Co. to throw out a $260 million suit against it by the British government for allegedly negligent audits after the collapse of Delorean Motor Co.'s Irish unit. That the U.S. courts will have jurisdiction in such cases spells more trouble for American accounting firms, as U.S. courts are known to be far tougher on accountants than are English and European courts.[71]

In March 1988 the liability exposure took a different dimension when the Supreme Court made it easier for shareholders to file class-action lawsuits against companies that issue misleading information. In its ruling the Supreme Court endorsed the efficient market hypothesis, which maintains that all publicly available information is reflected in the market price. Therefore, shareholders

who allege misleading information and security fraud don't have to prove that
they have relied on the misleading information. Basically, nobody can hide
anymore behind a white collar.[72]

Those developments put the accounting profession in a dangerous situation,
as all business failures could be blamed on the accountant and as the normal
risks of investment may be shifted from the investor to the accountant. Frivolous
litigation may arise, leading the accounting profession to avoid serving riskier
industries and to avoid innovations in its own practice. A case in point is the
review of earnings forecasts. Minow explains:

Accountants would be discouraged from innovations within their own practice, such as
review of earnings forecasts, which, though potentially highly useful to the investing
public, are necessarily speculative and, in the current climate, pose obvious litigation
risks to accountants.[73]

Fraud Engagement: The Issues

Fraud as the intentional deception, misappropriation of resources, or distortion
of data to the advantage of the perpetrator may involve either a manager or an
employee. Management fraud is the most difficult to detect and can cause ir-
reparable damage. The conduct of an audit in accordance with generally accepted accounting principles does not anticipate deceit and may fail to detect
fraud. The key to fraud prevention could be effective and functioning internal
controls. However, some fraud schemes may be effectively designed to work
within the framework of an effective internal control system. The level of assurance of these controls becomes the key, even though fraud is most associated
with a problem of integrity and, therefore, not easily quantifiable. What may be
needed besides the audit is a fraud engagement. This is different from an audit
based on a generally accepted auditing standard in the following way:

In short, the fraud engagement requires a specialized program that is singularly designed
for discovery. It is ideally concerned with what lies behind transactions, with regard to
materiality, and is not concerned with the application of generally accepted accounting
principles unless misapplication has led to fraudulent statements. In its purest form,
therefore, it is a hybrid of auditing and management advisory services. And the individual
searching for fraud must have a detection mentality that is tempered with a high level
of innovation and skepticism.[74]

Fraud engagement should be looking for specifically recurring fraud schemes
and watch for specific indicators of fraud. Recurring fraudulent schemes include
the following:

• Petty cash embezzlement, generally camouflaged by false or inadequate documentation
• Accounts payable fraud involving the formation of a dummy corporation to invoice
  the payer and receive the funds

- Cash inventory schemes in which inventory is purchased with cash or its equivalent, rather than by check, and is not placed on the books
- False payroll schemes involving the creation of a fictitious employee, with management cashing his or her spurious payroll checks
- Lapping schemes in which employees steal from one customer's account and attempt to cover the theft by applying to that account later collections from another customer
- Kickback schemes[75]

All of these schemes involve some diversion of assets or information followed by the prevention or deferral of the activities' disclosure. They can be detected if certain indicators or indicia are carefully watched, especially those indicators or indicia that are present time and again when fraud occurs. The following irregularities deserve closer scrutiny:

1. High rates of employee turnover, particularly in the accounting or bookkeeping departments
2. Refusal to use serially numbered documents or the undocumented destruction of missing numbers
3. Excessive and unjustified cash transactions
4. Excessive and unjustified use of exchange items, such as cashier's checks, traveler's checks, and money orders
5. Failure to reconcile checking accounts
6. Excessive number of checking accounts with a true business purpose
7. The existence of liens and other financial encumbrances before a bankruptcy, which may indicate that the bankruptcy was planned
8. Photocopies of invoices in files
9. A manager or employee who falls in debt
10. Excessive number of unexplained corporate checks bearing second endorsements
11. Excessive or material changes in bad-debt write-off
12. Inappropriate freight expenses in relation to historical sales or industry norms
13. Inappropriate ratio of inventory components
14. Business dealings with no apparent economic purpose
15. Assets apparently sold but possession maintained
16. Assets sold for much less than they are worth
17. Continuous rollover of loans to management or loans to employees not normally included in the loans accounts
18. Questionable changes in financial ratios, such as net income and inventory
19. Questionable leave practices, such as the failure or refusal of an employee to take leave[76]

It follows that auditors have to expand their role to that of police officers and engage in detecting and reporting fraud and financial weaknesses in the firms

that they audit. The three-year examination of the auditing profession by the House Subcommittee on Oversight and Investigations that ended in 1988 had a nonnegotiable item for the profession, which is to be the voluntary protector of the investor or face legislation that will make this role mandatory.[77] For that, Congress will use the Treadway findings as a basis for the legislation and increase the SEC power to impose sanctions and push for criminal prosecution. One would not blame Congress, as the typical situation now shows a failure of auditing standards when they allow auditors to wait until a company has failed before notifying the SEC of possible fraud. A case in point is the ZZZZ Best One, in which Ernst and Whinney had good reason to believe long before ZZZZ Best collapsed that many of the statements made by the carpet cleaning company were fraudulent. It was over and of no use to anyone when Ernst and Whinney decided to make its knowledge of fraud public. Only after the bankruptcy did Ernst and Whinney file documents with the SEC indicating that it had been tipped off that ZZZZ Best really was little more than a giant Ponzi scheme, costing investors more than $70 million.

Fraud auditing is then one solution to the problem of fraudulent financial reporting and fraud in general. It was referred to as the creation of an environment that encourages the detection and prevention of fraud in commercial transactions.[78] The advent of federal, criminal, and regulatory statutes involving business calls for some form of fraud auditing. When fraud auditing fails to connect the problems and frauds do happen, is there a role for forensic and investigative accounting? Forensic auditing deals with the relation and application of financial facts to legal problems.[79] What, then, is the difference between forensic accounting, fraud auditing, investigative auditing, and financial auditing? The answer to a survey among the staff members of Peat Marwick Lindquist Holmes, a Toronto-based firm of chartered accountants, is illustrative of the difference:

Forensic accounting is a general term used to describe any investigation of a financial nature that can result in some matter that has legal consequence.

Fraud auditing is a specialized discipline within forensic accounting, which involves the investigation of a particular criminal activity, namely fraud.

Investigative auditing involves the review of financial documentation for a specific purpose, which could relate to litigation support and insurance claims as well as criminal matters.[80]

Forensic accounting goes beyond routine auditing. It specializes in uncovering fraud in the ledger of business contracts and bank statements. Forensic auditors prepare a written profile of every key person involved with the company, including corporate officers, employees, and vendors. Keeping track of everything is the objective. The following comment by Douglas Carmichael illustrates the extent of the investigation under forensic auditing:

When the death of a company [occurs] under mysterious circumstances, forensic accountants are essential. . . . Other accountants may look at the charts. But forensic accountants actually dig into the body.[81]

THE POSITION OF THE ACCOUNTANTS IN THE COURTS

Do CPAs, because of their credentials as professionals, have special privileges in the legal system? The answer is that both as witnesses in the conduct of legal inquiry and as defendants in the law of torts, the accountants face a difficult and awkward situation.

Loss of Technical Privilege

The court requires of all witnesses that all relevant information be brought to court on pain of a charge of contempt. The best-known exception is the lawyer–client privilege. The general rule of privilege of Federal Rule of Evidence 503 reads as follows:

A client has a privilege to refuse to disclose and to prevent any other person from disclosing confidential communications made for the purpose of facilitating the rendition of professional [sic] legal services to the client, (1) between himself or his representative and his lawyer or his lawyer's representative, or (2) between his lawyer and the lawyer's representative, or (3) by him or his lawyer to a lawyer representing another in a matter of common interest, or (4) between representatives of the client or between the client and a representative of the client, or (5) between lawyers representing the client.

The same privilege has also been given to the psychologist and the physician (Supreme Court Standard 504) and the clergyman (Supreme Court Standard 506). How about accountants? Do they function or rate sufficiently high to overweigh the value of requiring them to reveal their secrets to the court? The official decision of the courts is that accountants cannot join the privileged few.

As part of the audit process, accountants review *contingencies* that could affect a company's financial conditions as reflected in its financial statements. They are guided in their analysis by Statement of Financial Accounting Standards (SFAS) No. 5, "Accounting for Contingencies." One of the important contingencies examined is that the Internal Revenue Service (IRS) will audit the company's tax return and make material adjustments to it. The auditor is assumed to estimate the probabilities of such adjustments and their magnitude. In the process the auditor prepares a number of papers, including an audit program, reports to management, and tax accrual work papers. The tax accrual papers, which are the subject of a controversy, usually consist of (1) a summary analysis of the transactions recorded in the taxpayer's income tax accounts, (2) a computation of the tax provision for the current year, and (3) a memorandum that discusses items reflected in the financial statements as income or expense, when the ultimate tax treatment is unclear.

The controversy is that the IRS policy states that its agents may seek access to both audit and tax work papers of independent accountants. Section 7602 of the Internal Revenue Code gives the commissioner of internal revenue sweeping authority to summons relevant documents in an investigation of income tax liability. In fact, the section gives the IRS the power to (1) examine any books, papers, records, or other data that may be relevant or material to such inquiry; (2) summon people to produce such books, papers, records, or other data; and (3) give such testimony, under oath, as may be relevant or material to such inquiry.

Would the access of the IRS to the tax accrual papers threaten an accountant's ability to perform an effective audit of a company's financial statements? Most concerned accountants would view the IRS review of their work papers as a fishing expedition and a mind-scam. Most would expect the courts to give them the same treatment as attorneys and reject the mind-scam of accountants. In effect, in *Hickman v. Taylor* (1947) the Supreme Court rejected a mind-scam of attorneys because it destroys the mental privacy that a professional needs to work effectively. The accountants used the mind-scam argument to argue against the IRS' use of the auditor's work papers. The Court's decisions, for some cases, were favorable to the accounting profession. This was true in *United States v. Humble Oil* (1974), *United States v. Powell* (1964), *SEC v. Arthur Young & Co.* (1979), *United States v. Matras* (1973), and *United States v. Coopers & Lybrand* (1977). Not all of the Court's decisions were favorable to accountants. This was true in *United States v. Arthur Young & Co.* (1981) and *United States v. Coopers & Lybrand* (1975). In fact, the Supreme Court, in March 1984, overruled the Second Circuit of Appeals and said that the IRS was entitled to see the tax accrual work papers of Arthur Young & Co. in the IRS' probe of Amerada Hess Corp. for 1972 through 1974. The company was accused of setting up a slush fund for political contributions and payments to foreign officials. Arthur Young and Amerada Hess argued that the work papers were irrelevant to any IRS investigation because they were not used in preparing the tax returns. Moreover, they argued that accountants and clients are protected by the same privilege of confidentiality as lawyers. Both arguments were rejected. The Court maintained, first, that the papers were relevant and, second, that lawyers are "advocates" and "advisers" for their clients, but accountants play a "public watchdog" role as auditors. Chief Justice Burger wrote:

By certifying the public reports that collectively depict a corporation's financial status, the independent auditor assumes a public responsibility transcending any employment relationship with the client. The independent public accountant performing this special function owes ultimate allegiance to the corporations' creditors and stockholders, as well as to the investing public.

The decision is not a cause for joy in the accounting profession despite assurance from the IRS that it will seek work papers only in unusual cases and

when it cannot get the information from the taxpayer. But will the IRS stick to the policy in the future? The decision raises many questions:

1. Will the decision lead companies to be less candid with their outside auditors about their tax pictures?
2. Should not the accountants be protected from disclosure by the privilege of confidentiality that applies to work done by accountants in much the same way that it applies to lawyers' work?
3. Are the outside auditors "watchdogs" or "advocates and advisers" to their clients?
4. Will the relationship between the auditors and their clients change toward less communication and more distortion?
5. Will the companies continue to self-disclose if they know that the CPA may have to give the contents of the disclosure to the IRS? Will it lead to less forthright disclosure?
6. Will the discovery of tax accrual work papers provide the IRS with a road map to the corporation's most aggressive interpretations of the Revenue Code?
7. Is the auditor's work-product privilege analogous to the attorney's work-product doctrine?
8. If candid communications between the taxpayer and the auditor are essential to ensure adequate reserves for tax contingencies, would it not be more appropriate that records of communications stating why a tax position was taken by the taxpayer and the settlement posture on that position should seldom, if ever, be discovered by the IRS?
9. Is the full disclosure of questionable positions required for effective revenue collection?
10. Why should corporations provide the IRS with the substance of the case against them?
11. Is the IRS at a disadvantage in its examination of tax returns because the taxpayer, or his or her agent, possesses the sources of information that the IRS needs to audit the return?
12. Without client cooperation and self-disclosure, can the auditor review contingencies as required by SFAS No. 5 and be able to give an unqualified opinion, or is the auditor limited now to give only a qualified or adverse opinion or a disclaimer?

The Accountant as Defendant in the Law of Torts

The U.S. society is a litigious society. The price tag is enormous, with evidence showing that many civil cases that go to trial—with or without a jury—can easily cost the taxpayers more money than is at stake for any of the litigants. In a speech to the American Bar Association on February 12, 1984, Chief Justice Warren Burger observed: "Our system is too costly, too painful, too destructive, too inefficient for a truly civilized people." As a result, accountants find themselves affected in many ways by the litigation explosion.

What is affecting accountants started with prudent liability and the notion of strict liability, whereby "strict liability means that whenever a particular product emerges from an assembly line in a defective condition, the manufacturer will be liable for any injury that the defect causes."[82] The notion of strict product liability was later expanded to the area of professional liability affecting, in the process, architects, doctors, lawyers, accountants, and so on. In the case of the accountants, it meant that they should be held responsible for a business that does not function properly. This action has generated a flood of lawsuits against accountants. Each time a company fails, its independent auditors become one of the few potential defendants that are solvent and, therefore, likely targets for a suit. Given this situation, the first step is to identify the five potential sources of legal liability of accountants.

The first source of legal liability is the common liability to clients. This involves contractual liability, negligence liability, and problems of independence.

With respect to contractual liability, the auditor is bound by a contract with the client and an engagement letter specifying the scope of the audit, that his or her audit examination is to be performed with due care and in accordance with professional standards, and that an opinion is to be issued regarding the quality of the client's financial statement. Without this, the accountant would be subjected to legal liability.

With respect to negligence liability, it would arise not only from a breach of contract but also from a failure to observe professional standards and from lapses such as the following: (1) inadequate preparation by failing to prepare or revise the audit program for a client to take into account internal or external changes; (2) lapses in examination by omission or misapplication of a procedure required by the generally accepted standards; (3) inadequate supervision, review, and training of the audit staff; (4) shortcomings of evaluation and judgment; and (5) failure in reporting the right opinion. The accountant can avoid negligent liability if he or she can prove that (1) the client's own negligence contributed to the problem in the company; (2) the client failed to supervise the company's personnel, which contributed to the accountant's failure to fulfill his or her contract and to report the truth; (3) the client disregarded the auditor's recommendations; and (4) the client knew that reliance on the auditor's opinion is unjustified and that such reliance is a form of contributory negligence.

Problems of independence arise when the auditor issues an opinion on the financial statements while acting as an advocate for the client or as unjustifiably deferential to the client management's judgment. This usually happens when the accountant is also performing nonaudit accounting services for the client.

The second source of liability for accountants is the common liability to third parties. For a long time accountants were liable at common law for negligence in the performance of their professional engagements only to their clients. This

is known as the *privity of contract doctrine*. The test of the privity of contract doctrine involving auditors came in *Ultramares Corp. v. Touche*.[83] In that case the defendant certified the accounts of a firm, knowing that banks and other lenders were guilty of negligence and fraudulent misrepresentation in not detecting fictitious amounts included in accounts receivable and accounts payable. In his opinion Justice Cardozo drew a sharp distinction between fraudulent conduct and merely negligent conduct, holding that the auditor would not be liable to third parties for the latter:

If liability for negligence exists, a thoughtless slip or blunder, the failure to detect a theft or forgery beneath the cover of deceptive entries, may expose accountants to a liability in an indeterminate amount for an indeterminate time to an indeterminate class. The hazards of a business conducted on these terms are so extreme as to rekindle doubt whether a flaw may not exist in an implication of a duty that espouses to these consequences. The court also stated, however, that if the degree of negligence is so gross as to amount to "constructive fraud," accountants' liability extends to third parties.

Then the defense of lack of privity eroded as the work of the auditors became more and more the subject of lawsuits by nonclient plaintiffs.

An accountant may be liable for ordinary negligence to third parties for whom the accountant knows the client has specifically engaged him or her to produce the accounting product. This type of third party is known as the *primary beneficiary*. An accountant may also be liable for ordinary negligence to third parties, those known or reasonably foreseen by the accountant, as well as those who the accountant knows will rely on his or her work product in making a particular business decision. This type of third party is known as the *foreseen party*. This liability may extend to all third parties, including merely foreseeable third parties. In other words, users of financial statements beyond those actually foreseen could hold a CPA liable.

In addition, accountants may be found liable to third parties for actual or constructive fraud that is inferred from evidence of gross negligence. The plaintiff is required, in this case, to prove that the auditor knew the falsity (or its equivalent) of a representation. This knowledge is known as the *scienter*, and the requirement of its proof is the *scienter requirement*. In any case, fraud consists of the following elements: (1) false representation, (2) knowledge of a wrong and acting with the intent to deceive, (3) intent to induce action in reliance, (4) justifiable reliance, and (5) resulting damage.

The third source of liability for accountants arises under the federal securities laws. Everybody relies on accountants to play a role in producing accurate information. This main responsibility lies in making an independent verification of a company's financial statements. The Securities and Exchange Commission (SEC) perceives the purpose of an audit as a public accountant's examination intended to be an independent check on management's account-

ing of its stewardships. Thus, the accountant has a direct and unavoidable responsibility, particularly where his or her engagement relates to a company that makes filings with the commission or where there is a substantial public interest. That audit responsibility is exactly the reason for the potential legal liability of a CPA under the federal securities laws, specifically under Section 11 of the Securities Act of 1933; Section 10(b) of the Securities Exchange Act of 1934 and related Rule 10b-5; Section 12(2) of the 1933 act; Sections 9 and 18 of the 1934 act; Section 17(a) of the 1933 act; and Section 14 of the 1934 act.

Section 11 of the 1933 act defines the rights of third parties and auditors as follows:

In case any part of the registration statement . . . contained an untrue statement of a material fact or omitted to state a material fact required to be stated therein or necessary to make the statements therein not misleading, any person acquiring such security . . . may . . . sue . . . every accountant . . . who has with his consent been named as having . . . certified any part of the registration statement . . . with respect to the statement in such registration . . . which purports to have been . . . certified by him.

Section 11 lists among potential defendants every accountant who helps to prepare any part of the registration statement or any financial statement used in it. It imposes a civil inability on accountants for misrepresentations or omissions of material facts in a registration statement. The leading Section 11 case, *Escott v. Barchris Construction Corp.*,[84] was a class action against a bowling alley construction corporation that had issued debentures and subsequently declared bankruptcy. The court ruled that the accountants were liable for not meeting the minimum standard of "due diligence" in their review of subsequent events occurring to the effective date of the registration statement.

Section 10(b) of the 1934 act states:

It shall be unlawful for any person directly or indirectly, by the use of any means or instrumentality of interstate commerce, or of the mails or of any facility of any national securities exchange, a) to employ any device, scheme, or artifice to defraud, b) to make any untrue statement of a material fact or omit to state a material fact necessary in order to make the statements made, in the light of the circumstances under which they are made, not misleading, or c) to engage in any act, practice, or course of business which operates or would operate as a fraud or deceit upon any person in connection with the purchase or sale of any security.[85]

The elements of Section 10(b) violations are, therefore, (1) a manipulative or deceptive practice, (2) in connection with a purchase or sale, (3) which results in a loss to the plaintiff. Unlike the case in Section 11 of the 1933 act, here the plaintiff carries the burden of proof under Section 10(b). For a while the courts disagreed on the standard of performance to enforce against an accountant under

Rule 10b-5. Then in 1976 the Supreme Court resolved the controversy in *Ernst & Ernst v. Hochfelder*[86] by ruling that some knowledge and intent to deceive are required before accountants can be held liable for violation of Rule 10b-5. In other words, the private suit must require the allegation of a scienter. Most lower courts have held that "recklessness" by a defendant is sufficient to satisfy the scienter requirement of Section 10(b), although mere negligence is not.

Section 12(2) of the 1933 act provides that any person who offers or sells a security by means of a prospectus or by oral statements that contain untrue statements or misleading opinions shall be liable to the purchaser for the damages sustained. Some courts have taken a broad view by implicating accountants as liable for aiding and abetting Section 12(2) violations.

Section 18(a) of the 1934 act imposes civil liability on accountants for filing a false or misleading statement. To escape liability, the defendant must prove that "he acted in good faith and had no knowledge that such statement was false or misleading."

Section 17(a) of the 1933 act states that it should be unlawful for any person in the offer or sale of securities (1) to defraud, (2) to obtain money or property by means of an untrue statement or misleading omission, or (3) to engage in any transaction, practice, or course of business that deceives a purchaser. This section does not state, however, whether a party violating the law is liable. The issue remains to be solved by the Supreme Court.

Section 14 of the 1934 act sets forth a comprehensive scheme governing solicitation of proxies. Rule 14a-9 outlaws proxy solicitation by use of false statements or misleading omissions.

The fourth source of liability for accountants arises under the Foreign Corrupt Practices Act (FCPA) of 1977. This act makes it illegal to offer a bribe to an official of a foreign country. It also requires SEC registrants under the 1934 act to maintain reasonably complete and accurate records and an adequate system of internal control to prevent bribery. Until now the SEC has refused to take any action against perceived violations of the accounting provisions of the FCPA unless those violations are linked to breaches of other securities.

The fifth source of liability is the criminal liability under both federal and state laws. The criminal provisions are in the Uniform Mail Fraud Statute and the Federal False Statements Statute. All of these statutes make it a criminal offense to defraud another person through knowingly being involved with false financial statements. Four of the most widely publicized criminal prosecutions were the *Continental Vending*, *Four Seasons*, *National Student Marketing*, and *Equity Funding* cases, in which errors of judgment on the part of the auditors resulted in criminal liabilities. The SEC position on bringing criminal charges against auditors was once stated as follows:

While virtually all Commission cases are civil in character, on rare occasions it is concluded that a case is sufficiently serious that it should be referred to the Department of

Justice for consideration of criminal prosecution. Referrals in regard to accountants have only been made when the Commission and the staff believed that the evidence indicated that a professional accountant certified financial statements that he knew to be false when he reported on them. The Commission does not make criminal references in cases that it believes are simply matters of professional judgment even if the judgments appear to be bad ones.[87]

CONCLUSIONS

The increase of fraud in the accounting environment is definitely an emerging problem for the accounting profession. The credibility of the profession and the field as a guarantor of the integrity of the financial recording system will suffer more unless drastic measures are taken to make the accountant and the auditor face the fraud problem as a major concern. The immorality of the phenomenon should be accentuated in special courses in the ethical problems of the profession. The education community should take the lead in sensitizing students to the existence, the gravity, the immorality, and the consequences of the problem. The short term-oriented management style that may account for a large proportion of corporate fraud needs to be de-emphasized because of its myopic view of the environment.

NOTES

1. *Michigan Law Review*, chap. 66, sect. 1529.

2. J. Bologna, *Corporate Fraud: The Basics of Prevention and Detection* (Boston: Butterworth Publishers, 1984).

3. Ibid., 10.

4. "Ethics 101," *U.S. News and World Report*, March 14, 1988, p. 76.

5. National Commission on Fraudulent Financial Reporting, *Report of the National Commission on Fraudulent Financial Reporting* (Washington, DC, April 1987), p. 2.

6. Bologna, *Corporate Fraud*, p. 63.

7. S. Lilien and V. Pastena, "Intermethod Comparability: The Case of the Oil and Gas Industry," *The Accounting Review* (July 1981), pp. 690–703.

8. D.S. Dhaliwal, G.L. Salamon, and E.D. Smith, "The Effect of Owner versus Management Control on the Choice of Accounting Methods," *Journal of Accounting and Economics* 1 (1982), pp. 41–53.

9. P.M. Healy, "The Effect of Bonus Schemes on Accounting Decisions," *Journal of Accounting and Economics* 1–3 (1985), pp. 85–107.

10. K.B. Schwartz, "Accounting Changes by Corporations Facing Possible Insolvency," *Journal of Accounting, Auditing and Finance* (Fall 1982), pp. 32–43; K.A. Merchant, *Fraudulent and Questionable Financial Reporting: A Corporate Perspective* (Morristown, NJ: Financial Executives Research Foundation, 1987), p. 105.

11. J.M. Fedders and L.G. Perry, "Policing Financial Disclosure Fraud: The SEC's Top Priority," *Journal of Accountancy* (July 1984), p. 59.

12. B. Lietbag, "Profile: James C. Treadway, Jr.," *Journal of Accountancy* (September 1986), p. 80.

13. Merchant, *Fraudulent and Questionable Financial Reporting*, p. 38.

14. E. Durkheim, *The Division of Labor in Society*, translated by George Simpson (New York: Free Press, 1964), p. 2.

15. E.A. Ross, *Sins and Society* (Boston: Houghton Mifflin, 1907).

16. Ibid., p. 7.

17. E. Sutherland, "White-Collar Criminality," *American Sociological Review* 5 (February 1940), pp. 110–123.

18. E. Sutherland, *White Collar Crime* (New York: Dryden Press, 1949), p. 9.

19. M.B. Clinard and R.F. Reier, *Sociology of Deviant Behavior* (New York: Holt, Rinehart, and Winston, 1979), p. viii.

20. F.E. Hartung, "White Collar Offenses in the Wholesale Meat Industry in Detroit," *American Journal of Sociology* 56 (1950), p. 25.

21. S. Wheeler and M.L. Rothman, "The Organization as Weapon in White-Collar Crime," *Michigan Law Review* (June 1982), pp. 1403–1476.

22. L.S. Shrager and O.F. Short Jr., "How Serious a Crime? Perceptions of Organizational and Common Crimes," in G. Geis and E. Stotland (eds.), *White-Collar Crime: Theory and Research* (London: Sage, 1980), p. 26.

23. V. Aubert, "White Collar Crime and Social Structure," *American Journal of Sociology* (November 1952), p. 265.

24. Ibid., p. 266.

25. H. Edelhertz, E. Stotland, M. Walsh, and J. Weimberg, *The Investigation of White Collar Crime: A Manual for Law Enforcement Agencies* (Washington, DC: U.S. Government Printing Office, 1970).

26. A. Bequai, *White-Collar Crime: A 20th Century Crisis* (Lexington, MA: Lexington Books, 1978), p. 13.

27. Z.V. Palmrose, "An Analysis of Auditor Litigation and Audit Service Quality," *The Accounting Review* (January 1988), p. 56.

28. L.E. DeAngelo, "Auditor Size and Audit Quality," *Journal of Accounting and Economics* (December 1981), pp. 183–199.

29. American Institute of Certified Public Accountants, *Professional Standards*, Vol. 1 (New York: AICPA, 1985), SAS no. 47.

30. Palmrose, "Analysis of Auditor Litigation," p. 72.

31. Z.-V. Palmrose, "Litigation and Independent Auditors: The Role of Business Failures and Management Fraud," *Auditing: A Journal of Practice and Theory* (Spring 1987), pp. 90–103.

32. J.E. Connor, "Enhancing Public Confidence in the Accounting Profession," *Journal of Accountancy* (July 1986), p. 83.

33. K. St. Pierre and J. Anderson, "An Analysis of Audit Failures Based on Documented Legal Cases," *Journal of Accounting, Auditing and Finance* (Spring 1988), pp. 229–247.

34. R.K. Elliott and J.J. Willingham, *Management Fraud: Detection and Deterrence* (New York: Petrocelli Books, 1980), p. 10.

35. K.A. Merchant, *Fraudulent and Questionable Financial Reporting* (New York: Financial Executives Research Foundation, 1987), p. 12.

36. J.T. Carey, *Introduction to Criminology* (Englewood Cliffs, NJ: Prentice-Hall, 1978), p. 8.

37. D.L. Gibbons, "Crime and Punishment: A Study in Social Attitudes," *Social Forces* (June 1969), pp. 391–397.

38. Carey, *Introduction to Criminology*, pp. 36–41.

39. Sutherland, *White Collar Crime*, p. 240.

40. W.B. Miller, "Lower Class Culture as a Generating Milieu of Gang Delinquency," *Journal of Social Issues* 14, 3 (1958), pp. 5–19.

41. Sutherland, "White Collar Criminality," p. 12.

42. Durkheim, *The Division of Labor in Society*.

43. R.K. Merton, "Social Structure and Anomie," *American Sociological Review* (October 1938), pp. 672–682.

44. R.K. Merton, *Social Theory and Social Structure* (New York: Free Press, 1957), pp. 31–60.

45. Ibid., p. 144.

46. Ibid., p. 150.

47. Ibid., p. 146.

48. R.K. Merton, "Priorities in Scientific Discovery: A Chapter in the Sociology of Science," *American Sociological Review* (December 1957), pp. 635–659.

49. A.K. Cohen, *Delinquent Boys: The Culture of the Gang* (New York: Free Press, 1955).

50. R.A. Cloward and L.E. Ohlin, *Delinquency and Opportunity* (New York: Free Press, 1960).

51. A.K. Cohen, "The Study of Social Disorganization and Deviant Behavior," in R.K. Merton, L. Boorm, and L.S. Cottrell Jr. (eds.), *Sociology Today: Problems and Prospects* (New York: Harper & Bros., 1959).

52. Cloward and Ohlin, *Delinquency and Opportunity*, p. 72.

53. R.J. Gomley, "RICO and the Professional Accountant," *Journal of Accounting, Auditing and Finance* (Fall 1982), pp. 51–60.

54. "AICPA Testifies at RICO Hearings: Support Boucher Proposal," *Journal of Accountancy* (January 1988), p. 82.

55. R.S. Banick and D.C. Broeker, "Arbitration: An Option for Resolving Claims Against CPAs," *Journal of Accountancy* (October 1987), p. 124.

56. Ibid., p. 126.

57. S.H. Collins, "Professional Liability: The Situation Worsens," *Journal of Accountancy* (November 1985), p. 66.

58. American Institute of Certified Public Accountants, Special Committee on Accountants' Legal Liability, *Alternative Dispute Resolution* (New York: AICPA, 1987).

59. Ibid., pp. 2, 8.

60. Ibid., p. 726.

61. J.D. Steward, "Arbitration," *Journal of Accountancy* (February 1988), p. 1213.

62. Collins, "Professional Liability," p. 57.

63. Ibid., p. 57.

64. *Leeds Estate, Building & Investment Co. v. Shepherd*, 36, Ch. D. 787 (18F7).

65. *Ultramares Corp. v. Torche*, 225 N.Y. 170, 174 N.E. 441 (1931).

66. See D.Y. Causey Jr., *Duties and Liabilities of Public Accountants* (Homewood, IL: Dow Jones–Irwin, 1982), pp. 16–17.

67. *Ultramares Corp. v. Torche*, 225 N.Y. 170, 179–180, 174 N.E. 441, 444 (1931).

68. N.N. Minow, "Accountants' Liability and the Litigation Explosion," *Journal of Accountancy* (September 1984), p. 72.

69. *Rosenblaum v. Adler*, Slip Op. A-39/85 (N.J., June 9, 1983), 21.

70. V. Earle, "Accountants on Trial in a Theater of the Absurd," *Fortune* (May 1972), p. 227.

71. L. Berton, "Accounting Firms Can Be Sued in U.S. over Audits Done Abroad, Judge Rules," *Wall Street Journal* (March 10, 1988), p. 2.

72. L.J. Tell, "Giliam's Legacy: Nobody Can Hide behind a White Collar," *Business Week* (February 8, 1988), p. 69.

73. Minow, "Accountants' Liability and the Litigation Explosion," p. 80.

74. M.M. Levy, "Financial Fraud: Schemes and Indicia," *Journal of Accountancy* (August 1985), p. 79.

75. Ibid., pp. 79–86.

76. Ibid., pp. 86–87.

77. S. Gaines, "From Balance Sheet to Fraud Beat," *Chicago Tribune* (February 28, 1988), sect. 7, p. 5.

78. J.G. Bologna and R.J. Lindquist, *Fraud Auditing and Forensic Accounting* (New York: John Wiley & Sons, 1987), p. 22.

79. Ibid., p. 85.

80. Ibid., p. 91.

81. D. Akst and L. Berton, "Accountants Who Specialize in Detecting Fraud Find Themselves in Great Demand," *Wall Street Journal* (February 26, 1988), sect. 2, p. 17.

82. J. Weberman, *The Litigious Society* (New York: Basic Books, 1981), p. 42.

83. *Ultramares Corp. v. Touche*, 255 N.Y. 170, 174, N.E. 441 (1931).

84. *Escott v. Barchis Construction Corp.* 283 F.Supp. 643 (S.D.N.Y. 1968).

85. Securities Act 1934, 17 C.F.R. Section 240. 10b-5 (1971).

86. *Ernst & Ernst v. Hochfelder*, 425 U.S. 185, 965 Ct. 1375, 47 L. Ed. 2d 668 (2nd ed.).

87. J.C. Burtow, "SEC Enforcement and Professional Accountants: Philosophy, Objectives and Approaches." *Vanderbilt Law Review* 78 (January 1975), p. 88.

SELECTED REFERENCES

"AICPA Testifies at RICO Hearings: Support Boucher Proposal." *Journal of Accountancy* (January 1988), p. 82.

Akst, D., and L. Berton. "Accountants Who Specialize in Detecting Fraud Find Themselves in Great Demand." *Wall Street Journal* (February 26, 1988), sect. 2, p. 17.

American Institute of Certified Public Accountants. *Professional Standards*, Vol. 1. New York: AICPA, 1985, SAS no. 47.

American Institute of Certified Public Accountants, Special Committee on Accountants' Legal Liability. *Alternative Dispute Resolution*. New York: AICPA, 1987.

Aubert, V. "White Collar Crime and Social Structure." *American Journal of Sociology* (November 1952), p. 265.

Banick, R.S., and D.C. Broeker. "Arbitration: An Option for Resolving Claims against CPAs." *Journal of Accountancy* (October 1987), p. 124.

Bequai, A. *White-Collar Crime: A 20th Century Crisis*. Lexington, MA: Lexington Books, 1978, p. 13.

Berton, L. "Accounting Firms Can Be Sued in U.S. over Audits Done Abroad, Judge Rules." *Wall Street Journal* (March 10, 1988), p. 2.

Bologna, J. *Corporate Fraud: The Basics of Prevention and Detection*. Boston: Butterworth Publishers, 1984, p. 39.

Bologna, J., and R.J. Lindquist. *Fraud Auditing and Forensic Accounting*. New York: John Wiley & Sons, 1987, pp. 22, 91.

Carey, J.T. *Introduction to Criminology*. Englewood Cliffs, NJ: Prentice-Hall, 1978, pp. 8, 36–41.

Causey, D.Y., Jr. *Duties and Liabilities of Public Accountants*. Homewood, IL: Dow Jones–Irwin, 1982, pp. 16–17.

Clinard, M.B., and R.F. Reier. *Sociology of Deviant Behavior*. New York: Holt, Rinehart, and Winston, 1979.

Cloward, R.A., and L.E. Ohlin. *Delinquency and Opportunity*. New York: Free Press, 1960.

Cohen, A.K. *Delinquent Boys: The Culture of the Gang*. New York: Free Press, 1955, pp. 77–82.

———. "The Study of Social Disorganization and Deviant Behavior." In Robert K. Merton, Leonard Boorm, and Leonard S. Cottrell Jr. (eds.), *Sociology Today: Problems and Prospects*. New York: Harper & Bros., 1959.

Collins, S.H. "Professional Liability: The Situation Worsens." *Journal of Accountancy* (November 1985), pp. 57, 66.

Connor, J.E. "Enhancing Public Confidence in the Accounting Profession." *Journal of Accountancy* (July 1986), p. 83.

Durkheim, E. *The Division of Labor in Society*, translated by George Simpson. New York: Free Press, 1964, p. 2.

Earle, V. "Accountants on Trial in a Theater of the Absurd." *Fortune* (May 1972), p. 227.

Edelhertz, H., E. Stotland, M. Walsh, and J. Weimberg. *The Investigation of White Collar Crime: A Manual for Law Enforcement Agencies*. U.S. Department of Justice, LEAH. Washington, DC: Government Printing Office, 1970.

"Ethics 101." *U.S. News and World Report* (March 14, 1988), p. 76.

Fedders, J.M., and L.G. Perry. "Policing Financial Disclosure Fraud: The SEC's Top Priority." *Journal of Accountancy* (July 1984), p. 59.

Gaines, S. "From Balance Sheet to Fraud Beat." *Chicago Tribune* (February 28, 1988), sect. 7, p. 5.

Gibbons, D.L. "Crime and Punishment: A Study in Social Attitudes." *Social Forces* (June 1969), pp. 391–397.

Gomley, R.J. "RICO and the Professional Accountant." *Journal of Accounting, Auditing and Finance* (Fall 1982), pp. 51–60.

Hartung, F.E. "White Collar Offenses in the Wholesale Meat Industry in Detroit." *American Journal of Sociology* 56 (1950), p. 25.

Leeds Estate, Building & Investment Co. v. Shepherd, 36, Ch. D. 787 (1887).

Levy, M.M. "Financial Fraud: Schemes and Indicia." *Journal of Accountancy* (August 1985), p. 79.

Lietbag, B. "Profile: James C. Treadway, Jr." *Journal of Accountancy* (September 1986), p. 80.

Merchant, K.A. *Fraudulent and Questionable Financial Reporting*. New York: Financial Executives Research Foundation, 1987, p. 12.

Merton, R.K. "Social Structure and Anomie." *American Sociological Review* (October 1938), pp. 672–682.

———. "Priorities in Scientific Discovery: A Chapter in the Sociology of Science." *American Sociological Review* (December 1957), pp. 635–659.

———. *Social Theory and Social Structure*. New York: Free Press, 1957, pp. 131–60.

Michigan Law Review, ch. 66, sect. 1529.

Miller, W.B. "Lower Class Culture as a Generating Milieu of Gang Delinquency." *Journal of Social Issues* 14, 3 (1958), pp. 5–19.

Minow, N.N. "Accountants' Liability and the Litigation Explosion." *Journal of Accountancy* (September 1984), pp. 72, 80.

National Commission on Fraudulent Financial Reporting. *Report of the National Commission on Fraudulent Financial Reporting*. Washington, DC: Author, April 1987, p. 2.

Palmrose, Z.-V. "Litigation and Independent Auditors: The Role of Business Failures and Management Fraud." *Auditing: A Journal of Practice and Theory* (Spring 1987), pp. 90–103.

————. "An Analysis of Auditor Litigation and Audit Service Quality." *The Accounting Review* (January 1988), pp. 56, 72.

Rosenblaum v. Adler, Slip Op. A-39/85. N.J. June 9, 1983, 21.

Ross, E.A. *Sins and Society*. Boston: Houghton Mifflin, 1907.

Russell, H.F. *Foozles and Fraud*. Altamonte Springs, FL: Institute of Internal Auditors, 1977.

Schwartz, K.B. *White Collar Crime*. New York: Dryden Press, 1949, p. 240.

————. "Accounting Changes by Corporations Facing Possible Insolvency." *Journal of Accounting, Auditing and Finance* (Fall 1982), pp. 32–43.

Schwartz, K.B., and K. Merton. "Auditor Switches by Failure Firms." *The Accounting Review* (April 1985), pp. 248–261.

Shrager, L.S., and O.F. Short Jr. "How Serious a Crime? Perceptions of Organizational and Common Crimes." In G. Geis and E. Stotland (eds.), *White-Collar Crime: Theory and Research*. London: Sage, 1980, p. 26.

Steward, J.D. "Arbitration." *Journal of Accountancy* (February 1988), pp. 12–13.

St. Pierre, K., and J. Anderson. "An Analysis of Audit Failures Based on Documented Legal Cases." *Journal of Accounting, Auditing and Finance* (Spring 1982), pp. 229–247.

Sutherland, E. "White-Collar Criminality." *American Sociological Review* (February 1940), pp. 210–231.

————. *White Collar Crime*. New York: Dryden Press, 1949, p. 9.

Tell, L. "Giliam's Legacy: Nobody Can Hide behind a White Collar." *Business Week* (February 8, 1988), p. 69.

Uecker, W.C., A.P. Brief, and W.R. Kinney Jr. "Perception of the Internal and External Auditor as a Deterrent to Corporate Irregularities." *The Accounting Review* (July 1981), pp. 465–478.

Ultramares Corp. v. Torche, 225 N.Y. 170, 179–180, 174 N.E. 441, 444 (1931).

Wheeler, S., and M.L. Rothman. "The Organization as Weapon in White-Collar Crime." *Michigan Law Review* (June 1982), pp. 1403–1476.

Chapter 5

Slack in Accounting

INTRODUCTION

Rational principles of management and accounting would dictate the planning and use of company resources in a manner emphasizing truth and accuracy in planning and optional efficiency in use. In reality, the prevailing principles of "designed" management and accounting favor the creation of organizational slack in the use of resources[1] and information distortion through slack budgeting in the planning and budgeting for the same resources.[2] Accordingly, this chapter reviews the research of this opportunistic behavior in management and accounting known as slack by differentiating between organizational slack and budgetary slack.

SLACK BEHAVIOR

Slack behavior refers to the tendency to deviate from principled management and accounting to designed management and accounting. It is a clear manifestation of opportunistic behavior by organizations and individuals.

Slack arises from the tendency of organizations and individuals to refrain from using all the resources available to them. It describes a tendency not to operate at peak efficiency. In general, two types of slack have been identified in the literature, organizational slack and budgetary slack. Organizational slack basically refers to an unused capacity, in the sense that the demands put on the resources of the organization are less than the supply of these resources. Budgetary slack is found in the budgetary process and refers to the intentional distortion of information that results from an understatement of budgeted sales and an overstatement of budgeted costs.

The concepts of organizational slack and budgetary slack appear in other literature under different labels. Economists refer to an X-inefficiency in instances where resources are either not used to their full capacity or effectiveness or are used in an extremely wasteful manner, as well as in instances where managers fail to make costless improvements. X-inefficiency is to be differentiated from allocative inefficiency, which refers to whether or not prices in a market are of the right kind, that is, whether they allocate input and output to those users who are willing to pay for them.[3] Categories of inefficiency of a nonallocative nature, or X-inefficiency, include inefficiency in (1) labor utilization, (2) capital utilization, (3) time sequence, (4) extent of employee cooperation, (5) information flow, (6) bargaining effectiveness, (7) credit availability utilization, and (8) heuristic procedures.[4]

Agency theory also refers to slack behavior. The problem addressed by the agency theory literature is how to design an incentive contract such that the total gains can be maximized, given (1) information asymmetry between principal and agent, (2) pursuit of self-interest by the agent, and (3) environmental uncertainty affecting the outcome of the agent's decisions.[5] Slack can occur when managers dwell in an "excess consumption of perquisites" or in a "tendency to shrink." Basically, slack is the possible "shrinking" behavior of an agent.[6]

The literature in organizational behavior refers to slack in terms of defensive, tactical responses and deceptive behavior. By viewing organizations as political environments, the deceptive aspects of individual power-acquisition behavior become evident.[7] A variety of unobtrusive tactics in the operation of power,[8] covert intents and means of those exhibiting power-acquisition behaviors,[9] and a "wolf in sheep's clothing"[10] phenomenon, whereby individuals profess a mission or goal strategy while practicing an individual-maximization strategy, characterize these deceptive behaviors, which are desired to present an illusionary or false impression. V.E. Schein has provided the following examples of deceptive behaviors in communication, decision making, and presentation of self.

Communication. With regard to written or oral communications, there may be an illusion that these communications include all the information or that these communications are true, which masks the reality either of their consisting of only partial information or of their actually distorting the information.

Decision making. A manager may present the illusion that he or she is actually compromising or giving in with regard to a decision, whereas in reality he or she is planning to lose this particular battle with the long-range objective of winning the war. Or a manager or a subunit may initiate a particular action and then work on plans and activities for implementing a program. This intensive planning and studying, however, may in reality be nothing more than a delaying tactic, during which the actual program will die or be forgotten. Underlying this illusion that one is selecting subordinates, members of boards of directors, or successors on the basis of their competence may be the reality that these indi-

viduals are selected for loyalty, compliance, or conformity to the superior's image.

Presentation of self. Many managers exude an apparent confidence, when in reality they are quite uncertain. Still other managers are skilled in organizing participatory group decision-making sessions, which in reality have been set up to produce a controlled outcome.[11]

Schein then hypothesized that the degree to which these behaviors are deceptive seems to be a function of both the nature of the organization and of the kinds of power exhibited (work-related or personal).[12] She relied on Cyert and March's dichotomization of organizations as either low- or high-slack systems.[13]

Low-slack systems are characterized by a highly competitive environment that requires rapid and nonroutine decision making on the part of its members and a high level of productive energy and work outcomes to secure an effective performance. High-slack systems are characterized by a reasonably stable environment that requires routine decision making to secure an effective performance.

Given these dichotomizations, Schein suggested that:

1. The predominant form of power acquisition behavior is personal in a high-slack organization and work-related in a low-slack organization.

2. The underlying basis of deception is the inherently overt nature of personal power acquisition behaviors in a high-slack organization and an organization's illusion as to how work gets done in a low-slack organization.

3. The benefits of deception to members are the provisions of excitement and personal rewards in a high-slack organization and the facilitation of work accomplishment and organizational rewards in a low-slack organization.

4. The benefits of deception to organization are to foster [the] illusion of a fast-paced, competitive environment in a high-slack organization and to maintain an illusion of workability of the formal structure in a low-slack organization.[14]

ORGANIZATIONAL SLACK

Nature of Organizational Slack

There is no lack of definitions for organizational slack, as can be seen from the definitions provided by Cyert and March,[15] Child,[16] Cohen, March, and Olsen,[17] March and Olsen,[18] Dimmick and Murray,[19] Litschert and Bonham,[20] and March.[21]

What appears from these definitions is that organizational slack is a buffer created by management in its use of available resources to deal with internal as well as external events that may arise and threaten an established coalition. Slack, therefore, is used by management as an agent of change in response to changes in both the internal and external environments.

Cyert and March's model explains slack in terms of cognitive and structural

factors.[22] It provides the rationale for the unintended creation of slack. Individuals are assumed to "satisfice," in the sense that they set aspiration levels for performance rather than a maximization goal. These aspirations adjust upward or downward, depending on actual performance, and in a slower fashion than actual changes in performance. This lag in adjustment allows excess resources from superior performance to accumulate in the form of an organizational stabilizing force to absorb excess resources in good times without requiring a revision of aspirations and intentions regarding the use of these excess resources. "By absorbing excess resources it retards upward adjustment of aspirations during relatively good times . . . by providing a pool of emergency resources, it permits aspirations to be maintained during relatively bad times."[23]

Oliver E. Williamson has proposed a model of slack based on managerial incentives.[24] This model provides the rationale for managers' motivation and desire for slack resources. Under conditions where managers are able to pursue their own objectives, the model predicts that the excess resources available after target levels of profit have been reached are not allocated according to profit-maximization rules. Organizational slack becomes the means by which a manager achieves his or her personal goals, as characterized by four motives: income, job security, status, and discretionary control over resources.

Williamson makes the assumption that the manager is motivated to maximize his or her personal goals subject to satisfying organizational objectives and that the manager achieves this by maximizing slack resources under his or her control.

Williamson has suggested that there are four levels of profits: (1) a maximizing profit equal to the profit that the firm would achieve when marginal revenue equals marginal cost, (2) actual profit equal to the true profit achieved by the firm, (3) reported profit equal to the accounting profit reported in the annual report, and (4) minimum profit equal to the profit needed to maintain the organizational coalition. If the market is noncompetitive, various forms of slack emerge: (1) *slack absorbed as staff* equal to the difference between maximum and actual profit, (2) *slack in the form of cost* equal to the difference between reported and minimum profits, and (3) *discretionary spending for investment* equal to the difference between reported and minimum profits.

Income smoothing can be used to substantiate the efforts of management to neutralize environmental uncertainty and to create organizational slack by means of an accounting manipulation of the level of earnings. J.Y. Kamin and J. Ronen have related organizational slack to income smoothing by reasoning that what often results in slack accumulation is aimed at smoothing earnings.[25]

They hypothesized that management-controlled firms were more likely to be engaged in smoothing as a manifestation of managerial discretion and slack. "Accounting" and "real" smoothing were tested by observing the behavior of discretionary expenses vis-à-vis the behavior of income numbers. Their results showed (1) that a majority of the firms behaved as if they were income smoothers and (2) that a particularly strong majority was found among management-

controlled firms with high barriers to entry. This line of reasoning was pursued by Ahmed Belkaoui and R.D. Picur.[26] Their study tested the effects of the dual economy on income-smoothing behavior. It was hypothesized that a higher degree of smoothing of income numbers would be exhibited by firms in the periphery sector than by firms in the core sector in reaction to different opportunity structures and experiences. Their results indicated that a majority of the firms may have been resorting to income smoothing. A higher number were found among firms in the periphery sector.

Lewin and Wolf proposed the following statements as a theoretical framework for understanding the concept of slack:

1. Organizational slack depends on the availability of excess resources.

2. Excess resources occur when an organization generates or has the potential to generate resources in excess of what is necessary to maintain the organizational coalition.

3. Slack occurs unintentionally as a result of the imperfection of the resource allocation decision-making process.

4. Slack is created intentionally because managers are motivated to maximize slack resources under their control to ensure achievement of personal goals subject to the achievement of organizational goals.

5. The disposition of slack resources is a function of a manager's expense preference function.

6. The distribution of slack resources is an outcome of the bargaining process-setting organization and reflects the discretionary power of organization members in allocating resources.

7. Slack can be present in a distributed or concentrated form.

8. The aspiration of organizational participants for slack adjusts upward as resources become available. The downward adjustment of aspirations for slack resources, when resources become scarce, is resisted by organizational participants.

9. Slack can stabilize short-term fluctuations in the firm's performance.

10. Beyond the short term, the reallocation of slack requires a change in organizational goals.

11. Slack is directly related to organizational size, maturity, and stability of the external environment.[27]

Functions of Organizational Slack

Because the definition of slack is often intertwined with a description of the functions that slack serves, L.J. Bourgeois discussed these functions as a means of making palpable the ways of measuring slack.[28] From a review of the administrative theory literature, he identified organizational slack as an independent variable that either "causes" or serves four primary functions: "(1) as an inducement for organizational actors to remain in the system, (2) as a resource for conflict resolution, (3) as a buffering mechanism in the work flow process,

or (4) as a facilitator of certain types of strategic or creative behavior within the organization."[29]

The concept of slack as an inducement to maintain the coalition was first introduced by C.I. Barnard in his treatment of the inducement/contribution ratio (VC) as a way of attracting organizational participants and sustaining their membership.[30] March and H.A. Simon later described slack resources as the source of inducements through which the inducement/contribution ratio might exceed a value of 1, which is equivalent to paying an employee more than would be required to retain his or her services.[31] This concept of slack was then explicitly introduced by Cyert and March as consisting of payments to members of the coalition in excess of what is required to maintain the organization.[32]

Slack as a resource for conflict resolution was introduced in L.R. Pondy's goal model.[33] In this model subunit goal conflicts are resolved partly by sequential attention to goals and partly by adopting a decentralized organizational structure. A decentralized structure is made possible by the presence of organizational slack.

A notion of slack as a technical buffer from the variances and discontinuities caused by environmental uncertainty was proposed by J.D. Thompson.[34] It was also acknowledged in Pondy's system model, which described conflict as a result of the lack of buffers between interdependent parts of an organization.[35] Jay Galbraith saw buffering as an information-processing problem:

Slack resources are an additional cost to the organization or the customer. . . . The creation of slack resources, through reduced performance levels, reduces the amount of information that must be processed during task execution and prevents the overloading of hierarchical channels.[36]

According to Bourgeois, slack facilitates three types of strategic or creative behavior within the organization: (1) providing resources for innovative behavior, (2) providing opportunities for a satisficing behavior, and (3) affecting political behavior.[37]

First, as a facilitator of innovative behavior, slack tends to create conditions that allow the organization to experiment with new strategies[38] and introduce innovation.[39] Second, as a facilitator of suboptimal behavior, slack defines the threshold of acceptability of a choice, or "bounded search,"[40] by people whose bounded rationality leads them to satisfice.[41] Third, the notion that slack affects political activity was advanced by Cyert and March, who argued that slack reduces both political activity and the need for bargaining and coalition-forming activity.[42] Furthermore, W.G. Astley has argued that slack created by success results in self-aggrandizing behavior by managers who engage in political behavior to capture more than their fair share of the surplus.[43]

W. Richard Scott argued that lowered standards create slack—unused resources—that can be used to create ease in the system.[44] Notice the following comment:

Of course, some slack in the handling of resources is not only inevitable but essential to smooth operations. All operations require a margin of error to allow for mistakes, waste, spoilage, and similar unavoidable accompaniments of work.[45]

But the inevitability of slack is not without consequences:

The question is not whether there is to be slack but how much slack is permitted. Excessive slack resources increase costs for the organization that are likely to be passed on to the consumer. Since creating slack resources is a relatively easy and painless solution available to organizations, whether or not it is employed is likely to be determined by the amount of competition confronting the organization in its task environment.[46]

Measurement of Organizational Slack

One problem in investing empirically in the presence of organizational slack relates to the difficulty of securing an adequate measurement of the phenomenon. Various methods have been suggested. In addition to these methods, eight variables that appear in public data, whether they are created by managerial actions or made available by environment, may explain a change in slack.[47] The model, suggested by Bourgeois, is as follows:

$$Slack = f(RE, DP, G\&A, WC/S, D/E, CR, I/P, P/E)$$

where

RE = Retained earnings

DP = Dividend payout

G&A = General and administrative expense

WC/S = Working capital as a percentage of sales

D/E = Debt as a percentage of equity

CR = Credit rating

I/P = Short-term loan interest compared to prime rate

P/E = Price/earnings ratio

Here RE, G&A, WC/S, and CR are assumed to have a positive effect on changes and DP, D/E, P/E, and I/P are assumed to have a negative effect on changes in slack.

Some of these measures have also been suggested by other researchers. For example, Martin M. Rosner used profit and excess capacity as slack measures,[48] and Lewin and Wolf used selling, general, and administrative expenses as surrogates for slack.[49] Bourgeois and Jitendra V. Singh refined these measures by suggesting that slack could be differentiated on an "ease-of-recovery" dimension.[50] Basically, they considered excess liquidity to be available slack, not yet

earmarked for particular uses. Overhead costs were termed recoverable slack, in the sense that they are absorbed by various organizational functions but can be recovered when needed elsewhere. In addition, the ability of a firm to generate resources from the environment, such as the ability to raise additional debt or equity capital, was considered potential slack. All of these measures were divided by sales to control for company size.

Building on Bourgeois and Singh's suggestions, Theresa K. Lant opted for the four following measures:

1. Administrative Slack = (General and Administrative Expenses)/Cost of Goods Sold
2. Available Liquidity = (Cash + Marketable Securities − Current Liabilities)/Sales
3. Recoverable Liquidity = (Accounts Receivable + Inventory)/Sales
4. Retained Earnings = (Net Profit − Dividends)/Sales[51]

Lant used these measures to show empirically (1) that available liquidity and general and administrative expenses have significantly higher variance than profit across firms and across time and (2) that the mean change in slack is significantly greater than the mean change in profit. She concluded as follows:

These results are logically consistent with the theory that slack absorbs variance in actual profit. They also suggest that the measures used are reasonable measures for slack. Thus, it supports prior work which has used these measures and implies that further large sample models using slack as a variable are feasible since financial information is readily available for a large number of firms. Before these results can be generalized however, the tests conducted here should be replicated using different samples of firms from a variety of industries.[52]

Organizational Slack and Competition

The line of research studying the impact of market competition on internal efficiency of firms suggested results about competition reducing slack. Hart[53] and Scharfstein[54] use a hidden information model with a common shock transmitted via the market price to show that the (informational) effect of an increase in competition by entrepreneurial (profit-maximizing) firms on the internal efficiency of managerial firms depends on the specification of managers' preferences. This informational effect of competition was also confined in a hidden action model.[55] Similarly, when the strategic value of incentive contracts under much different market conditions is examined, it will appear that the increase in the intensity of completion leads to more X-inefficiency.[56] A similar negative relation between the intensity of completion and the degree of internal efficiency was observed in a Cournot principal-agent model, where the principal's managerial benefit of including the agent to minimize cost becomes smaller when competition increases.[57] In the case of multinational firms with multiple plants in different locations, the in-home competition may have an impact on slack

under different economic conditions. For example, Kerschbamer and Tournas evaluated the impact of variations of product demand on the amount of internal slack in multiplant firms in a model in which facilities can produce output at a privately known cost up to a previously determined capacity level.[58] Their model shows the amount of slack to be pro-cyclical in the sense that as capacity constraints become tighter in booms, slack increases in booms, because the power of in-house competition is reduced, while the opposite is true in downturns.

BUDGETARY SLACK

Nature of Budgetary Slack

The literature on organizational slack shows that managers have the motives necessary to desire to operate in a slack environment. The literature on budgetary slack considers the budget as the embodiment of that environment and, therefore, assumes that managers will use the budgeting process to bargain for slack budgets. As stated by Michael Schiff and Lewin, "managers will create slack in budgets through a process of understating revenues and overstating costs."[59] The general definition of budgetary slack, then, is the understatement of revenues and the overstatement of costs in the budgeting process. A detailed description of the creation of budgetary slack by managers was reported by Schiff and Lewin in their study of the budget process of three divisions of multidivision companies.[60] They found evidence of budgetary slack through underestimation of gross revenue, inclusion of discretionary increases in personnel requirements, establishment of marketing and sales budgets with internal limits on funds to be spent, use of manufacturing costs based on standard costs that do not reflect process improvements operationally available at the plant, and inclusion of discretionary "special projects."

Evidence of budgetary slack has also been reported by others. A.E. Lowe and R.W. Shaw found a downward bias, introduced through sales forecasts by line managers, which assumed good performance where rewards were related to forecasts.[61] M. Dalton reported various examples of department managers' allocating resources to what they considered justifiable purposes, even though such purposes were not authorized in their budgets.[62] G. Shillinglaw noted the extreme vulnerability of budgets used to measure divisional performance given the great control exercised by divisional management in budget preparation and the reporting of results.[63]

Slack creation is a generalized organizational phenomenon. Many different organizational factors have been used to explain slack creation, in particular, organizational structure, goal congruence, control system, and managerial behavior. Slack creation is assumed to occur in cases where a Tayloristic organizational structure exists,[64] and it is also assumed to occur in a participative organizational structure.[65] It may be due to conflicts that arise between the individual and organizational goals, leading managers intentionally to create slack.

It may also be due to the attitudes of management toward the budget and to worst views of the budgets as a device used by management to manipulate them.[66] Finally, the creation of slack may occur whether or not the organization is based on a centralized or decentralized structure.[67] With regard to this last issue, Schiff and Lewin have reported that the divisional controller appears to have undertaken the tasks of creating and managing divisional slack and is most influential in the internal allocation of slack.

Using agency theory, budgetary slack can be attributed to four conditions: "1) information asymmetry between the superior (the principal) and the subordinate's effort or output potential, 2) uncertainty in the relation between effort and output, 3) conflicting goals between the superior and the subordinate, and 4) opportunism or self-interest on the part of the subordinate."[68]

Budgeting and the Propensity to Create Budgetary Slack

The budgeting system has been assumed to affect a manager's propensity to create budgetary slack, in the sense that this propensity can be increased or decreased by the way in which the budgeting system is designed or complemented. Mohamed Onsi was the first to investigate empirically the connections between the type of budgeting system and the propensity to create budgetary slack.[69] From a review of the literature, he stated the following four assumptions:

1. Managers influence the budget process through bargaining for slack by understating revenues and overstating costs.
2. Managers build up slack in "good years" and reconvert slack into profit in "bad years."
3. Top management is at a "disadvantage" in determining the magnitude of slack.
4. The divisional controller in decentralized organizations participates in the task of creating and managing divisional slack.[70]

Personal interviews of thirty-two managers of five large national and international companies and statistical analysis of a questionnaire were used to identify the important behavioral variables that influence slack buildup and utilization. The questionnaire's variables were grouped into the following eight dimensions:

1. Slack attitude, described by the variables indicating a manager's attitude to slack.
2. Slack manipulation, described by the variables indicating how a manager builds up and uses slack.
3. Slack institutionalization, described by the variables that make a manager less inclined to reduce his or her slack.
4. Slack detection, described by the variables indicating the superior's ability to detect slack based on the amount of information that he receives.

5. Attitude toward the top management control system, described by the variables indicating an authoritarian philosophy toward budgeting being attributed to top management by divisional managers.

6. Attitudes toward the divisional control system, described by variables on attitudes toward subordinates, sources of pressure, budget autonomy, budget participation, and supervisory uses of budgets.

7. Attitudes toward the budget, described by variables on attitude toward the level of standards, attitude toward the relevancy of budget attainment to valuation of performance, and the manager's attitude (positive or negative) toward the budgetary system in general, as a managerial tool.

8. Budget relevancy, described by variables indicating a manager's attitudes toward the relevancy of standards for his department's operation.[71]

Factor analysis reduced these dimensions to seven factors and showed a relationship between budgetary slack and what Onsi called "an authoritarian top management budgetary control system." Thus, he stated:

Budgetary slack is created as a result of pressure and the use of budgeted profit attainment as a basic criterion in evaluating performance. Positive participation could encourage less need for building up slack. However, the middle managers' perception of pressure was an overriding concern. The positive correlation between managers' attitudes and attainable level of standards is a reflection of this pressure.[72]

Cortland Cammann explored the moderating effects of subordinates' participation in decision making and the difficulty of subordinates' jobs based on their responses to different uses of control systems by their superiors.[73] His results showed that the use of control systems for contingent reward allocation produced defensive responses by subordinates under all conditions, which included the creation of budgetary slack. Basically, when superiors used budgeting information as a basis for allocating organizational rewards, their subordinates' responses were defensive. Allowing participation in the budget processes reduced this defensiveness.

Finally, Kenneth A. Merchant conducted a field study designed to investigate how managers' propensities to create budgetary slack are affected by the budgeting system and the technical context.[74] He hypothesized that the propensity to create budgetary slack is positively related to the importance placed on meeting budget targets and negatively related to the extent of participation allowed in budgeting processes, the degree of predictability in the production process, and the superiors' abilities to create slack. Unlike earlier studies drawn across functional areas, 170 manufacturing managers responded to a questionnaire measuring the propensity to create slack, the importance of meeting the budget, budget participation, the nature of technology in terms of work-flow integration and product standardization, and the ability of superiors to detect slack. The results suggested that managers' propensities to create slack (1) do vary with

the setting and with how the budgeting system is implemented; (2) are lower where managers actively participate in budgeting, particularly when technologies are relatively predictable; and (3) are higher when a tight budget requires frequent tactical responses to avoid overruns.

The three studies by Onsi, Cammann, and Merchant provide evidence that participation may lead to positive communication between managers so that subordinates feel less pressure to create slack. This result is, in fact, contingent on the amount of information asymmetry existing between the principals (superiors) and the agents (the subordinates). Although participation in budgeting leads subordinates to communicate or reveal some of their private information, agents may still misrepresent or withhold some of their private information, leading to budgetary slack. Accordingly, Alan S. Dunk proposed a link between participation and budgetary slack through two variables: superiors' budget emphasis in their evaluation of subordinate performance and the degree of information asymmetry between superiors and subordinates:[75] "When participation, budget emphasis, and information asymmetry are high (low), slack will be high (low)."[76] The results, however, showed that low (high) slack is related to high (low) participation, budget emphasis, and information asymmetry. The results are stated as follows:

The results of this study show that the relation between participation and slack is contingent upon budget emphasis and information asymmetry, but in a direction contrary to expectations. The results provide evidence for the utility of participative budgeting, and little support for the view that high participation may result in increased slack when the other two predictors are high. Although participation may induce subordinates to incorporate slack in budgets, the results suggest that participation alone may not be sufficient. The findings suggest that slack reduction results from participation, except when budget emphasis is low.[77]

Budgetary Slack, Information Distortion, and Truth-Inducing Incentive Schemes

Budgetary slack involves a deliberate distortion of input information. Distortion of input information in a budget setting arises, in particular, from the need of managers to accommodate their expectations about the kinds of payoffs associated with different possible outcomes. Several experiments have provided evidence of such distortion of input information. Cyert, March, and W.H. Starbuck showed in a laboratory experiment that subjects adjusted the information that they transmitted in a complex decision-making system to control their payoffs.[78] Similarly, Lowe and Shaw have shown that in cases where rewards were linked to forecasts, sales managers tended to distort the input information and to induce biases in their sales forecast.[79] Dalton also provided some rich situational descriptions of information distortion in which lower-level managers distorted the budget information and allocated resources to what were perceived to

be justifiable objectives.[80] Finally, a payoff structure can induce a forecaster to bias intentionally his or her forecast. R.M. Barefield provided a model of forecast behavior that showed a "rough" formulation of a possible link between a forecaster's biasing and the quality of the forecaster as a source of data for an accounting system.[81]

Taken together, these studies suggest that budgetary slack, through systematic distortion of input information, can be used to accommodate the subjects' expectations about the payoffs associated with various possible outcomes. They fail, however, to provide a convincing rationalization of the link between distortion of input information and the subjects' accommodation of their expectations. Agency theory and issues related to risk aversion may provide such a link. Hence, given the existence of divergent incentives and information asymmetry between the controller (or employer) and the controlee (or employee) and the high cost of observing employee skill or effort, a budget-based employment contract (i.e., where employee compensation is contingent on meeting the performance standard) can be Pareto-superior to fixed pay or linear sharing rules (where the employer and employee split the output).[82] However, these budget-based schemes impose a risk on the employee, as job performance can be affected by a host of uncontrollable factors. Consequently, risk-averse individuals may resort to slack budgeting through systematic distortion of input information. In practice, moreover, any enhanced (increased) risk aversion would lead the employee to resort to budgetary slack. One might hypothesize that, without proper incentives for truthful communication, the slack budgeting behavior could be reduced. One suggested avenue is the use of truth-inducing, budget-based schemes.[83] These schemes, assuming risk neutrality, motivate a worker to reveal truthfully private information about future performance and to maximize performance regardless of the budget.

Accordingly, Mark S. Young conducted an experiment to test the effects of risk aversion and asymmetric information on slack budgeting.[84] Five hypotheses related to budgetary slack were developed and tested using a laboratory experiment. The hypotheses were as follows:

Hypothesis 1: A subordinate who participates in the budgeting process will build slack into the budget.

Hypothesis 2: A risk-averse subordinate will build in more budget slack than a non-risk-averse subordinate.

Hypothesis 3: Social pressure not to misrepresent productive capability will be greater for a subordinate whose information is known by management than for a subordinate having private information.

Hypothesis 4: As social pressure increases for the subordinate, there is a lower degree of budgetary slack.

Hypothesis 5: A subordinate who has private information builds more slack into the budget than a subordinate whose information is known by management.[85]

The results of the experiment confirmed the hypotheses that a subordinate who participates builds in budgetary slack and that slack is, in part, attributable to a subordinate's risk preferences. Given state uncertainty and a worker-manager information asymmetry about performance capability, the subjects in the experiment created slack even in the presence of a truth-inducing scheme. In addition, risk-averse workers created more slack than non-risk-averse workers did. Similarly, C. Chow, J. Cooper, and W. Waller provided evidence that, given a worker-manager information asymmetry about performance capability, slack is lower under a truth-inducing scheme than under a budget-based scheme with an incentive to create slack.[86]

Both Young's and Chow, Cooper, and Waller's studies were found to have limitations.[87] With regard to Young's study, William S. Waller found three limitations:

First, unlike the schemes examined in the analytical research, the one used in his study penalized outperforming the budget, which limits its general usefulness. Second, there was no manipulation of incentives, so variation in slack due to incentives was not examined. Third, risk preferences were measured using the conventional lottery technique of which the validity and reliability are suspect.[88]

With regard to Chow, Cooper, and Waller's study, Waller found the limitations to be the assumption of state certainty and the failure to take risk preference into account. Accordingly, Waller conducted an experiment under which subjects participatively set budgets under either a scheme with an incentive for creating slack or a truth-incentive scheme like those examined in the analytical research. In addition, risk neutrality was induced for one-half of the subjects, and constant, absolute risk aversion for the rest, using a technique discussed by J. Berg, L. Daley, J. Dickhaut, and T. O'Brien that allows the experimenter to induce (derived) utility functions with any shape.[89] The results of the experiment show that when a conventional truth-inducing scheme is introduced, slack decreases for risk-neutral subjects but not for risk-averse subjects. Added to the evidence provided by the other studies, this study indicates that risk preference is an important determinant of slack, especially in the presence of a truth-inducing scheme.

Basically, there is preliminary evidence that risk-averse workers create more budgetary slack than risk-neutral ones. In addition, "truth-inducing incentive schemes" reduce budgetary slack for risk-neutral subjects but not for risk-averse subjects. It seems that resource allocations within organizations are mediated by perceptions of risk, where risk is a stable personal trait. Accordingly, D.C. Kim tested whether risk preferences are domain-specific, that is, whether latent risk preferences translate into differing manifest risk preferences according to the context.[90] He relied on an experiment simulating the public accountants' budgeting of billable bonus to test the hypothesis that subject preference for tight or safe budget behavior depends on the performance of coworkers and

domain-specific risk preferences. The results supported the view that subordinates' risk preferences are influenced by a situation-dependent variable. As stated by Kim:

The reversal of risk preferences around a neutral reference point is statistically significant for both dispositionally risk-averse and dispositionally risk-seeking subjects. The dispositional variable also contributes to the explanation of variations in subjects' manifest risk preferences. Thus the propensity to induce budgetary slack seems to be a joint function of situations and dispositions.[91]

Budgetary Slack and Self-Esteem

The enhancement of risk aversion and the resulting distortion of input information can be more pronounced when self-esteem is threatened. It was found that persons who have low opinions of themselves are more likely to cheat than persons with higher self-esteem.[92] A situation of dissonance was created in an experimental group by giving out positive feedback about a personality test to some participants and negative feedback to others. All of the participants were then asked to take part in a competitive game of cards. The participants who received a blow to their self-esteem cheated more often than those who had received positive feedback about themselves. Could it also be concluded that budgetary slack through information distortion may be a form of dishonest behavior, arising from the enhancement of risk aversion caused by a negative feedback on self-esteem? A person's expectations can be an important determinant of his or her behavior. A negative impact on self-esteem can lead an individual to develop an expectation of poor performance. At the same time, the individual who is given negative feedback about his or her self-esteem would be more risk-averse than others and would be ready to resort to any behavior to cover the situation. Consequently, the person may attempt to distort the input information in order to have an attainable budget. Belkaoui accordingly tested the hypothesis that individuals given negative feedback about their self-esteem would introduce more bias into estimates than individuals given positive or neutral feedback about their self-esteem.[93] One week after taking a self-esteem test, subjects were provided with false feedback (either positive or negative) and neutral feedback about their self-esteem score.

They were then asked to make two budgeting decisions, first one cost estimate and then one sales estimates for a fictional budgeting decision. The results showed that, in general, the individuals who were provided with information that temporarily caused them to lower their self-esteem were more apt to distort input information than those who were made to raise their self-esteem. It was concluded that, whereas slack budgeting may be consistent with generally low self-esteem feedback, it is inconsistent with generally high or neutral self-esteem feedback.

Toward a Theoretical Framework for Budgeting

A theoretical framework aimed at structuring knowledge about biasing behavior was proposed by Kari Lukka.[94] It contains an explanatory model for budgetary biasing and a model for budgetary biasing at the organizational level.

The explanatory model of budgetary biasing at the individual level draws from the management accounting and organizational behavior literature and related behavioral research to suggest a set of intentions and determinants of budgetary biasing. Budgetary biasing is at the center of many interrelated and sometimes contradictory factors with the actor's intentions as the synthetic core of his or her behavior.

The model for budgetary biasing at the organizational level shows that the "bias contained in the final budget is not the result of one actor's intentional behavior, but rather the result of the dialectics of the negotiations."[95] Whereas budgetary biases 1 and 2 are the original biases created in the budget by the controlling unit and the controlled unit, biases 3 and 4 are the final biases to end up in the budget after the budgetary negotiations, which are characterized by potential conflicts and power factors. The results of semistructured interviews at different levels of management of a large decentralized company verified the theoretical framework. The usefulness of this theoretical framework rests on further refinements and empirical testing.

Positive versus Negative Slack

Although the previous sections have focused on budgetary, or positive, slack, budgetary bias is, in fact, composed of both budgetary slack and an upward bias, or a negative slack. Whereas budgetary slack refers to bias in which the budget is designed intentionally so as to make it easier to achieve the forecast, upward bias refers to overstatement of expected performance in the budget. David T. Otley has described the difference as follows: "Managers are therefore likely to be conservative in making forecasts when future benefits are sought (positive slack) but optimistic when their need for obtaining current approval dominates (negative slack)."[96]

Evidence for negative slack was first provided by W.H. Read, who showed that managers distort information to prove to their superiors that all is well.[97] He cited several empirical studies of budgetary control that indicated that managers put a lot of effort and ingenuity into assuring that messages conveyed by budgetary information serve their own interests.[98] Following earlier research by Barefield, Otley argued that forecasts may be the mode, rather than the means, of people's intuitive probability distributions.[99] Given that the distribution of cost and revenue is negatively skewed, there will be a tendency for budget forecasts to become unintentionally biased in the form of negative slack. Data collected from two organizations verified the presence of negative slack.

REDUCING BUDGETARY SLACK: A BONUS-BASED TECHNIQUE

In general, firms use budgeting and bonus techniques to overcome slack budgeting. One such approach consists of paying higher rewards when budgets are set high and achieved and lower rewards when budgets are either set high but not met or set low and achieved. G.S. Mann presented a bonus system that gave incentives for managers to set budget estimates as close to achievable levels as possible.[100] The following two formulas were proposed:

Formula 1 applies for bonus if actual performance is equal to or greater than budget.

> (multiplier no. 2 × budget goal) + [multiplier no. 1 × (actual level achieved − budget goal)]

Formula 2 applies for bonus if actual performance is less than budget.

> (multiplier no. 2 × budget goal) + [multiplier no. 3 × (actual level achieved − budget goal)]

The three multipliers set by management served as factors in calculating different components of bonuses. They were defined as follows:

Multiplier no. 1 (which must be less than multiplier no. 2, and which in turn must be less than multiplier no. 3) is used when actual performance is greater than budget. It provides a smaller bonus per unit for the part of actual performance that exceeds the budgeted amount.

Multiplier no. 2 is the rate per unit used to determine the basic bonus component. It is based on the budgeted level of activity which equals multiplier no. 2 times the budgeted level.

Multiplier no. 3 is the rate used to reduce the bonus when the achieved level is less than the budget (multiplier no. 3 times work of units by which actual performance fell short of budget).[101]

Figure 5.1 shows an illustration of the application of the method and the effect of variations in multipliers or bonuses. As the figure shows, the manager will be rewarded for accurate estimation of the level of rates. In addition, the multipliers can be set with greater flexibility for controlling the manager's estimates.

CONCLUSION

Organizational slack and budgetary slack are two hypothetical constructs to explain organizational phenomena that are prevalent in all forms of organiza-

Figure 5.1
Reducing Slack through a Bonus System

(1)	(2)	(3)	(4) Bonus I	(5) Bonus II
Budget Slacks	Actual Slacks	State of Nature	Multiple No. 1 = $.05 Multiple No. 2 = $.10 Multiple No. 3 = $.15	Multiple No. 1 = $.01 Multiple No. 2 = $.10 Multiple No. 3 = $.30
200,000	180,000	Overestimation	$17,000	$14,000
200,000	200,000	Actual = Budget	20,000	20,000
200,000	220,000	Underestimation	21,000	22,000

tions. Evidence linking both constructs to organizational, individual, and contextual factors is growing and in the future may contribute to an emerging theoretical framework for an understanding of slack. Further investigation into the potential determinants of organizational and budgetary slack remains to be done. This effort is an important one because the behavior of slack is highly relevant to the achievement of internal economic efficiency in organizations. Witness the following comment:

The effective organization has more rewards at its disposal, or more organizational slack to play with, and thus can allow all members to exercise more discretion, obtain more rewards, and feel that their influence is higher.[102]

NOTES

1. R.M. Cyert and J.G. March (eds.), *A Behavioral Theory of the Firm* (Englewood Cliffs, NJ: Prentice-Hall, 1963).

2. A.Y. Lewin and C. Wolf, "The Theory of Organizational Slack: A Critical Review," *Proceedings: Twentieth International Meeting of TIMS* (1976), pp. 648–654.

3. H. Leibenstein, "Allocative Efficiency vs. X-Efficiency," *American Economic Review* (June 1966), pp. 392–415.

4. H. Leibenstein, "X-Efficiency: From Concept to Theory," *Challenge* (September–October 1979), pp. 13–22.

5. N. Choudhury, "Incentives for the Divisional Manager," *Accounting and Business Research* (Winter 1985), pp. 11–21.

6. S. Baiman, "Agency Research in Managerial Accounting: A Survey," *Journal of Accounting Literature* (Spring 1982), pp. 154–213.

7. D. Packard, *The Pyramid Climber* (New York: McGraw-Hill, 1962); E.A. Butler, "Corporate Politics-Monster or Friend?" *Generation* 3 (1971), pp. 54–58, 74; A.N. Schoomaker, *Executive Career Strategies* (New York: American Management Association, 1971).

8. J. Pfeffer, "Power and Resource Allocation in Organizations," in B.M. Shaw and G.R. Salancik (eds.), *New Directions in Organizational Behavior* (Chicago: St. Clair Press, 1977).

9. V.E. Schein, "Individual Power and Political Behaviors in Organizations: An Inadequately Explored Reality," *Academy of Management Review* (January 1977), pp. 64–72.

10. B. Bowman and W. Malpive, "Goals and Bureaucratic Decision-Making: An Experiment," *Human Relations* (June 1977), pp. 417–429.

11. V.E. Schein, "Examining an Illusion: The Role of Deceptive Behaviors in Organizations," *Human Relations* (October 1979), pp. 288–289.

12. Ibid., p. 290.

13. Cyert and March, *A Behavioral Theory of the Firm*.

14. Schein, "Examining an Illusion," p. 293.

15. Cyert and March, *A Behavioral Theory of the Firm*.

16. J. Child, "Organizational Structure, Environment, and Performance: The Role of Strategic Choice," *Sociology* 6, 1 (1972), pp. 2–22.

17. M.D. Cohen, J.G. March, and J.P. Olsen, "A Garbage Can Model of Organizational Choice," *Administrative Science Quarterly* 17, 1 (1972), pp. 1–25.

18. J.G. March and J.P. Olsen, *Ambiguity and Choice* (Bergen: Universitetsforlagt, 1976).

19. D.E. Dimmick and V.V. Murray, "Correlates of Substantive Policy Decisions in Organizations: The Case of Human Resource Management," *Academy of Management Journal* 21, 4 (1978), pp. 611–623.

20. R.J. Litschert and T.W. Bonham, "A Conceptual Model of Strategy Formation," *Academy of Management Review* 3, 2 (1978), pp. 211–219.

21. J.G. March, interview by Stanford Business School Alumni Association, *Stanford GSB* 47, 3 (1978–1979), pp. 16–19.

22. Cyert and March, *A Behavioral Theory of the Firm*.

23. Ibid., p. 38.

24. O.E. Williamson, "A Model of Rational Managerial Behavior," in Cyert and March, *A Behavioral Theory of the Firm*; O.E. Williamson, *The Economics of Discretionary Behavior: Managerial Objectives in a Theory of the Firm* (Englewood Cliffs, NJ: Prentice-Hall, 1964).

25. J.Y. Kamin and J. Ronen, "The Smoothing of Income Numbers: Some Empirical Evidence on Systematic Differences among Management-Controlled and Owner-Controlled Firms," *Accounting, Organizations and Society* (October 1978), pp. 141–157.

26. A. Belkaoui and R.D. Picur, "The Smoothing of Income Numbers: Some Empirical Evidence on Systematic Differences between Core and Periphery Industrial Sector," *Journal of Business Finance and Accounting* (Winter 1984), pp. 527–545.

27. Lewin and Wolf, "The Theory of Organizational Slack," p. 653.

28. L.J. Bourgeois, "On the Measurement of Organizational Slack," *Academy of Management Review* 6, 1 (1981), pp. 29–39.

29. Ibid., p. 31.

30. C.I. Barnard, *Functions of the Executive* (Cambridge, MA: Harvard University Press, 1938).

31. J.G. March and H.A. Simon, *Organizations* (New York: John Wiley and Sons, 1958).

32. Cyert and March, *A Behavioral Theory of the Firm*, p. 36.

33. L.R. Pondy, "Organizational Conflict: Concepts and Models," *Administrative Science Quarterly* 12, 2 (1967), pp. 296–320.

34. J.D. Thompson, *Organizations in Action* (New York: McGraw-Hill, 1967).

35. Pondy, "Organizational Conflict."

36. J. Galbraith, *Designing Complex Organizations* (Reading, MA: Addison-Wesley, 1973), p. 15.

37. Bourgeois, "On the Measurement of Organizational Slack," p. 34.

38. D.C. Hambrick and C.C. Snow, "A Contextual Model of Strategic Decision Making in Organizations," in R.L. Taylor, J.J. O'Connell, R.A. Zawaki, and D.D. Warrick (eds.), *Academy of Management Proceedings* (1977), pp. 109–112.

39. Cyert and March, *A Behavioral Theory of the Firm.*

40. March and Simon, *Organizations.*

41. H.A. Simon, *Administrative Behavior* (New York: Free Press, 1957).

42. Cyert and March, *A Behavioral Theory of the Firm.*

43. W.G. Astley, "Sources of Power in Organizational Life" (Ph.D. diss., University of Washington, 1978).

44. W.R. Scott, *Organizations: Rational, Natural and Open Systems* (Englewood Cliffs, NJ: Prentice-Hall, 1981), p. 216.

45. Ibid.

46. Ibid.

47. Bourgeois, "On the Measurement of Organizational Slack," p. 38.

48. M.M. Rosner, "Economic Determinant of Organizational Innovation," *Administrative Science Quarterly* 12 (1968), pp. 614–625.

49. A.Y. Lewin and C. Wolf, "Organizational Slack: A Test of the General Theory," *Journal of Management Studies* (forthcoming).

50. L.J. Bourgeois and J.V. Singh, "Organizational Slack and Political Behavior within Top Management Teams," Working paper, Graduate School of Business, Stanford University, 1983.

51. T.K. Lant, "Modeling Organizational Slack: An Empirical Investigation," Stanford University Research Paper no. 856, July 1986.

52. Ibid., p. 14.

53. O. Hart, "The Market Mechanism as an Incentive Scheme," *Bell Journal of Economics* 14 (1983), pp. 366–382.

54. D. Scharfstein, "Product Market Competition and Managerial Slack," *Rand Journal of Economics* 14 (1988), pp. 147–153.

55. B. Hermalin, "The Effects of Competition on Executive Behavior," *Rand Journal of Economics* 23 (1992), pp. 350–365.

56. H. Horn, H. Lang, and S. Lundgren, "Competition, Long Run Contracts and Inefficiencies in Firms," *European Economic Review* 38 (1994), pp. 213–233.

57. S. Martin, "Endogenous Firm Efficiency in a Cournot Principal-Agent Model," *Journal of Economic Theory* 59 (1993), pp. 445–450.

58. R. Kerschbamer and Y. Tournas, "In-House Competition, Organizational Slack and the Business Cycle," Working paper, Department of Economics, University of Vienna, July 2000.

59. M. Schiff and A.Y. Lewin, "The Impact of People on Budgets," *Accounting Review* (April 1970), pp. 259–268.

60. M. Schiff and A.Y. Lewin, "Where Traditional Budgeting Fails," *Financial Executive* (May 1968), pp. 51–62.

61. A.E. Lowe and R.W. Shaw, "An Analysis of Managerial Biasing: Evidence from a Company's Budgeting Process," *Journal of Management Studies* (October 1968), pp. 304–315.

62. M. Dalton, *Men Who Manage* (New York: John Wiley and Sons, 1961), pp. 36–38.

63. G. Shillinglaw, "Divisional Performance Review: An Extension of Budgetary Control," in C.P. Bonini, R.K. Jaedicke, and H.M. Wagner (eds.), *Management Controls: New Directors in Basic Research* (New York: McGraw-Hill, 1964), pp. 149–163.

64. C. Argyris, *The Impact of Budgets on People* (New York: Controllership Foundation, 1952), p. 25.

65. E.H. Caplan, *Management Accounting and Behavioral Sciences* (Reading, MA: Addison-Wesley, 1971).

66. Argyris, *The Impact of Budgets on People*.

67. Schiff and Lewin, "Where Traditional Budgeting Fails," pp. 51–62.

68. Stevens, D.E. "Determinants of Budgetary Slack in the Laboratory: An Investigation of Contracts for Self-Interested Behavior." Working paper, Syracuse University, March 2000, p. 1.

69. M. Onsi, "Factor Analysis of Behavioral Variables Affecting Budgetary Slack," *Accounting Review* (July 1973), pp. 535–548.

70. Ibid., p. 536.

71. Ibid., p. 539.

72. Ibid., p. 546.

73. C. Cammann, "Effects of the Use of Control Systems," *Accounting, Organizations and Society* (January 1976), pp. 301–313.

74. K.A. Merchant, "Budgeting and the Propensity to Create Budgetary Slack," *Accounting, Organizations and Society* (May 1985), pp. 201–210.

75. A.S. Dunk, "The Effect of Budget Emphasis and Information Asymmetry on the Relation between Budgetary Participation and Slack," *The Accounting Review* (April 1993), pp. 400–410.

76. Ibid., p. 400.

77. Ibid., pp. 408–409.

78. R.M. Cyert, J.G. March, and W.H. Starbuck, "Two Experiments on Bias and Conflict in Organizational Estimation," *Management Science* (April 1961), pp. 254–264.

79. Lowe and Shaw, "An Analysis of Managerial Biasing."

80. Dalton, *Men Who Manage*.

81. R.M. Barefield, "A Model of Forecast Biasing Behavior," *Accounting Review* (July 1970), pp. 490–501.

82. J.S. Demski and G.A. Feltham, "Economic Incentives in Budgetary Control Systems," *Accounting Review* (April 1978), pp. 336–359.

83. Y. Ijiri, J. Kinard, and F. Putney, "An Integrated Evaluation System for Budget Forecasting and Operating Performance with a Classified Budgeting Bibliography," *Journal of Accounting Research* (Spring 1968), pp. 1–28; M. Loeb and W. Magat, "Soviet Success Indicators and the Evaluation of Divisional Performance," *Journal of Accounting Research* (Spring 1978), pp. 103–121; P. Jennergren, "On the Design of Incentives in Business Firms—A Survey of Some Research," *Management Science* (February 1980), pp. 180–201; M. Weitzman, "The New Soviet Incentive Model," *Bell Journal of Economics* (Spring 1976), pp. 251–257.

84. M.S. Young, "Participative Budgeting: The Effects of Risk Aversion and Asymmetric Information on Budgetary Slack," *Journal of Accounting Research* (Autumn 1985), pp. 829–842.

85. Ibid., pp. 831–832.

86. C. Chow, J. Cooper, and W. Waller, "Participative Budgeting: Effects of a Truth-Inducing Pay Scheme and Information Asymmetry on Slack and Performance," Working paper, University of Arizona, Tucson, 1986.

87. W.S. Waller, "Slack in Participative Budgeting: The Joint Effect of a Truth-Inducing Pay Scheme and Risk Preferences," *Accounting, Organizations and Society* (December 1987), pp. 87–98.

88. Ibid., p. 88.

89. J. Berg, L. Daley, J. Dickhaut, and J. O'Brien, "Controlling Preferences for Lotteries on Units of Experimental Exchange," *Quarterly Journal of Economics* (May 1986), pp. 281–306.

90. D.C. Kim, "Risk Preferences in Participative Budgeting," *The Accounting Review* (April 1992), pp. 303–318.

91. Ibid., p. 304.

92. E. Aronson and D.R. Mettee, "Dishonest Behavior as a Function of Differential Levels of Induced Self-Esteem," *Journal of Personality and Social Psychology* (January 1968), pp. 121–127.

93. A. Belkaoui, "Slack Budgeting, Information Distortion and Self-Esteem," *Contemporary Accounting Research* (Fall 1985), pp. 111–123.

94. K. Lukka, "Budgetary Biasing in Organizations: Theoretical Framework and Empirical Evidence," *Accounting, Organizations and Society* (February 1988), pp. 281–301.

95. Ibid., p. 292.

96. D.T. Otley, "The Accuracy of Budgetary Estimates: Some Statistical Evidence," *Journal of Business Finance and Accounting* (Fall 1985), p. 416.

97. W.H. Read, "Upward Communication in Industrial Hierarchies," *Human Relations* (1962), pp. 3–16.

98. G.H. Hofstede, *The Game of Budget Control* (London: Tavistock, 1968); A.G. Hopwood, "An Empirical Study of the Role of Accounting Data in Performance Evaluation," *Journal of Accounting Research* (Supplement, 1972), pp. 156–182; D.T. Otley, "Budget Use and Managerial Performance," *Journal of Accounting Research* (Spring 1978), pp. 122–149.

99. R.M. Barefield, "Comments on a Measure of Forecasting Performance," *Journal of Accounting Research* (Autumn 1969), pp. 324–327; Otley, "The Accuracy of Budgetary Estimates."

100. G.S. Mann, "Reducing Budget Slack," *Journal of Accountancy* (August 1988), pp. 118–122.

101. Ibid., p. 119.

102. C. Perrow, *Complex Organizations: A Critical Essay* (Glenview, IL: Scott, Foreman, and Company, 1972), p. 140.

SELECTED REFERENCES

Antle, R., and G. Eppen. "Capital Rationing and Organizational Slack in Capital Budgeting." *Management Science* (February 1985), pp. 163–174.

Argyris, C. *The Impact of Budgets on People.* New York: Controllership Foundation, 1952.

Aronson, E., and D.R. Mettee. "Dishonest Behavior as a Function of Differential Levels of Induced Self-Esteem." *Journal of Personality and Social Psychology* (January 1968), pp. 121–127.

Barefield, R.M. "A Model of Forecast Biasing Behavior." *Accounting Review* (July 1970), pp. 490–501.

Barnea, A., J. Ronen, and S. Sadan. "Classifactory Smoothing of Income with Extraordinary Items." *Accounting Review* (January 1976), pp. 110–122.

Belkaoui, A. *Conceptual Foundations of Management Accounting.* Reading, MA: Addison-Wesley, 1980.

———. "The Relationships between Self-Disclosure Style and Attitudes to Responsibility Accounting." *Accounting, Organizations and Society* (December 1981), pp. 281–289.

———. *Cost Accounting: A Multidimensional Emphasis.* Hinsdale, IL: Dryden Press, 1983.

———. "Slack Budgeting, Information Distortion and Self-Esteem." *Contemporary Accounting Research* (Fall 1985), pp. 111–123.

Belkaoui, A., and R.D. Picur. "The Smoothing of Income Numbers: Some Empirical Evidence of Systematic Differences between Core and Periphery Industrial Sectors." *Journal of Business Finance and Accounting* (Winter 1984), pp. 527–545.

Bourgeois, L.J. "On the Measurement of Organizational Slack." *Academy of Management Review* 6, no. 1 (1981), pp. 29–39.

Bourgeois, L.J., and J.V. Singh. "Organizational Slack and Political Behavior within Top Management Teams." *Academy of Management Proceedings* (1983), pp. 43–47.

———. "Organizational Slack and Political Behavior within Top Management Teams." Working paper, Graduate School of Business, Stanford University, 1983.

Bourgeois, L.J., and W.G. Astley. "A Strategic Model of Organizational Conduct and Performance." *International Studies of Management and Organization* 9, 3 (1979), pp. 40–66.

Brownell, P. "Participation in the Budgeting Process—When It Works and When It Doesn't." *Journal of Accounting Literature* (Spring 1982), pp. 124–153.

Caplan, E.H. *Management Accounting and Behavioral Sciences.* Reading, MA: Addison-Wesley, 1971.

Carter, E. "The Behavioral Theory of the Firm and Top-Level Corporate Decisions." *Administrative Science Quarterly* 16, 4 (1971), pp. 413–428.

Child, J. "Organizational Structure, Environment, and Performance: The Role of Strategic Choice." *Sociology* 6, 1 (1972), pp. 2–22.

Chow, D. "The Effects of Job Standard Tightness and Compensation Scheme on Performance: An Exploration of Linkages." *Accounting Review* (October 1983), pp. 667–685.

Christensen, J. "The Determination of Performance Standards and Participation." *Journal of Accounting Research* (Autumn 1982), pp. 589–603.

Cohen, M.D., J.G. March, and J.P. Olsen. "A Garbage Can Model of Organizational Choice." *Administrative Science Quarterly* 17, 1 (1972), pp. 1–25.

Collins, F. "Managerial Accounting Systems and Organizational Control: A Role Perspective." *Accounting, Organizations and Society* (May 1982), pp. 107–122.

Conn, D. "A Comparison of Alternative Incentive Structures for Centrally Planned Economic Systems." *Journal of Comparative Economics* (September 1979), pp. 261–278.

Cyert, R.M., and J.G. March. "Organizational Factors in the Theory of Oligopoly." *Quarterly Journal of Economics* (April 1956), pp. 44–66.

———— (eds.). *A Behavioral Theory of the Firm.* Englewood Cliffs, NJ: Prentice-Hall, 1963.

Cyert, R.M., J.G. March, and W.H. Starbuck. "Two Experiments on Bias and Conflict in Organizational Estimation." *Management Science* (April 1961), pp. 254–264.

Dalton, M. *Men Who Manage.* New York: John Wiley and Sons, 1961.

Demski, J.S., and G.A. Feltham. "Economic Incentives in Budgetary Control Systems." *Accounting Review* (April 1978), pp. 336–359.

Dunk, A.S. "The Effect of Budget Emphasis and Information Asymmetry on the Relation between Budgetary Participation and Slack." *The Accounting Review* (April 1993), pp. 400–410.

Gonik, J. "Tie Salesmen's Bonuses to Their Forecasts." *Harvard Business Review* (May–June 1978), pp. 116–123.

Hopwood, A.G. "An Empirical Study of the Role of Accounting Data in Performance Evaluation." *Journal of Accounting Research* (Supplement, 1972), pp. 156–182.

Irjiri, Y., J. Kinard, and F. Putney. "An Integrated Evaluation System for Budget Forecasting and Operating Performance with a Classified Budgeting Bibliography." *Journal of Accounting Research* (Spring 1968), pp. 1–28.

Itami, H. "Evaluation Measures and Goal Congruence under Uncertainty." *Journal of Accounting Research* (Spring 1975), pp. 163–180.

Jennergren, P. "On the Design of Incentives in Business Firms—A Survey of Some Research." *Management Science* (February 1980), pp. 180–201.

Karpik, P., and A. Riahi-Belkaoui. "A Comparison of the Financial Characteristics of Companies in the Core and Periphery Economies." *Advances in Quantitative Analysis in Finance and Accounting* 2 (1993), pp. 105–139.

Kerr, S., and W. Slocum Jr. "Controlling the Performances of People in Organizations." In W. Starbuck and P. Nystrom (eds.), *Handbook of Organizational Design*, Vol. 2. New York: Oxford University Press, 1981, pp. 116–134.

Kim, D.C. "Risk Preferences in Participative Budgeting." *The Accounting Review* (April 1992), pp. 303–319.

Lecky, P. *Self-Consistency.* New York: Island Press, 1945.

Leibenstein, H. "Allocative Efficiency vs. X-Efficiency." *American Economic Review* (June 1966), pp. 392–415.

————. "X-Efficiency: From Concept to Theory." *Challenge* (September–October 1979), pp. 13–22.

Levinthal, D., and J.G. March. "A Model of Adaptive Organizational Search." *Journal of Economic Behavior and Organization* (May 1981), pp. 307–333.

Lewin, A.Y., and C. Wolf. "The Theory of Organizational Slack: A Critical Review." *Proceedings: Twentieth International Meeting of TIMS* (1976), pp. 648–654.

Litschert, R.J., and T.W. Bonham. "A Conceptual Model of Strategy Formation." *Academy of Management Review* 3, 2 (1978), pp. 211–219.

Locke, E., and D. Schweiger. "Participation in Decision Making: One More Look." In B. Staw (ed.), *Research in Organizational Behavior.* Greenwich, CT: JAI Press, 1979, pp. 265–339.

Loeb, M., and W. Magat. "Soviet Success Indicators and the Evaluation of Divisional Performance." *Journal of Accounting Research* (Spring 1978), pp. 103–121.

Lowe, A.E., and R.W. Shaw. "An Analysis of Managerial Biasing: Evidence from a Company's Budgeting Process." *Journal of Management Studies* (October 1968), pp. 304–315.

March, J.G., and H.A. Simon. *Organizations*. New York: John Wiley and Sons, 1958.

Mezias, S.J. "Some Analytics of Organizational Slack." Working paper, Graduate School of Business, Stanford University, November 1985.

Miller, J., and J. Thornton. "Effort, Uncertainty, and the New Soviet Incentive System." *Southern Economic Journal* (October 1978), pp. 432–446.

Mitroff, I.I., and J.R. Emshoff. "On Strategic Assumption-Making: A Dialectical Approach to Policy and Planning." *Academy of Management Review* 4, 1 (1979), pp. 1–12.

Moch, M.K., and L.R. Pondy. "The Structure of Chaos: Organized Anarchy as a Response to Ambiguity." *Administrative Science Quarterly* 22, 2 (1977), pp. 351–362.

Parker, L.D. "Goal Congruence: A Misguided Accounting Concept." *Abacus* (June 1976), pp. 3–13.

Riahi-Belkaoui, A. *The New Foundations of Management Accounting*. Westport, CT: Quorum Books, 1992.

Schein, V.E. "Examining an Illusion: The Role of Deceptive Behaviors in Organizations." *Human Relations* (October 1979), pp. 287–295.

Schiff, M. "Accounting Tactics and the Theory of the Firm." *Journal of Accounting Research* (Spring 1966), pp. 62–67.

Schiff, M., and A.Y. Levin. "Where Traditional Budgeting Fails." *Financial Executive* (May 1968), pp. 51–62.

———. "The Impact of People on Budgets." *Accounting Review* (April 1970), pp. 259–268.

———. *Behavioral Aspects of Accounting*. Englewood Cliffs, NJ: Prentice-Hall, 1974.

Simon, H.A. *Administrative Behavior*. New York: Free Press, 1957.

Singh, J.V. "Performance, Slack and Risk Taking in Strategic Decisions: Test of a Structural Equation Model." Ph.D. diss., Stanford Graduate School of Business, 1983.

———. "Performance, Slack, and Risk Taking in Organizational Decision Making." *Academy of Management Journal* (September 1986), pp. 562–585.

Stolzenberg, R.M. "Bringing the Boss Back In: Employer Size, Employee Schooling, and Socioeconomic Achievement." *American Sociological Review* 43 (1978), pp. 42–53.

Swieringa, R.J., and R.H. Moncur. "The Relationship between Managers' Budget Oriented Behavior and Selected Attitudes, Position, Size and Performance Measures." *Journal of Accounting Research* (Supplement, 1972), p. 19.

Thompson, J.D. *Organizations in Action*. New York: McGraw-Hill, 1967.

Waller, W.S., and C. Chow. "The Self-Selection and Effort of Standard-Based Employment Contracts: A Framework and Some Empirical Evidence." *Accounting Review* (July 1985), pp. 458–476.

Watchel, H.M. "The Impact of Labor Market Conditions on Hard-Core Unemployment." *Poverty and Human Resources* (July–August 1970), pp. 5–13.

Weitzman, M. "The New Soviet Incentive Model." *Bell Journal of Economics* (Spring 1976), pp. 251–257.

Williamson, O.E. "A Model of Rational Managerial Behavior." In Richard M. Cyert and James G. March (eds.), *A Behavioral Theory of the Firm*. Englewood Cliffs, NJ: Prentice-Hall, 1963, pp. 113–128.

———. *The Economics of Discretionary Behavior: Managerial Objectives in a Theory of the Firm*. Englewood Cliffs, NJ: Prentice-Hall, 1964.

Winter, S.G. "Satisficing, Selection, and the Innovating Remnant." *Quarterly Journal of Economics* 85 (1971), pp. 237–257.

Young, M.S. "Participative Budgeting: The Effects of Risk Aversion and Asymmetric Information on Budgetary Slack." *Journal of Accounting Research* (Autumn 1985), pp. 829–842.

Appendix 5A. Slack Budgeting, Information Distortion and Self-Esteem

INTRODUCTION

Psychological variables are very helpful in explaining some of the accountant's behavioral patterns and can contribute to the development of better management accounting systems (Belkaoui, 1980; Collins, 1982). Personality traits and behavioral factors may be indicative of different accounting behavior and effectiveness. For example, self-disclosure was found to be positively related to attitudes to responsibility accounting (Belkaoui, 1981), and Gordon's Personality Profile and the Ohio State Leadership Behavior Description Questionnaire were found to be a predictor of budgeting behavior (Hopwood, 1972; Swieringa and Moncur, 1972). Slack creation is another important managerial behavior in need of explanation, correction, and/or control. An evaluation of the effectiveness of a firm's control system requires, among other things, the identification of the behavioral factors that lead to slack creation (Onsi, 1973, p. 535). Accordingly, this appendix reports on research designed to provide insights into the relationships between individual characteristics and slack creation. More specifically, it examines slack budgeting as a case of information distortion and investigates empirically the effects of self-esteem feedback on information distortion.

THEORY

Slack Budgeting and Information Distortion

The literature on the behavioral implications of budgets as instruments of planning and control has found its way into most cost accounting textbooks (Belkaoui, 1983). It is suggested that the budget in its dual role of being a planning tool and a control device may give rise to slack. Cyert and March (1963) defined organizational slack as the difference between "the total resources available to the firm and the total necessary to maintain the organizational coalition" (p. 36). Slack arises from imperfections in the organizational process of resource allocation. Slack may be distributed in the form of additional dividends and excessive wages beyond the minimum required to obtain a healthy coalition

Source: A. Riahi-Belkaoui, "Slack Budgeting, Information Distortion and Self-Esteem," *Contemporary Accounting Research* (Fall, 1985), pp. 11–123. Reprinted with permission.

of all the participants in the organization or be undistributed as idle cash and securities. In examining the relationships between the controller and the controlled within the organization, Schiff and Lewin (1970) argued that these relationships revolved around the budget process and that the "controlled" exercise significant influence on the outcome of the budgets by the incorporation of slack into their budgets.[1] In brief, since the budget is an expression of the performance criteria and because managers bargain and participate in its formation, the budget process may become the vehicle for slack. Thus, organizational slack is a general organizational phenomenon that may be reflected in slack budgeting behavior. In an accounting framework, slack budgeting is, in general, operationally defined as the process of understating revenues and overstating costs. Lowe and Shaw (1968) report also on downward and upward bias introduced in sales forecasts by line managers that may indicate the existence of negative slack in some cases.

Slack creation is a generalized organizational phenomenon. Various organizational factors have been used to explain slack creation, namely, organizational structure, goal congruence, control system, and managerial behavior. Basically (1) it is assumed to occur in cases where a Tayloristic organizational structure exists (Argyris, 1952, p. 25), although it is also assumed to occur in a participative organization structure (Caplan, 1971, p. 85); (2) it may be due to conflicts arising between the individual and organizational goals leading managers to intentionally create slack (March and Simon, 1958, p. 84; Williamson, 1964; Parker, 1976, p. 12); (3) it may be due to the attitudes of management toward the budget and to the workers' views of budgets as devices used by management to manipulate them (Argyris, 1952); and (4) it may occur whether or not the organization is based on a centralized or decentralized structure (Schiff and Lewin, 1970, p. 264).

Whatever the sources or causes of slack creation, slack involves a deliberate distortion of input information. Distortion of input information in a budget setting in particular arises from a need by managers to accommodate their expectations about the kinds of payoff associated with different possible outcomes. For example, Cyert, March, and Starbuck (1961) (hereafter referred to as CMS) showed in a laboratory experiment that subjects adjusted the information that they transmitted in a complex decision-making system to control their payoffs. Similarly, Lowe and Shaw (1968) have shown that in cases where rewards were related to forecast, sales managers tended to distort the input information and to induce biases in their sales forecasts. Dalton (1961) also provided some rich situational descriptions of information distortion in which lower-level managers distorted the budget information and allocated resources to what were perceived to be justifiable objectives. Finally, given the existence of a payoff structure that may induce a forecaster to intentionally bias his or her forecast, Barefield (1970) provides a model of forecast behavior that shows a "rough" formulation of a possible link between a forecaster's biasing and the quality of the forecaster as a source of data for an accounting system. All these studies seem to suggest that slack budgeting through systematic distortion of input information may be

used to accommodate the subject's expectations about the payoffs associated with various possible outcomes. They fail, however, to provide a better rationalization of the link between distortion of input information and the subject's accommodation of expectations. Agency theory- and risk aversion-related issues may provide such a link. Hence, given the existence of divergent incentives and information asymmetry between controller (or employer) and controllee (or employee) and the high cost of observing employee skill or effort, a budget-based employment contract (i.e., employee compensation is contingent on meeting the performance standard) can be Pareto-superior to fixed pay or linear sharing rules (where the employer and employee split the output) (Demski and Feltham, 1978). However, these budget-based schemes impose a risk on the employee (since job performance may be affected by a host of uncontrollable factors). Consequently, risk-averse individuals may resort to slack budgeting through systematic distortion of input information. Moreover, any enhanced (increased) risk aversion would, in practice, lead the employee to resort to slack budgeting.

Self-Esteem

The enhancement of risk aversion and the resulting distortion of input information may be more pronounced when self-esteem is threatened. It was found that persons who have low opinions of themselves are more likely to cheat than persons with high self-esteem (Aronson and Mettee, 1968). A situation of dissonance was created in an experimental group by giving out positive feedback about a personality test to some participants and negative feedback to others. Then, all the participants were asked to take part in a competitive game of cards. The participants who received a blow to their self-esteem cheated more than those who had received positive feedback about themselves. Could it also be concluded that slack budgeting through information distortion may be a form of dishonest behavior arising from enhancement of risk aversion caused by negative feedback on self-esteem? A person's expectations may be an important determinant of his or her behavior. Negative feedback on self-esteem may lead an individual to develop an expectation of poor performance. At the same time the individual who is given negative feedback about his or her self-esteem would be more risk-averse than others and would be ready to resort to any behavior to cover the situation. Consequently, he or she may attempt to distort the input information in order to have an attainable budget. Accordingly, one hypothesis may be stated as follows: *Individuals given negative feedback about their self-esteem will introduce more bias into estimates than individuals given positive or neutral feedback about their self-esteem.*

METHOD

A laboratory experiment was used to investigate the impact of self-esteem feedback on input information distortion in a budgeting task. The subjects were

sixty male and female students drawn from the fourth-year undergraduate accounting theory class, the second-year graduate managerial accounting class, and the introductory undergraduate accounting class in the Faculty of Administration at the University of Ottawa who agreed to cooperate and participate in the experiment. Students rather than managers were used in order to better isolate the impact of self-esteem on input information distortion, given that managers may be influenced by a host of other organizational factors to create slack. The subjects were told that they were participating in a study concerned with the correlation between self-esteem scores and "estimation aptitudes." They were told that the Tennessee Self-Concept Scale (TSCS) would be used to measure their self-esteem, and the "estimation aptitudes" would be ascertained upon the completion of a budgeting test (Fitts, 1965).

All subjects were given the TSCS and were informed of its nature and intent. The test belongs to a wide variety of instruments that have been employed to measure the self-concept. The instrument is simple for the subject to understand, which explains its popularity as a means of studying and understanding human behavior. Sociologists, psychiatrists, theologians, philosophers, educators, and psychologists have increasingly come to view the self-concept as a central construct for the understanding of people and their behavior. Consequently, a whole theoretical school, known as self-theory, has evolved, as evidenced by works of people like Rogers (1951), Snygg and Combs (1949), Lecky (1945), Wylie (1961), and others. Self-theory is strongly phenomenological in nature and is based on the general principle that people react to their phenomenal world in terms of the way that they perceive this world. Self-theory holds that people's behavior is always meaningful and that we understand each person's behavior only if we can perceive his or her phenomenal world as he or she does. The TSCS was devised for the purpose of measuring the self-concept. Although subject to the limitations of any verbal or pencil-and-paper type of scale, the TSCS is nevertheless applicable to a broad range of people and situations (Fitts and Hammer, 1969; Fitts, 1970, 1972a, 1972b, 1972c; Fitts et al., 1971; Thompson, 1972). It yields a number of measures and scores and is well standardized. Among these scores are:

The self-criticism score (SC): High scores indicate a normal, healthy openness and capacity for self-criticism.

The positive score (P): Scores on ninety items are summed to provide a total *P* score, which reflects general esteem. In general, people with high scores tend to like themselves, feel that they are persons of value and worth, have confidence in themselves, and act accordingly. People with low scores are doubtful about their own worth and unhappy and have little faith or confidence in themselves (Fitts, 1965, p. 1).

Other scores are provided by the TSCS. To avoid any confusion, only the positive score is used in this study. The subjects were provided with sufficient

information about the TSCS and the positive score to consider it relevant and important.

A week after the administration of the TSCS and before participating in a budgeting paper-and-pencil test, subjects were assigned to one of three experimental conditions: positive, neutral, and negative feedback on self-esteem scores. This manipulation of self-esteem was done by disclosing the highest, lowest, and average scores in the class and by either (1) communicating the right score, (2) having the subject's score equal to the highest score in the class, or (3) having the subject's score equal to the lowest score in the class. In general, the first alternative was communicated to those whose right score was around the average score in the class, the second alternative to those with low scores, and the third alternative to those with high scores. The last two alternatives were aimed at temporarily inducing either an increase in self-esteem or a decrease in self-esteem. *The first alternative, where no change in self-esteem was sought, was intended for control purposes.*[2]

The highest scores were 405 for the positive score and 46 for the self-criticism score. The lowest scores were 261 for the positive score and 23 for the self-criticism score. The average scores were 310 for the positive score and 32 for the self-criticism score. The provision of such a range of scores for the false feedback groups was assumed to be high enough to generate a blow to the self-esteem of the subject.[3] To avoid any confusion, the subjects were provided with only the positive scores.

The experimental material included four pages: one page for instructions; one page for the positive, neutral, or negative feedback on their self-esteem scores; and the last two pages for a paper-and-pencil test requiring the subject to make cost and sales estimates.

The instructions stated:

The purpose of this experiment is to correlate the estimation ability with self-esteem characteristics. In order to get a true measure of a person's estimation ability, it is necessary to keep in mind the estimation's objective function which is first, to insure that the budget is attainable and, second, that the budget is accurate. In order to accomplish this, I am having you engage in the estimation of both cost and sales for a fictional situation. It is important that you keep the estimation's objective function in mind when making your decision. The second page gives your self-esteem score. The last two pages constitute the budgeting situation.

The second page for the feedback on the self-esteem scores stated:

In the middle of the semester, you were asked to complete the Tennessee Self-Concept Scale. The test belongs to a wide variety of instruments which have been employed to measure the self-concept. The test gives a measure of self-esteem. Persons with high scores tend to like themselves, feel that they are persons of value and worth, have confidence in themselves, and act accordingly. Your score was _____. The highest, the lowest, and the average scores in your class were respectively _____, _____, _____.

The last two pages of the experimental material included a paper-and-pencil budgeting test requiring each subject to make ten estimates on the basis of the estimates of others. Two versions of the budgeting test were presented: a cost version and a sales version. The cost version reads as follows:

Assume that you are the controller of a manufacturing company considering the production of a new product. You are required to submit your estimate of the unit cost of the product if 500,000 units are produced. Your two assistants A and B, in whom you have equal confidence, presented you with preliminary estimates. For each of the cases below, indicate your estimate of costs you would submit.

The sales version reads as follows:

Assume that you are the marketing manager of a manufacturing concern considering the production of a new product. You are required to submit your estimate of the sales volume of the product if the price is set at $10.80. Your two assistants A and B, in whom you have equal confidence, presented you with preliminary estimates. For each of the cases below, indicate what estimates of sales you would submit.

Each question was followed by a list of ten pairs of numbers, representing the ten pairs of estimates by the two subordinates. The experiment involved in each case the choice between two estimates of cost and two estimates of sales. The cost estimates are indicated below:

Cost Estimates Presented to Participants

Cases	A's Estimate	B's Estimate	Your Estimate
(1)	$1.54	$6.75	$____
(2)	$8.42	$4.56	$____
(3)	$3.25	$7.52	$____
(4)	$1.25	$4.35	$____
(5)	$6.54	$4.70	$____
(6)	$1.80	$7.30	$____
(7)	$6.89	$1.65	$____
(8)	$3.25	$7.52	$____
(9)	$4.74	$1.54	$____
(10)	$3.20	$5.35	$____

The sales estimates were similar in value except that the cost estimates are expressed in dollars, and those for sales in units. However, the sales estimates were presented in various different orders to obscure the similarities in values. One such order of sales estimates is indicated below:

Sales Estimates Presented to Participants

Cases	A's Estimate	B's Estimate	Your Estimate
(1)	320,000 units	535,000 units	___ units
(2)	474,000	154,000	___
(3)	325,000	752,000	___
(4)	689,000	165,000	___
(5)	180,000	730,000	___
(6)	654,000	470,000	___
(7)	125,000	435,000	___
(8)	325,000	752,000	___
(9)	842,000	456,000	___
(10)	154,000	675,000	___

The three types of feedback on self-esteem scores (negative, neutral, and positive) and the two types of budgeting decisions (cost and sales estimates) resulted in the $2 \times 3 \times N$ factorial design in Table 5A.1. The group receiving the correct and hence neutral feedback was intended to be the control group in this experiment.

The nature of the task is assumed to lead the subjects to build in slack. First, it asks for an attainable budget. Second, the courses being taken by the subjects and taught by the experimenter emphasize the notion of a biased payoff schedule within an organization. Therefore, following the argumentation provided by CMS (1961, p. 254), if the payoffs are perceived to be biased or if they are perceived to depend on considerations other than the relations between the estimate and the true value, the tactical decision on biasing the estimate becomes important to the estimator.

RESULTS

Each subject's cost and sales estimates, E, were transformed into a summary statistic, x, which represented the weight assigned to the larger of the two given numbers in the pair presented to the subject such that

$$E = xU + (1 - x)L$$

where U is the upper number, and L the lower number.

Upper and lower limits of the ten pairs ranged from 125 to 842 and included two pairs in which the difference was approximately 200; two pairs in which the difference was approximately 300: two pairs in which the difference was approximately 400; two pairs in which the difference was approximately 550; one pair in which the difference was 521; and one pair in which the difference was 386.

Table 5A.1
Diagram of the Two-Factor Sample Experiment

		Types of feedback sample experiment		
		Negative	Correct	Positive
Types of budgeting	Cost	n = 20	n = 20	n = 20
decisions	Sales	n = 20	n = 20	n = 20

The use of a linear combination of the two estimates was considered superior to a single reliance on the mean. In effect, the summary statistic, x, highlights the bias brought by the subject to his or her estimates better than a single use of the mean estimate. It is used in the study as the database for the analysis of variance. The mean estimate does not highlight the bias because it gives equal weight to the observations.

The analysis of variance is summarized in Table 5A.2. The main effects were significant. The nature of the feedback on self-esteem had an impact on the weight assigned to the largest estimate ($F_{obs} = 6.71 > F_{.95} (2, 54) = 3.20$), and the nature of the budgeting decision had an impact on the weight assigned by the subject to the highest estimate ($F_{obs} = 5.71 > F_{.95} (1, 54) = 4.00$). The interaction effects were also significant ($F_{obs} = 5.44 = F_{.95} (1, 54) = 3.20$). The nature of the interaction effects is indicated by an inspection of the cell means. These means are shown in Table 5A.3. A geometric representation of these means is also given in Figure 5A.1. This figure presents the profiles corresponding to the simple main effects of the type of feedback on self-esteem for each of the budgeting decisions. A response of 0.5 is unbiased, and responses of > 0.5 for cost estimates and $< .05$ for sales estimates represent slack creation. The profiles for the cost and sales decisions appear to have different slopes indicating that an analysis of the simple effects is warranted. Only one simple effect is significant. Given negative feedback on self-esteem, the impact of the budgeting decision on the weights assigned to the highest estimate is different ($F_{obs} = 14.2 > F_{.95} (1, 54) = 4.00$). In fact, in the case of negative feedback, thirteen of the cost response points were superior to 0.5, and fourteen of the sales response points were inferior to 0.5.

However, the experimental data do not indicate a difference in the weights assigned given a neutral ($F_{obs} = 0.9$) or positive ($F_{obs} = 1.01$) feedback on self-esteem. Although the results are not significant, the positive feedback caused slack to be incorporated with cost estimation. If the positive feedback were significant, the evidence in this study would have been consistent with a curvilinear hypothesis that invalid feedback on self-esteem causes the incorporation of slack. Given the results of this study, however, the evidence seems more

Table 5A.2
Summary ANOVA for Gain and Simple Effects

Source of variation	SS	Y	MS	F
A (Budgeting decision)	0.68	1	0.68	5.71*
A for b_1 (negative feedback)	$(1.690)^1$	(1)	(1.690)	(14.2)*
A for b_2 (neutral feedback)	(0.115)	(1)	(0.115)	(0.9)
A for b_3 (positive feedback)	(0.221)	(1)	(.0221)	(1.01)
B (feedback on self-esteem)	1.6	2	0.8	6.71*
B for a_1 (cost decision)	(0.546)	(2)	(0.273)	(2.29)
B for a_2 (sales decision)	(0.955)	(2)	(0.473)	(3.9)
AB	1.336	2	0.668	5.44*
Within cell	6.474	54	0.119	
Total	10.090	59		

Notes:
*significant at .05 level.
[1]data for simple effects are in parentheses.
Legend: SS = Sum of squares; Y = Degrees of freedom; MS = Mean square; F = F statistic.

Table 5A.3
Mean of Cells Summary Table

	Negative Feedback	Neutral Feedback	Positive Feedback
Cost	0.81	0.50	0.75
Sales	0.23	0.65	0.54

consistent with the linear hypothesis that negative feedback on self-esteem causes the incorporation of slack.

DISCUSSION

The above results suggest that inaccurate but neutral or positive feedback on self-esteem may not result in observed differences in the cost of sales budgeting decisions. An inaccurate but favorable feedback on self-esteem does not seem to lead to a slack budgeting behavior and distortion of input information. Similarly, negative but inaccurate feedback does lead to a difference in the type of budgeting decision, cost or sales. The inaccurate and negative feedback of self-esteem seems to result in the distortion of input information. An examination

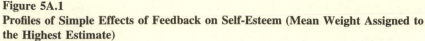

Figure 5A.1
Profiles of Simple Effects of Feedback on Self-Esteem (Mean Weight Assigned to the Highest Estimate)

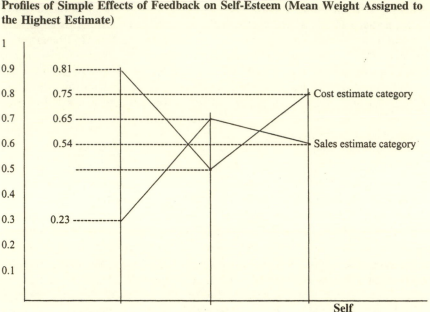

of Figure 5A.1 shows that given negative feedback on self-esteem, subjects tend to overestimate cost and underestimate sales.

These results seem to support the findings of CMS in part. They support the same idea that "cost and sales would tend to be estimated with a bias even though the bias might be in a different direction for each type of estimate." They also support their main proposition that "estimates within a complex decision making system involve attempts by the estimators to control their payoffs." Two differences arise, however, when comparing the scope of both results. First, the differences in the cost and sales estimation decisions result, in our study, in the creation of slack. Our subjects tend to overestimate cost and underestimate sales. Second, our results show that the bias introduced by the estimators is caused by the inaccurate and negative feedback on self-esteem.

One possible interpretation consistent with the observed effect may be related to the cognitive dissonance theory. Inaccurate and negative feedback on self-esteem may lead to enhanced risk aversion and increased dissonance, and since dissonance and risk aversion lead to an effort to reduce them, and since the only means of reduction in this experiment is the budget, slack budgeting behavior is expected.[4]

Another possible interpretation is that slack budgeting behavior occurs as a result of being consistent with an enhanced risk aversion due to a negative self-

concept. The inaccurate and negative feedback on self-esteem apparently accentuates the risk aversion, leading to a distortion of input information. In other words, a shock to one's self-esteem will cause one to be willing to be a party to cheating to achieve success. Given the nature of the task, the behavior is similar to that which would be exhibited by an increase in one's risk aversion. Two words of caution to qualify this conclusion are necessary. First, this study did not assess risk aversion directly, and, therefore, one cannot infer from the analysis that individuals with negative feedback on self-esteem are indeed risk averters. Second, future research should incorporate an incentive scheme; otherwise, the effects in the negative case may be overstated.

To be consistent with the work of Rogers (1951), the slack budgeting behavior may be altered by first changing the self-concept in a positive direction and thereby reducing the risk aversion. Clearly, any planning or control system within a firm must take into account the predisposition and biases created in the planner by the nature of the feedback on his or her performance and consequently on his or her self-esteem: an inaccurate and negative feedback on self-esteem may induce slack. So, the control of slack during the budget-setting period should be emphasized in the case of those employees who had previously received invalid feedback on their performance and self-esteem. In short, if an individual in an organization is tempted to use slack budgeting, it may be easier for him or her to yield to this temptation if his or her self-esteem has been lowered by inaccurate negative feedback. It is, however, appropriate to caution that the suggestions derived from the findings are tentative pending replication and further demonstrations of the external validity of this experiment.

One possible improvement would be to investigate whether the results of this study are due solely to the effects of negative and positive feedback on the subjects or are due to their perceived level of self-esteem. A second possible improvement would be to investigate the effects on estimation of accurate information concerning high and low self-esteem. To do so, the experiment should include individuals with high and low levels of self-esteem who either receive no feedback concerning their self-esteem levels (additional control group) or who receive accurate feedback concerning their self-esteem (additional experimental group). Another possible improvement would be to design an experiment dealing with more than the two budgetary items examined in this experiment, namely, cost and sales volume.

CONCLUSION

Certain hypotheses on slack budgeting were deduced from an examination of the nature of the feedback of self-esteem on the distortion of input information. Three main results appear. First, it can be said that the nature of the feedback on self-esteem has an impact on organizational estimation decisions. Second, the experiment also indicates that the nature of the budgeting decision leads to

a different estimation figure. Finally, the negative and inaccurate feedback of self-esteem appears to accentuate the distortion of input information and the creation of slack. Until the impact of accurate feedback of self-esteem is investigated, this study's findings indicate that negative feedback should not be released before it has been categorically proven to be accurate.

NOTES

1. Various organizational processes grounded in the development and maintenance of coalitions as well as a variety of group and political behaviors may constitute other cases in which these relationships may be either successfully resolved or not.

2. Parametric and nonparametric tests ($\alpha = .10$) failed to reject the hypothesis of no differences in the TSCS scores of the three types of subjects (fourth-year undergraduate, first-year undergraduate, and second-year graduate).

3. At the end of the experiment the subjects were debriefed and given their correct TSCS scores.

4. In other words, to reduce the risk aversion and to reach more consonance, subjects reverted to a slack budgeting behavior.

REFERENCES

Argyris, C. *The Impact of Budgets on People*. New York: The Controllership Foundation, 1952.

Aronson, E., and D.R. Mettee. "Dishonest Behavior as a Function of Differential Levels of Induced Self-Esteem." *Journal of Personality and Social Psychology* (January 1968), pp. 121–127.

Barefield, R.M. "A Model of Forecast Biasing Behavior." *The Accounting Review* (July 1970), pp. 490–501.

Belkaoui, A. *Conceptual Foundations of Management Accounting*. Reading, MA: Addison-Wesley, 1980.

———. "The Relationships between Self-Disclosure Style and Attitudes to Responsibility Accounting." *Accounting, Organizations and Society* (December 1981), pp. 281–289.

———. *Cost Accounting: A Multidimensional Emphasis*. Hinsdale, IL: Dryden Press, 1983.

Caplan, E.H. *Management Accounting and Behavioral Sciences*. Reading, MA: Addison-Wesley, 1971.

Collins, F. "Managerial Accounting Systems and Organizational Control: A Role Perspective." *Accounting, Organizations and Society* (May 1982), pp. 107–122.

Cyert, R.M., and J.G. March. *A Behavioral Theory of the Firm*. Englewood Cliffs, NJ: Prentice-Hall, 1963.

Cyert, R.M., J.G. March, and W.H. Starbuck. "Two Experiments on Bias and Conflict in Organizational Estimation." *Management Science* (April 1961), pp. 254–264.

Dalton, M. *Men Who Manage*. New York: John Wiley, 1961.

Demski, J.S., and G.A. Feltham. "Economic Incentives in Budgetary Control Systems." *The Accounting Review* (April 1978), pp. 336–359.

Fitts, W.F. *Manual for the Tennessee Self-Concept Scale.* Nashville, TN: Counselor Recording and Tests, 1965.

―――. *Interpersonal Competence: The Wheel Model.* Nashville, TN: Counselor Recording and Tests, 1970.

―――. *The Self-Concept and Behavior: Overview and Supplement.* Nashville, TN: Counselor Recording and Tests, 1972a.

―――. *The Self-Concept and Performance.* Nashville, TN: Counselor Recording and Tests, 1972b.

―――. *The Self-Concept and Psychopathology.* Nashville, TN: Counselor Recording and Tests, 1972c.

Fitts, W.F., J.L. Adams, G. Radford, W.C. Richard, B.K. Thomas, M.M. Thomas, and W. Thompson. *The Self-Concept and Self-Actualization.* Nashville, TN: Counselor Recording and Tests, 1971.

Fitts, W.F., and W.T. Hammer. *The Self-Concept and Delinquency.* Nashville, TN: Counselor Recording and Tests, 1969.

Hopwood, A.G. "An Empirical Study of the Role of Accounting Data in Performance Evaluation." *Empirical Research in Accounting: Selected Studies*, suppl. to *Journal of Accounting Research* 10 (1972), pp. 194–209.

Lecky, P. *Self-Consistency.* New York: Island Press, 1945.

Lowe, A.E., and R.W. Shaw. "An Analysis of Managerial Biasing: Evidence from a Company's Budgeting Process." *The Journal of Management Studies* (October 1968), pp. 304–315.

March, J.G., and H.A. Simon. *Organizations.* New York: John Wiley, 1958.

Onsi, M. "Factor Analysis of Behavioral Variables Affecting Budgetary Slack." *The Accounting Review* (July 1973), pp. 535–548.

Parker, L.D. "Goal Congruence: A Misguided Accounting Concept." *Abacus* (June 1976), pp. 3–13.

Rogers, C.R. *Client Centered Therapy.* Boston: Houghton Miffin, 1951.

Schiff, M., and A.Y. Lewin. "The Impact of People on Budgets." *The Accounting Review* (April 1970), pp. 259–268.

Snygg, D., and A.W. Combs. *Individual Behavior.* New York: Harper and Row, 1949.

Swieringa, R.J., and R.H. Moncur. "The Relationship between Managers' Budget Oriented Behavior and Selected Attitudes, Position, Size and Performance Measures." *Empirical Research in Accounting: Selected Studies*, suppl. to *Journal of Accounting Research* 10 (1972), p. 19.

Thompson, W. *Correlates of the Self-Concept.* Nashville, TN: Counselor Recording and Tests, 1972.

Williamson, O.E. *The Economy of Discretionary Behavior: Managerial Objectives in the Theory of the Firm.* Englewood Cliffs, NJ: Prentice-Hall, 1964.

Wylie, R.C. *The Self-Concept: A Critical Survey of Pertinent Research Literature.* Lincoln: University of Nebraska Press, 1961.

Appendix 5.B. The Association between Performance Plan Adoption and Organizational Slack

INTRODUCTION

Recent accounting research has argued that managerial compensation contracts influence managerial decision making (Watts and Zimmerman, 1978; Hagerman and Zmijewski, 1979; Dukes et al., 1981; Horwitz and Kolodny, 1981) and motivate executives to improve firm performance by working harder, lengthening their decision horizons, and becoming less risk-averse in their investment decisions (Smith and Watts, 1982; Larcker, 1983; Baril, 1988). The evidence shows that performance plan adoption was associated with an increase in capital expenditures (Larcker, 1983; Gaver, Gaver, and Furze, 1989).[1] The resources used for the increased capital expenditures are derived from organizational slack.

Organizational slack is a cushion of actual resources used by organizations to adapt successfully either to internal pressures for adjustments or to external pressures for change in policy (March, 1979; Bourgeois, 1981).[2] A review of the concept of organizational slack and its use in theory indicates that there are two measures (Bourgeois, 1978; Singh, 1983, pp. 37–49). Organizational slack is conceptualized as *unabsorbed slack*, which corresponds to the excess, uncommitted resources in organizations. It is also conceptualized as *absorbed slack*, which corresponds to excess costs in organizations (Williamson, 1964). This distinction raises the following question: How does performance plan adoption affect changes in absorbed and unabsorbed slack? The question is investigated here. The empirical results indicate that firms adopting performance plans (relative to similar nonadopting firms) decreased the amount of unabsorbed slack that they were holding.

These results make a significant contribution to research for two reasons. First, they demonstrate a relationship between performance plan adoption and unabsorbed slack. It suggests that some of the resources needed for investment following the adoption of performance plans, as shown by Larcker (1983), come from the organization's unabsorbed slack. Second, they show that the adoption of performance plan is not sufficient to reduce absorbed slack. This means that managers have incentives to invest unused resources but that the plan is insufficient to get them to give up perks.

The remainder of this appendix consists of four sections. First is the introduction of the concept of organizational slack, followed by discussion of the theoretical linkages between performance plan adoption and organizational slack and description of the methodology used. The next section presents the empirical results. Finally, the research findings are discussed and summarized.

Source: A. Riahi-Belkaoui, "The Association between Performance Plan Adoption and Organizational Slack," *Indian Accounting Review* (December 1999): 13–27. Reprinted with permission.

ORGANIZATIONAL SLACK

Slack arises from the tendency of organizations and individuals to refrain from using all the resources available to them. It describes a tendency not to operate at peak efficiency. In general, two types of slack have been identified in the literature: organizational slack and budgetary slack. Organizational slack refers to an unused capacity, in the sense that the demands put on the resources of the organization are less than the supply of these resources. Budgetary slack is found in the budgetary process and refers to the intentional distortion of information that results from an understatement of budgeted sales and overstatement of budgeted costs. The interest in this study is with organizational slack. It is a buffer created by management in its use of available resources to deal with internal as well as external events that may arise and threaten an established coalition. Organizational slack, therefore, is used by management as an agent of change in response to changes in both the internal and external environments.

Cyert and March (1963) explain organizational slack in terms of cognitive and structural factors. They provide a rationale for the unintended creation of organizational slack. Individuals are assumed to "satisfice," in the sense that they set aspiration levels for performance rather than a maximization goal. The aspirations adjust upward or downward, depending on actual performance, and in a slower fashion than actual changes in performance. This lag in adjustment allows excess resources from superior performance to accumulate in the form of organizational slack. This form is then used as a stabilization force to absorb excess resources in good times without requiring a revision of aspiration and intentions regarding the use of these excess resources.

O.E. Williamson (1964) proposed a model of slack based on managerial incentives. This model provides the rationale for managers' motivation and desire for slack resources. Under conditions in which managers are able to pursue their own objectives, the model predicts that excess resources available after target levels of profit have been reached are not allocated according to profit maximization rules. Organizational slack becomes the means by which a manager achieves his or her personal goals, as characterized by four motives: income, job security, status, and discretionary control over resources. Williamson makes the assumption that the manager is motivated to maximize his or her personal goals subject to satisfying organizational objectives and that the manager achieves this by maximizing slack resources under his or her control.

The slack, as identified by Cyert and March and/or Williamson, can be conceptualized as unabsorbed, corresponding to the excess uncommitted resources, or absorbed, corresponding to the excess costs in the organization (Bourgeois, 1981). They are assumed in this study to be affected by the adoption of performance plans. A rationale for this thesis follows.

PERFORMANCE PLANS AND ORGANIZATIONAL SLACK

In essence, organizational slack is the difference between resources available to management and the resources used by management. Management uses it as a buffer to deal with internal as well as external events that may arise and/ or threaten an established coalition (Cyert and March, 1963, p. 36). The performance plan adoptions motivate management to improve firm performance as evidenced by the increase in capital expenditures reported by Larcker (1983). The resources needed by management for such endeavors can be easily provided by the excess resources of organizational slack. The use of organizational slack may, however, depend on whether the slack is absorbed or unabsorbed.

First, performance plans are based on accounting measures of corporate performance. The adoption of performance plans will encourage managers to allocate their efforts to the improvement of the short-term accounting performance measure through reduction of costs. Accordingly, absorbed slack, also labeled administrative slack, is expected to decrease following the adoption of the performance plan.

Second, the adoption of the performance plan will encourage the managers to allocate their efforts to the improvement of long-term accounting performance measures by searching, and spending for, new investment opportunities. Some of the resources needed for the new investment may come from unabsorbed slack. Accordingly, unabsorbed slack is expected to decrease following the adoption of a performance plan.

The following research hypotheses are examined in the subsequent empirical study.

H1: The adoption of a performance plan is associated with a decrease in absorbed slack.

H2: The adoption of a performance plan is associated with a decrease in unabsorbed slack.

METHODS

This study uses a longitudinal design because the relationship between performance plan adoption and organizational slack occurs over time.

Sample and Data Collection

A list of corporate incentive plans was obtained from previous research (Larcker, 1983) and through independent historical research. Each experimental firm was required to satisfy two criteria. First, the performance plan adoption must have occurred during the 1971–1982 period. Second, a firm passing the criterion must have a matching control firm.

Seventy experimental firms were identified. The control firms were required to satisfy the following criteria:

1. same industry as the experimental firms.[3]
2. similar size as the experimental firm measured by corporate sales in the year prior to performance plan adoption by the experimental firm.
3. similar fiscal year as the experimental firm.

The sample of companies is shown in Table 5B.1. The plans were all long-term plans consisting of forty-four performance unit plans and twenty-six performance share plans. To measure the effect of the performance plan, organizational slack is analyzed before and after the change while controlling for one categorical variable and two covariates.

Independent Variables

Financial statement data for years -5 to $+5$ (relative to the year of adoption of the performance plan by the experimental company) for each firm were collected from Compustat. Year 0, the year of adoption of the performance plan, was excluded from the analysis to avoid confounding the slack measures with outcomes during the transition. The data collected were on absorbed slack and unabsorbed slack. Various measures of slack have been used. Rosner (1968) used profit and excess capacity as slack measures. Lewin and Wolf (1976) suggested selling, general, and administrative expenses as surrogates for slack.

A case for financially derived measures of slack was made by Bourgeois (1981) and Bourgeois and Singh (1983). A two-component concept of slack was proposed that made the distinction between absorbed slack, referring to slack absorbed as costs in organizations, and unabsorbed slack, referring to uncommitted resources. Analogously, absorbed slack was measured by (1) the ratio of selling, general, and administrative expenses to cost of goods sold in order to capture slack absorbed in salaries, overhead expenses, and various administrative costs and (2) the ratio of working capital to sales in order to capture the absorption of slack related to capital utilization. Unabsorbed slack was computed as (cash plus marketable securities minus current liabilities) divided by sales, in order to capture the amount of liquid resources uncommitted to liabilities in the near future (Singh, 1986).

Control Variable and Covariates

One control variable and two covariates were used to control for possible intervening effects. First, to control for size and profitability, total assets and

Table 5B.1
Sample of Companies

Experimental Firm	Year	Control Firm	Experimental Firm	Year	Control Firm
A.E. Staley	1980	Hormel	Intl. Harvester	1975	Borg Warne
Akzona	1971	Lowenstein	Koopers	1979	Phelps Dodge
Allied Corp.	1980	Halliburton	Manville	1978	U.S. Gypsum
AMF	1980	General Tire	Merck	1982	Sterling Drug
Armstrong Rubber	1982	Cooper Tire	Minnesota Mining & Mfg. Co.	1981	TRW
Ashland Oil	1979	Standard Oil (Ohio)	Monsanto	1974	Dow Chemical
Atlantic Richfield	1976	Cities Service Co.	Nabisco	1976	Campbell Taggert
			Nalco	1977	Schering-Plough
Baxter Travenol	1982	Schering-Plough	Nashua	1981	Dennison
Beatrice Foods	1978	Quaker Oats	NCR	1982	Deere
Bemis	1974	Great Northern Nekoosa	NL Industries	1978	Schlumberger
			Outboard Marine	1982	Briggs & Stratton
Bendix	1974	Fruehauf	Owens-Corning	1980	Libby Owens Food
Black & Decker	1980	Baker Intl.	Owens-Illinois	1975	Owens-Corning
Bristol Myers	1978	Avon Products	Phillips Petroleum	1978	Cities Service Co.
Burroughs	1982	Digital Equipment	Pillsbury	1975	Intl. Multifoods
Cabot	1972	Handy & Harman	Ralston-Purina	1975	Carnation
Celanese	1980	Hercules	Rexnord	1982	Smith Intl.
Central Soya	1981	Anderson Clayton	Roblin	1977	Midland-Ross
Cincinnati Milacron	1979	Ametek	Rockwell Intl.	1977	General Dynamics
			Sanders Associates	1980	Tracor
Combustion Eng.	1978	Gillette	Sealed Power	1978	Compugraphic
Cooper Labs	1978	ICN Pharm.	Shell	1979	Standard Oil (Indiana)
Corning Glass	1979	Norton			
Crown Zellerbach	1973	Diamond Intl.	Singer	1981	Martin Marietta
Datapoint	1979	Storage Technology	Squibb	1975	Pfizer
Diamond Shamrock	1980	Sherwin Williams	Sun Co.	1972	Royal Dutch Petroleum–N.Y.
Dover	1974	Harsichfeger	Sybron	1981	Becton Dickinson
Eaton	1974	Lockheed	Texas Instruments	1980	Raytheon
Emerson Electronic	1977	Whirlpool	Textron	1982	Dresser Inc.
			Toro	1976	Hesston
Ferro	1982	Syntex	Union Oil of California	1975	Conoco
FMC	1973	DuPont			
General Mills	1980	Carnation	United Technologies	1979	Boeing
General Motors	1982	Ford Motor Co.			
Hershey Foods	1978	Intl. Multifoods	Vulcan Materials	1973	Anchor Hocking
Hobart	1977	Scott & Fetzer	Warner Lambert	1982	American Home Products
Honeywell	1978	Litton			
Illinois Toolwork	1980	Hornsichfeger	Westinghouse	1979	RCA

Note: *Year in which the experimental firm adopted a performance plan.

rate of return on assets were used as covariates. Second, an influence on the use of slack may have advantages or disadvantages resulting from early or late adoption of performance plans with a set of competitors. Another argument is that imitators may learn from first adopters' mistakes and can benefit from the adoption of performance plans. To control for innovation effects, the experimental firms were coded into two groups, with the first thirty early adopters of performance plans classified as early adopters and the rest as late adopters.

Data Analysis

Analysis of covariance was used to test the overall relationship between (1) slack and firm effect, (2) slack and performance plan adoption, and (3) the interaction of firm effect and performance plan adoption on slack. The model's control variable was early/late adoption, and covariates included assets and rate of return on assets.

RESULTS

Tables 5B.2–5B.4 present overall results for the two measures of absorbed slack and the measure of unabsorbed slack. Table 5B.5 presents the means and standard deviations of each of the slack measures before and after the adoption of the performance plan for both the experimental and control groups of firms.

The first measure of absorbed slack is the ratio of selling, general, and administrative expenses as a percentage of cost of goods sold. It captures slack absorbed in salaries, overhead expenses, and various administrative costs. The results for this measure of absorbed slack are reported in Table 5B.2 and show that the main firm effects and performance plan adoption as well as the interactive effects on slack are both insignificant. The same result is found in Table 5B.5 for this measure. The second measure of absorbed slack is the ratio of working capital of sales, which is used to capture the absorption of slack related to capital utilization. Results regarding this second measure of absorbed slack are summarized in Table 5B.3 and show that the main effects of firm effects and performance plan adoption as well as the interaction effects on slack are all insignificant. The same result is found in Table 5B.5 for this measure.

The measure of unabsorbed slack is the ratio of cash plus marketable securities minus current liabilities to sales. This measure is used to capture the amount of liquid resources uncommitted to liabilities in the near future. Results regarding this measure of unabsorbed slack are summarized in Table 5B.4 and show that the following relationships are all significant at $\alpha = 0.05$: (1) between slack and firm effect, (2) between slack and performance plan adoption, and (3) between firm effect-performance plan adoption interactions and slack. An ex-

Table 5B.2
Results of Overall Analysis of Covariance for Absorbed Slack Computed as Selling, General, and Administrative Expenses/Cost of Goods Sold*

Sources	F	P
A: Firm effect (experimental control)	1.53	0.2170
B: Performance plan adoption (before/after)	0.92	0.3382
A x B interaction	0.89	0.3462
Control variables		
Early/late adoption	21.79	0.0001
Covariates		
Size	28.27	0.0001
Rate of return on assets	71.87	0.0001

Notes:
*R^2 = 0.1607.
Overall F = 20.88 (p = 0.0001).

Table 5B.3
Results of Overall Analysis of Covariance for Absorbed Slack Computed as Working Capital/Sales*

Sources	F	P
A: Firm effect (experimental control)	0.13	0.7152
B: Performance plan adoption (before/after)	3.19	0.0748
A x B interaction	0.06	0.8093
Control variables		
Early/late adoption	1.58	0.2094
Covariates		
Size	35.52	0.0001
Rate of return on assets	136.79	0.0001

Notes:
*R^2 = 0.2084.
Overall F = 29.54 (p = 0.0001).

amination of the mean results on absorbed slack in Table 5B.5 shows a significant reduction in unabsorbed slack taking place subsequent to the adoption of the performance plan. This result is consistent with hypothesis 2. That is, unabsorbed slack declines following the adoption of the performance plan. It suggests that following the implementation of compensation plans managers do seek

Table 5B.4
Results of Overall Analysis of Covariance for Unabsorbed Slack Computed as Cash + Marketable Securities − Current Liabilities/Sales*

Sources	F	P
A: Firm effect (experimental control)	5.09	0.0245
B: Performance plan adoption (before/after)	14.13	0.0002
A x B interaction	4.38	0.0368
Control variables		
Early/late adoption	0.01	0.9217
Covariates		
Size	7.11	0.0079
Rate of return on assets	165.10	0.0001

Notes:
*$R^2 = 0.2255$.
Overall $F = 32.67$ (p = 0.0001).

Table 5B.5
T-Tests and Slack Means by Firm Group before and after Performance Plan Adoption

	Before Adoption	After Adoption	T
Slack 1			
Experimental Group—Mean	0.2571	0.30571	1.4962
Control Group—Mean	0.3216	0.3215	0.0021
Slack 2			
Experimental Group—Mean	0.1928	0.21166	1.3015
Control Group—Mean	0.1992	0.2135	0.9486
Slack 3			
Experimental Group—Mean	−0.1881	−0.1236	−2.1209
Control Group—Mean	−0.0713	−0.1252	−2.9442

new investment opportunities, as shown in Larcker (1983). It also suggests that some of the resources needed for the new investment come from the unabsorbed slack existing in the firms. The amount of liquid resources uncommitted to liabilities in the near future appears as the first resources to be invested by managers following the adoption of performance plans.

DISCUSSION AND SUMMARY

The hypothesis that changes in executive compensation contracts are associated with changes in managerial decisions is important to the incentive research taking place in management, accounting, and economics. One incentive question investigated in this study concerns the association between performance plan adoption and organizational slack. A differentiation was made between absorbed slack and unabsorbed slack. The results on absorbed slack were insignificant. However, the empirical results indicate that, when compared to similar non-adopting firms, those firms that adopt performance plans exhibit a significant reduction in unabsorbed slack following plan adoption. A logical interpretation is that the performance plan encourages managers to allocate their efforts toward improving accounting-based, long-term performance measures by increasing capital investment. That investment leads to a reduction of the unabsorbed slack. The unabsorbed slack is used to fund some of the increase in capital investment. Before these results can be generalized, future research should investigate the impact of the use of different measures of organizational slack, different firms, and different periods.

NOTES

1. Other related evidence indicates that the adoption of a performance plan was associated with (1) a decrease in corporate risk (Gaver, Gaver, and Furze, 1989), (2) mixed evidence on the stock market reaction to the announcement of performance plan adoption (Larcker, 1983; Brickley, Bhagat, and Lease, 1985; Gaver, Gaver, and Battistel, 1992; Kumar and Sopariwala, 1991), and (3) significant positive excess returns on announcements of earnings (Tehranian, Travlos, and Waegelein, 1987a, 1987b).

2. There is a clear differentiation between organizational slack, which refers to the difference between the available and used resources, and budgetary slack, which refers to the use of the budget process for the creation of attainable budgets.

3. For the seventy matched pairs, forty-six had the same two-digit SIC code, five had the same five-digit SIC code and nineteen had the same four-digit SIC code.

REFERENCES

Baril, C.P. 1988. "Long Term Incentive Compensation, Ownership and the Decision Horizon Problem." Working Paper, McIntyre School of Commerce, University of Virginia, Charlottesville.

Bourgeois, L.J. 1981. "Oil the Measurement of Organizational Slack." *Academy of Management Review* 6 (October): 29–39.

Bourgeois, L.J., and J.V. Singh. 1983. "Organizational Slack and Political Behavior within Top Management Teams." *Academy of Management Proceedings*: 43–47.

Brickley, J.A., S. Bhagat, and R.C. Lease. 1985. "The Impact of Long-Range Managerial Compensation Plans on Shareholder Wealth." *Journal of Accounting and Economics* 7 (April): 115–129.

Cyert, R.M., and J.G. March. 1963. *A Behavioral Theory of the Firm.* Englewood Cliffs, NJ: Prentice-Hall.

Dukes, R., T.R. Dyckman, and J. Elliot. 1981. "Accounting for Research and Development Costs: The Impact on Research and Development Expenditures." *Journal of Accounting Research* 18, Supplement: 1–26.

Gaver, J.J., K.M. Gaver, and G.P. Battistel. 1992. "The Stock Market Reaction to Performance Plan Adoptions." *The Accounting Review* 1 (January): 172–182.

Gaver, J.J., K.M. Gaver, and S. Furze. 1989. "The Association between Performance Plan Adoption and Corporate Investment Decisions." Working Paper, University of Oregon.

Hagerman, R.L., and M.E. Zmijewski. 1979. "Some Economic Determinants of Accounting Policy Choice." *Journal of Accounting and Economics* 1: 141–161.

Horwitz, B., and R. Kolodny. 1981. "The Economic Effects of Involuntary Uniformity in the Financial Reporting of R&D Expenditures." *Journal of Accounting Research* 18, Supplement: 38–74.

Kumar, R., and P.R. Sopariwala. 1991. "The Effect of Adoption of Long-Term Performance Plans on Stock Prices and Accounting Numbers." Working Paper, Virginia Polytechnic Institute and State University.

Larcker, D.F. 1983. "The Association between Performance Plan Adoption and Corporate Capital Investment." *Journal of Accounting and Economics* 5 (April): 9–30.

Lewin, A.Y., and C. Wolf. 1976. "The Theory of Organizational Slack: A Critical Review." *Proceedings: Twentieth International Meeting of ITMS*: 648–654.

March, J.G. 1978. "Bounded Rationality, Ambiguity and the Engineering of Choice." *Bell Journal of Economics* 9: 587–608.

Rosner, M.M. 1968. "Economic Determination of Organizational Innovation." *Administrative Science Quarterly* 12: 614–625.

Singh, J.V. 1983. "Performance, Slack and Risk Taking in Strategic. Decisions: Test of a Structural Equation Model." Unpublished doctoral diss., Graduate School of Business, Stanford University, Palo Alto, CA.

Singh, J.V. 1986. "Performance, Slack and Risk Taking in Organizational Decision Making." *Academy of Management Journal* 3 (September): 562–585.

Smith, C.W., and R.L. Watts. 1982. "Incentive and Tax Effects of U.S. Executive Compensation Plans." *Australian Journal of Management* 7 (December): 39–157.

Tehranian, H., T. Travlos, and J.F. Waegelein. 1985. "Market Reaction to Short-Term Executive Compensation Plan Adoption." *Journal of Accounting and Economics* 7 (April): 131–144.

Watts, R.L., and J.L. Zimmerman. 1978. "Towards a Positive Theory of the Determination of Accounting Standards." *The Accounting Review* (January): 112–134.

Williamson, O.E. 1964. *The Economics of Discretionary Behavior: Managerial Objectives in a Theory of the Firm.* Englewood Cliffs, NJ: Prentice-Hall.

Appendix 5.C. The Impact of the Multi-Divisional Structure on Organizational Slack: The Contingency of Diversification Strategy

INTRODUCTION

American corporations have been experimenting with various forms of organizational structure. The M-form or multi-divisional structure has evolved as the more popular solution to the problems of managing growth and diversity within a centralized structure. It is generally presented as providing information-processing advantages, as well as better performance in large multi-product firms (Teece, 1981). As a result the relationship between corporate diversification and firm performance has been at the forefront of issues relating to corporate strategy (Hoskisson, 1987). However, although implied by Williamson (1970) and Ezzamel (1985), the impact of the M-form implementation on organizational slack remains unexplored. This study examines the proposition that the impact of the implementation of such structure on organizational slack should vary with the diversification strategy adopted.[1] More specifically, given the trade-offs between control-system emphasis in various diversification strategies, certain controls are better suited to reducing certain types of slacks in certain strategies. The next sections cover the M-form hypothesis and organizational slack. Diversification strategy is then discussed, before a presentation of the central proposition. The next two sections set out the empirical results, and the appendix ends with a final discussion.

THE MULTI-DIVISIONAL FORM HYPOTHESIS

The multi-divisional form structure was adopted as a response to the increasingly complex administrative problems encountered within a centralized functional structure as firm size and diversity increased (Chandler, 1962). Building on Chandler's analysis, Williamson (1970) suggested that because of two problems encountered by expanding multi-product firms—cumulative control loss and confounding of strategic and operating decision making—there is the risk of failure to achieve least-cost profit maximization behavior. Basically, he maintained that as size increases, people reach their limits of control as a result of bounded rationality and start resorting to opportunism, thereby threatening efficiency and profitability. The M-form is presented as a unique structural framework that overcomes these difficulties and favors goal pursuits and least-cost behavior more nearly associated with the neoclassical profit-maximizing hypothesis.

Source: A. Riahi-Belkaoui, "The Impact of the Multi-Divisional Structure on Organizational Slack: The Contingency of Diversification Strategy." *British Journal of Management* 9, 1998, pp. 211–217. Reprinted with permission of Blackwell Publishing.

Based on the transaction-cost analysis, researchers investigated a hypothesis of links between the M-form structure and better performance.[2] Results to date provide either a support of the proposition that M-form implementation affects performance in large corporations regardless of other contingencies or mixed results (Cable and Dirrheimer, 1983; Ezzamel, 1985). These studies did not differentiate between the firms on the basis of their diversification strategy. Two studies provide evidence in support of a contingency view of the relationship between either performance (Hoskisson, 1987) or productivity (Riahi-Belkaoui, 1997) and implementation of the M-form structure. These studies examined considerations of return and risk, but not organizational slack.

ORGANIZATIONAL SLACK

Because the definition of slack is often intertwined with a description of the functions that slack serves, Bourgeois (1981) discussed these functions as a means of making palpable the ways of measuring slack.[3] From a review of administrative theory literature, he identified organizational slack as an independent variable that either "causes" or serves four primary functions:

1. as an instrument for organizational actors to remain in the system, a form of inducement (Barnard, 1938; March and Simon, 1958; Cyert and March, 1963);
2. as a resource for conflict resolution (Pondy, 1967);
3. as a technical buffer from the variances and discontinuities created by environmental uncertainty (Thompson, 1967; Galbraith, 1973);
4. as a facilitator of certain types of strategic or creative behavior, providing opportunities for a satisfying behavior and promoting political behavior (Hambrick and Snow, 1977).

One of the problems of empirically investigating the presence of organizational slack related to the difficulties of securing adequate measurement for the phenomenon. Various ad hoc measures based on questionnaires, interviews, or archival measures were proposed (Rosner, 1968; Bourgeois; 1981). Bourgeois and Singh (1983) refined these measures by suggesting that slack can be differentiated on an "ease of recovery dimension." A distinction is made between absorbed slack, slack that has been absorbed as cost in the organization, and unabsorbed slack, referring to excess liquidity not yet earmarked for particular uses.

Absorbed slack was measured by the level of general and administrative expenses divided by the cost of goods sold. This concept of absorbed slack, also referred to as administrative slack, captures slack absorbed as costs. It follows from Williamson's notion of slack as extra staff that can be reduced in difficult times (Williamson, 1970).

Unabsorbed slack was measured by the sum of cash and marketable securities

minus current liabilities divided by sales. It follows the notion of slack as readily accessible resources not absorbed by costs, thus giving the amount of liquid resources uncommitted to liabilities in the near future.

DIVERSIFICATION STRATEGY AND CONTROL

Galbraith and Nathanson (1979) traced the growth of firms to three major categories of corporate diversification strategy: vertical integration, related business diversification, and unrelated business diversification.

Vertical integration offers the firm economics owing to control of its supply/output markets. The firm's value-added margin for a chain of processing is increased because of increased control over raw materials and/or outlets (Pfeffer and Salancik, 1978; Scherer, 1980; Harrigan, 1985). Furthermore, market transaction costs—such as opportunistic actions by traders or the drafting and monitoring of contingent claims contracts to ensure harmonious trading relationships—can be either eliminated or reduced (Hill and Hoskisson, 1987).

Firms pursuing a strategy of related diversification can realize synergistic economies of scope through the joint use of inputs (Teece, 1981). Exploitation of this energy is achieved through both tangible and intangible interrelationships (Porter, 1985). Tangible interrelationships are created by such devices as joint procurement of raw materials, joint development of shared technologies or production process, joint sales force, and joint physical distribution systems. Intangible interrelationships arise from the sharing of know-how and capabilities.

An unrelated diversification strategy is assumed to yield financial economies. The risk of pooling of imperfectly correlated income streams created by unrelated diversification is, in principle, assumed to produce an asset with a superior risk/return relationship (Lewellen, 1971).

The differences in economic characteristics between the three types of strategies create situations that will call for different types of control. It is suggested that control arrangements within a basic M-form framework must be consistent with a firm's corporate diversification strategy if the firm is to realize the economic benefits associated with that strategy. Similarly, based on a review of a large body of research on strategy implementation, Baysingh and Hoskisson (1989) concluded that firms pursuing a dominant or vertical strategy place a higher emphasis on strategic control than related and unrelated diversification, in that order, and a lower emphasis on financial controls than related and unrelated diversifiers, in that order.

THEORY AND HYPOTHESES

The M-form hypothesis predicts that under the U-form structure, a fair degree of managerial slack would develop within each department, causing the creation

of discretionary investment projects to justify the extra staff (Ezzamel, 1985; Williamson, 1996). The implementation of the M-form structure is expected to reduce this managerial slack and channel the operation of the firm toward goal pursuit and least-cost behavior more nearly associated with the neoclassical profit maximization hypothesis (Williamson, 1970).

The reduction of slack following the implementation of the M-form differs, however, depending on whether slack refers to absorbed or unabsorbed slack and on the diversification strategy adopted.

If the diversification strategy adopted is a vertical integration or related diversification, a greater emphasis is placed on strategic control than on financial control. It eliminates the need for extra staff and discretionary investment projects, and the formulation of investment opportunities occurs at the top of the organization or at the level of strategic business units (Ackerman, 1976). Absorbed slack or administrative slack should therefore be expected to decrease following the implementation of the M-form by firms using either vertical integration or related diversification. The reduction of unabsorbed slack may be more difficult given the moderate or low reliance on financial controls.

If the diversification strategy adopted is an unrelated diversification, a higher emphasis is placed on financial control than on strategic control. It reduces the level of unabsorbed slack as cash flows are not automatically returned to their sources but, instead, are exposed to internal competition, and investment projects are evaluated on strict objective criteria. The reduction of absorbed slack may be more difficult because of the extra staff needed to manage the large accountability for divisional profits. This suggests the following two hypotheses:

H1: Implementation of the M-form structure in vertically integrated and in related diversified firms leads to a decrease in absorbed slack.

H2: Implementation of the M-form structure in unrelated diversified firms leads to a decrease in unabsorbed slack.

METHODS

Sample and Data Collection

Previous research has identified sixty-two firms that adopted the M-form during the period 1950–1978 (Armour and Teece, 1978). The sample used in this study consists of these firms. Each firm was diversified at the time of the restructuring and is classified by Rumelt's (1974) method as having been in one of three diversification classes: unrelated (sixteen firms), related (twenty-two firms), or vertical (twenty-four firms).

A longitudinal design is used to capture the effects over time of the implementation of the M-form.[4] Data for two measures of slack were collected for year -5 through year $+5$ (relative to the year of restructuring). In addition, three covariables (growth in gross national product [GNP], growth in total assets,

and firm size) and two control variables (early/late adoption of the M-form and industry classification) are used.

Dependent Variable

Financial statement data for years -5 to $+5$ (relative to the year of restructuring) for each firm were collected from Compustat. Year 0, relative to the year of restructuring, was excluded from the analysis to avoid the potential confounding of slack measures with events during the transition. The data collected were absorbed slack—computed as general and administrative costs divided by cost of goods sold—and unabsorbed slack—computed as cash plus marketable securities minus current liabilities divided by sales.

Control Variables and Covariables

The two control factors (early/late adoption of the M-form and industry classification) and three covariates (growth in GNP, growth in total assets, and firm size) are included to control for possible intervening effects.

The early/late adopter control factor is motivated by the belief that late adopters learn from the experience of early adopters and are thus able to restructure faster and more efficiently (Mansfield, 1985). Early/late adoption is measured by the year of restructuring relative to the sample median. Hence, firms adopting the M-form structure prior to 1967 are classified as early movers, and those adopting in 1967 or later are classified as late movers. The industry control factor is included to control for industry effects. Firm size, asset growth rate, and GNP growth rate are included as covariates. Their use is motivated by the suggestion that firms may sacrifice profitability in periods of growth and by the need to control for changes in organizational slack related to major external shifts in aggregate demands. Firm size is measured as the proportional change in total assets, and GNP growth is measured as the proportional change in GNP. Each of the covariates is measured for the same period as the dependent variable.

DATA ANALYSIS

To test the overall relationship between organizational structure and organizational slack, between diversification strategy and organizational slack, and between the interactive effect of organizational structure and diversification strategy on organizational slack, an analysis of covariance is used. Tables 5C.1 and 5C.2 present the results of the analysis of covariance for absorbed and unabsorbed slack for the sixty-two firms in the sample. The results of the overall analysis of the covariance in both exhibits are highly significant and suggest that organizational structure and organizational slack as well as diversification strategy and organizational slack are related. The significant interaction effect in both figures between strategic type and the implementation of the M-form

Table 5C.1
Results of Overall Analysis of Variance for the Absorbed Slack

Sources	F	P
Diversification strategy	760.32	0.0001*
M-form implementation (before/after)	432.25	0.0001*
M-form* diversification interaction	851.26	0.0001*
Control variable		
Early/late adopter	2.85	0.094**
Covariates		
Size	0.00	0.947
Total asset growth	0.16	0.685
Total growth in GNP	1.08	0.295
Industry	684.19	0.001*

Notes: *Significant at $\alpha = 0.01$; **Significant at $\alpha = 0.10$.

suggests that the M-form implementation had a differential impact on organizational slack, depending on the diversification strategy adopted.

The impact of the M-form implementation on organizational slack is further investigated by performing mean comparisons of absorbed and unabsorbed slack before and after the M-form by strategic type. Table 5C.3 presents the results. It indicates that following the implementation of the M-form, vertically integrated and related diversified firms decreased their absorbed slack while unrelated diversified firms decreased their unabsorbed slack, which is consistent with both H1 and H2.

DISCUSSION

The objective of this study was to show that the implementation of the M-form structure creates differences in organizational slack measures in firms that employ different diversification strategies. The slack measures used were absorbed or administrative slack, and unabsorbed slack or available liquidity. The diversification strategies were related diversification, vertical integration, and unrelated diversification. The results show that the implementation of the M-form structure was supported for both absorbed and unabsorbed slack.

H1 was confirmed, suggesting that the implementation of a multidivisional

Table 5C.2
Results of Overall Analysis of Variance for the Unabsorbed Slack

Sources	F	P
Diversification strategy	5.76	0.0061*
M-form implementation (before/after)	7.06	0.0110**
M-form* diversification interaction	2.33	0.0032*
Control variable		
Early/late adopter	2.87	0.094**
Covariates		
Size	0.00	0.945
Total asset growth	0.17	0.683
Total growth in GNP	1.09	0.299
Industry	2.29	0.0033*

Notes: *Significant at $\alpha = 0.01$; **Significant at $\alpha = 0.10$.

structure leads to a reduction of absorbed slack or administrative slack in both vertically integrated and related diversified firms. This result follows from the general thesis that the M-form reduces the organizational slack developed within each department under the U-form and from the particular thesis that vertically integrated and related diversified firms rely most on strategic controls that are most effective in monitoring expenditures on excess staff and discretionary expenses.

H2 was also confirmed, suggesting that the implementation of a multidivisional structure leads to reduction of unabsorbed slack or available liquidity in unrelated diversified firms. This result follows again from the slack reduction thesis of the M-form hypothesis and from the particular thesis that unrelated diversified firms rely mostly on financial controls that are most effective in monitoring cash flows within the firm.

The results suggest that the M-form implementation increases the firm's capacity to manage absorbed slack in the cases of vertically integrated and related diversified firms and unabsorbed slack in the case of unrelated diversified firms. It points to additional benefits of the M-form, when coupled with the appropriate control system, strategic controls for the vertically integrated and related diver-

Table 5C.3
T-Tests and Slack Measures, Means, and Standard Deviations by Strategy Types before and after M-form Implementation

Measures	Before M-form		After M-form		
	Mean	s.d.	Mean	s.d.	t
Vertically integrated firms					
Absorbed slack	0.16744	0.086100	0.14860	0.0674	0.8260
Unabsorbed slack	-0.05838	0.007711	-0.10210	0.0689	2.1339*
Related diversified firms					
Absorbed slack	0.28156	0.187870	0.29270	0.20022	-0.1859
Unabsorbed slack	-0.07611	0.147400	-0.14080	0.11942	1.5627**
Unrelated diversified firms					
Absorbed slack	2.66570	7.487400	0.20720	0.14642	1.2715**
Unabsorbed slack	-0.16067	0.108448	-0.14640	0.06373	-0.4394

Notes: *Significant at $\alpha = 0.05$; **Significant at $\alpha = 0.10$.

sified firms, and financial controls for the unrelated diversified firms. The efficient use of control systems is contingent on the nature of the diversification strategy. In general, benefits would result from an increase in the use of financial controls by the related diversified and vertically integrated firms and in the use of strategic controls by the unrelated diversified firms. In this particular case, a reduction in absorbed slack is possible through the implementation of strategic controls for vertically integrated and related diversified firms, and a reduction in unabsorbed slack is possible through the implementation of financial controls for the unrelated diversified firms. Obviously, more research is needed to verify these results using different measures of slack, and/or using different companies from different periods and from different countries.

NOTES

1. It follows from other studies showing the contingency of diversification strategy on the relationship between multi-divisional structure and performance (Hoskisson, 1987; Riahi-Belkaoui, 1997) and between multi-divisional structure and capital structure (Riahi-Belkaoui and Bannister, 1994).

2. Fligstein (1985) proposed five theories that may be used to explain the genesis of the multidivisional structure: (1) strategy-structure thesis (Chandler, 1962), (2) transaction-cost analysis (Williamson, 1970), (3) population-ecology theory (Hannan and Freeman, 1977, 1984), (4) control theory based on power (Pfeffer and Salancik, 1978; Pfeffer, 1981, 1982), and (5) organizational homogeneity theory (DiMaggio and Powell, 1983).

3. While this study examines the concept of organizational slack, most of the related accounting studies examined the concept of budgetary slack. The literature on organizational slack shows that managers have the motives necessary to operate in a slack environment. The literature on budgetary slack considers the budget as the embodiment of that environment and, therefore, assumes that managers will use the budgeting process to bargain for slack budgets (Schiff and Lewin, 1968; Merchant, 1985).

4. Various studies have evaluated various proxies of performance over several years following a major corporate policy (Healy and Palepu, 1988; Lakonishok and Vermaelen, 1990; Agrawal, Jaffe, and Mandelken, 1992; Cornett and Tehranian, 1992; Healy, Palepu, and Ruback, 1992; John, Lang, and Netter, 1992; Smith, 1990).

REFERENCES

Ackerman, R.W. (1976). "Influences of Integration and Diversity in the Investment Process." *Administrative Science Quarterly* 15, pp. 341–351.

Agrawal, A., F. Jaffe, and G. Mandelker. (1992). "The Post Merger Performance of Acquiring Firms: A Re-Examination of an Anomaly." *Journal of Finance* 47, pp. 1605–1622.

Armour, R.A., and D.J. Teece. (1978). "Organizational Structure and Economic Performance: A Test of the Multi Divisional Hypothesis." *Journal of Economics* 9, pp. 106–122.

Barnard, C.I. (1938) *Functions of the Executive*. Cambridge, MA: Harvard University Press.

Baysingh, B., and R.E. Hoskisson. (1989). "Diversification Strategy and R&D Intensity in Multi-Product Firms." *Academy of Management Journal* 12, pp. 310–322.

Bourgeois, L.J. (1981). "On the Measurement of Organizational Slack." *Academy of Management Review* 6, pp. 29–39.

Bourgeois, L.J., and J.V. Singh. (1983). "Organizational Slack and Political Behavior within Top Management." *Academy of Management Proceedings* 2(2), pp. 43–47.

Cable, J., and M.J. Dirrheimer. (1983). "Hierarchies and Markets: An Empirical Test of the Multidimensional Hypothesis in West Germany." *International Journal of Industrial Organization* 1, pp. 43–62.

Chandler, A.D., Jr. (1962). *Strategy and Structure: Chapters in the History of the American Industrial Enterprise*. Cambridge, MA: MIT Press.

Cornett, M.M., and H. Tehranian. (1992). "Change in Corporate Performance Associated with Bank Acquisitions." *Journal of Financial Economics* 31, pp. 211–234.

Cyert, R.M., and J.G. March. (1963). *A Behavioral Theory of the Firm*. Englewood Cliffs, NJ: Prentice-Hall.

DiMaggio, P., and W. Powell. (1983). "Institutional Isomorphism." *American Sociological Review* 48, pp. 142–160.

Ezzamel, M.A. (1985). "On the Assessment of the Performance Effects of Multidivisional Structures: A Synthesis." *Accounting and Business Research* 61, pp. 23–34.

Fligstein, N. (1985). "The Spread of the Multi Divisional Form among Large Firms, 1919–1979." *American Sociological Review* 3, pp. 377–391.

Galbraith, J.R. (1973). *Designing Complex Organizations*. Reading, MA: Addison-Wesley.

Galbraith, J.R., and D.A. Nathanson. (1979). "Role of Organizational Structure and Process." In D. Schendel and S. Hofer (eds.), *Strategic Management: A New View of Business Policy and Planning*. Boston: Little, Brown.

Hambrick, D.C., and C.C. Snow. (1977). "A Contextual Model of Strategic Decision Making in Organizations." *Academy of Management Proceedings* 3, pp. 109–112.

Hannan, M., and J. Freeman. (1977). "The Population Ecology of Organizations." *American Journal of Sociology* 92, pp. 929–964.

Hannan, M., and J. Freeman. (1984). "Structural Inertia and Organizational Change." *American Sociological Review* 49, pp. 149–164.

Harrigan, K.R. (1985). "Vertical Integration and Corporate Strategy." *Academy of Management Journal* 28, pp. 397–425.

Healy, P.M., and K.G. Palepu. (1988). "Earnings Information Conveyed by Dividend Initiations and Omissions." *Journal of Financial Economics* 21(2), pp. 149–175.

Healy, P.M., K.G. Palepu, and R.S. Ruback. (1992). "Does Corporate Performance Improve after Mergers?" *Journal of Financial Economics* 31(2), pp. 135–175.

Hill, C.W.L., and R.E. Hoskisson. (1987). "Strategy and Structure in the Multi Product Firm." *Academy of Management Review* 4, pp. 331–334.

Hoskisson, R.E. (1987). "Multi Divisional Structure and Performance: The Contingency of Diversification Strategy." *Academy of Management Journal* 3, pp. 625–644.

John, K., L.H.E. Lang, and J. Netter. (1992). "The Voluntary Restructuring of Large Firms in Response to Performance Decline." *Journal of Finance* 47(3), pp. 891–916.

Lakonishok, J., and T. Vermaelen. (1990). "Anomalous Price Behavior around Repurchase Tender Offers." *Journal of Finance* 45(2), pp. 455–477.

Lewellen, W. (1971). "A Pure Financial Rationale for the Conglomerate Merger." *Journal of Finance* 26, pp. 521–545.

Mansfield, E. (1985). "How Rapidly Does New Industrial Technology Leak Out?" *Journal of Industrial Economics* 34, pp. 217–255.

March, J.C., and H.A. Simon. (1958). *Organizations*. New York: John Wiley.

Merchant, K.A. (1985). "Budgeting and the Propensity to Create Budgetary Slack." *Accounting Organizations and Society* 10, pp. 201–210.

Pfeffer, J. (1981). *Power in Organizations*. Marshfield, MA: Pilman.

Pfeffer, J. (1982). *Organizations and Organizational Theory*. Marshfield, MA: Pilman.

Pfeffer, J., and G. Salancik. (1978). *The External Control of Organizations: A Resource Dependency Perspective*. New York: Harper and Row.

Pondy L.R. (1967). "Organizational Conflict: Concepts and Models." *Administrative Science Quarterly* 12(2), pp. 296–320.

Porter, L.R. (1985). *Competitive Advantage: Creating and Sustaining Superior Performance*. New York: Free Press.

Riahi-Belkaoui, A. (1997). "Multidivisional Structure and Productivity: The Contingency of Diversification Strategy." *Journal of Business Finance and Accountancy* 24, pp. 615–627.

Riahi-Belkaoui, A., and J. Bannister. (1994). "Multidivisional Structure and Capital

Structure: The Contingency of Diversification Strategy." *Managerial and Decision Economics* 15, pp. 267–276.

Rosner, M.M. (1968). "Economic Determinants of Organizational Innovation." *Administrative Science Quarterly* 12, pp. 614–625.

Rumelt, R.P. (1974). *Strategy, Structure and Economic Performance*. Cambridge, MA: Harvard University Press.

Scherer, F.M. (1980). *Industrial Market Structure and Economic Performance*. Chicago: Rand McNally.

Schiff, M., and A.Y. Lewin. (1968). "Where Traditional Budgeting Fails." *Financial Executive* (May), pp. 50–62.

Smith, A. (1990). "Corporate Ownership Structure and Performance: The Case of Management Buyouts." *Journal of Financial Economics* 27(1), pp. 143–164.

Teece, D.J. (1981). "Internal Organization and Economic Performance: An Empirical Analysis of the Profitability of Principal Firms." *Journal of Industrial Economics* 30, pp. 173–199.

Thompson, J.D. (1967). *Organizations in Action*. New York: McGraw-Hill.

Williamson, O.E. (1970). *Corporate Control and Business Behavior*. Englewood Cliffs, NJ: Prentice-Hall.

Williamson, O.E. (1996). *Mechanisms of Governance*. Oxford: Oxford University Press.

Index

About the Author

AHMED RIAHI-BELKAOUI is CBA Distinguished Professor of Accounting in the College of Business Administration, University of Illinois, Chicago. Author and coauthor of more than 40 Quorum books, he is an equally prolific contributor to the scholarly and professional journals of his field and has served on various editorial boards that oversee them. He is the editor of *Review of Accounting and Finance.*

DATE DUE

About the Author

Vernon L. Mogensen teaches and writes on the subjects of American politics and public policy. He is currently a Research Associate at the Michael Harrington Center, Queens College, the City University of New York.